INFECTIONS IN OUTPATIENT PRACTICE

Recognition and Management

INFECTIONS IN OUTPATIENT PRACTICE

Recognition and Management

Richard A. Gleckman, M.D., F.A.C.P.

Professor of Medicine
Department of Medicine
University of Massachusetts School of Medicine and
Chief
Division of Infectious Diseases
Saint Vincent Hospital
Worcester, Massachusetts

Nelson M. Gantz, M.D., F.A.C.P.

Professor of Medicine and Microbiology
Clinical Director
Division of Infectious Diseases
Department of Medicine
University of Massachusetts School of Medicine and
Hospital Epidemiologist
University of Massachusetts Medical Center
Worcester, Massachusetts

Richard B. Brown, M.D., F.A.C.P.

Associate Professor of Medicine
Department of Medicine
Tufts University School of Medicine
Boston, Massachusetts and
Chief
Infectious Disease Services
Baystate Medical Center
Springfield, Massachusetts

PLENUM MEDICAL BOOK COMPANY
NEW YORK AND LONDON

Library of Congress Cataloging in Publication Data

Gleckman, Richard Alan.
Infections in Outpatient Practice: recognition and management / Richard A. Gleckman, Nelson M. Gantz, and Richard B. Brown.
p. cm.
Includes bibliographies and index.
ISBN 0-306-42970-5
1. Communicable diseases. I. Gantz, Nelson Murray, 1941- . II. Brown, Richard B. III. Title.
RC111.G59 1988 88-23885
616.9—dc19 CIP

233 Spring Street, New York, N.Y. 10013

Plenum Medical Book Company is an imprint of Plenum Publishing Corporation

Printed in the United States of America

Preface

The intent of this book is to provide a practical approach to the recognition and therapy of selected outpatient problems faced by the internist, family practitioner, house officer, physician's assistant, and nurse. The topics selected were based on problems often encountered by clinicians in the outpatient setting, as well as by the interests of the authors. No attempt was made to write an all-encompassing textbook of infectious disease.

We want to thank Dr. John Czachor, infectious disease fellow, Saint Vincent Hospital, for his contributions to two chapters: mononucleosis and mononucleosislike syndromes and selective laboratory studies.

We want to thank Suzanne Hedstrom and Sharon Budzyna for typing and preparing the manuscript.

Finally, we would like to give special recognition to our wives, Brenda, Roberta, and Bonnie, for their support during the preparation of this book.

Richard A. Gleckman
Nelson M. Gantz
Richard B. Brown

Worcester and Springfield

Contents

2 Infectious Disease Problems for the Traveler

Richard B. Brown

3 Intestinal and Lymphatic Infectious Disorders in the Male Homosexual

Richard A. Gleckman

7 Management of Pneumonia in Outpatients

Richard B. Brown

8 Urethral Discharge

Nelson M. Gantz

9 Vaginal Discharge

Nelson M. Gantz

16 Endocarditis Prophylaxis

Nelson M. Gantz

17 Tuberculin Skin Testing and Managing a Positive Tuberculin Reactor

Nelson M. Gantz

18 Selective Laboratory Studies

Richard A. Gleckman and John S. Czachor

19 Home Intravenous Antibiotic Therapy

Richard B. Brown

1

Immunization in Adults

Richard B. Brown

Over the past several years renewed emphasis has been placed on the role of the prevention of infections. Reasons for this include the documentation of cost effectiveness and cost savings from this strategy[1,2] and the fact that several important infections such as tetanus, rabies, polio, and hepatitis B remain preventable but not specifically treatable. Indeed, much of the illness historically associated with childhood diseases is now seen in adults. For instance, for the year 1985, 100% of all cases of diphtheria, 93% of cases of tetanus, and almost 60% of cases of rubella occurred in patients over the age of 20.[3] Similarly, only 20% of persons considered at high risk for complications of viral influenza and 10% of those at risk for pneumococcal infection have been vaccinated.[3] Surveys demonstrate that at least 50% of persons over 60 years of age lack protective antibody to tetanus, and at least 40% lack antibody to diphtheria.[3] It has been suggested that up to seven million adults are suceptible to measles, and as many as 11 million women of childbearing age are not immune to rubella.[3]

Although the role of immunization for children has historically been well appreciated, less attention has been paid to this subject in adults. Increasing awareness is necessary because of the role of preventable "pediatric" infections in adults, travel as a source of unusual but preventable infection, and the potential for adults in unusual social or work-related situations to be at risk for potentially preventable but otherwise lethal infections. This chapter reviews the role of immunization in adults and provides data and strategies for the physician. Initial paragraphs deal with basic principles and definitions. Later discussions center on immunizations in various patient categories, and the last section focuses on specific vaccines that are useful in adults.

DEFINITIONS AND PRINCIPLES

Immunization is defined as the act of artificially inducing immunity or providing protection from disease.[4] Agents that can be employed include vac-

Table 1.1
Commonly Employed Immunobiologics

Live vaccines	Killed/inactivated vaccines	Toxoids
Measles	Viral	Diptheria
Mumps	Parenteral polio (IPV)	Tetanus
Rubella	Hepatitis B	
Oral polio (OPV)	Rabies	
Yellow fever		
	Bacterial	
	Cholera	
	Typhoid	
	Pneumococcal	

cines, toxoids, and specific antibody-containing agents. Vaccines are suspensions of attenuated live or killed microorganisms that can include bacteria, viruses, and rickettsiae and that are administered to induce immunity.[4] Toxoids represent modifications of bacterial toxins that have been rendered nontoxic but remain capable of inducing antitoxin production. Both of these groups of agents represent examples of active immunization, whereby the substances given induce an immune response that results in antibody production by the host. In general, this form of immunization is long-lived and is preferred when possible. Table 1.1 presents commonly employed immunobiologics by type of agent.

Nonspecific immune globulin represents a sterile solution that contains preformed antibody.[4] It contains 15–18% protein and is prepared by cold fractionation from large pools of human plasma. It can be utilized for immune maintenance of selected immunodeficient persons as well as for passive immunization against hepatitis A and possibly measles.[5] Other immune globulins are considered "specific" because they are prepared from sera of selected donor populations that contain high levels of antibody against specific pathogens that include hepatitis B, rabies, varicella–zoster, and tetanus. Administration of all immune globulins represents examples of passive immunization, where preformed antibody is given to the person at risk. This results in relatively short-lived immunity but can be useful for immediate protection of a person at risk. In selected circumstances (e.g., hepatitis B or rabies prevention), both active and passive immunization should be administered concomitantly.[6,7]

Immunobiologics contain constituents in addition to the immunizing agent. Suspending fluids are often saline or sterile water. However, in selected instances they may contain small amounts of materials utilized in the production of the biological material. These may include egg proteins or cell-culture-derived antigens. Other materials noted in selected materials can include antibiotics or stabilizers, which are utilized either to inhibit bacterial growth or to stabilize the antigen and may rarely be implicated as a source of severe allergic reactions. An adjuvant, typically an aluminum salt, may be added to selected vaccines such as hepatitis B vaccine and toxoids to enhance the efficacy of the antigen. All adjuvant-enhanced vaccines must be administered by deep intramuscular injection to prevent severe inflammation or necrosis.

Physicians caring for adults must become comfortable in obtaining a careful history of immunization, as this becomes the basis for determining future immunization needs. Although some persons may carry documentation of prior immunizations, many do not. Most authorities feel that it is wiser, if questions exist, to assume that they have not been immunized and to base needs on current risks.[5] Clues can be obtained from a history of prior military service, travel, and age. Current laws in most states require documentation of selected vaccinations of all school-age children. Occasionally, serological studies may be indicated if questions exist and vaccination is deemed necessary. A vaccination record should be kept by all persons and updated as necessary.

In general, the physician caring for adults is less comfortable with vaccine management than is the pediatrician, and immunobiologic usage is more sporadic. It is imperative that all physicians follow package intructions carefully with regard to storage and administration. Especial note should be taken with regard to refrigeration versus freezing, as some (e.g., tetanus and diphtheria toxoids and hepatitis B vaccine) cannot be safely frozen.[5,8] Most vaccines are administered either by intramuscular or subcutaneous injection. Some may also be given intradermally. Care should be taken that the latter are not inoculated subcutaneously; they should be given into the volar aspect of the forearm when feasible. Subcutaneous and intramuscular injections should usually be given into the deltoid rather than the anterior thigh except in infants. Inoculations into the buttock should be reserved for only those injections with extremely large volumes. Risk of nerve damage or poor uptake mitigates against the routine use of this site.[9] The recommended dose of most immunobiologics administered either by intramuscular or subcutaneous routes is 0.5–1.0 cc. In most instances the full dose, as recommended by the manufacturer, should be administered as one inoculation.

Although hypothetical reasons (related to failure to mount an adequate antibody response) exist for not simultaneously administering a variety of immunobiologics, most can be safely given together when warranted by circumstances such as impending travel or exposures.[10] Several caveats exist, however. First, some side effects such as fever and sore arm may be enhanced by the simultaneous administration of these agents. Additionally, some authorities feel that combinations of live vaccines not administered on the same day be best administered at least 1 month apart.[5] Some data exist that cholera and yellow fever vaccines not be coadministered.[11] Finally, live virus vaccines should not be given for at least 6 weeks after immune globulins.[1,4,10]

Routine childhood vaccination against common "pediatric" pathogens has been advocated for several decades and has resulted in precipitous declines in the

Table 1.2
Routine Immunization for Adults[a]

Age (years)	Recommended immunizations
18–24	Diphtheria–tetanus (primary), booster every 10 years
	Measles
	Rubella
	Mumps[b]
25–64	Diphtheria–tetanus (primary), booster every 10 years
	Rubella
	Measles[c]
≥65	Influenza
	Diphtheria–tetanus (primary), booster every 10 years
	Pneumococcus[d]

[a]Adopted from Committee on Immunizations.[5]
[b]Usually routinely administered as MMR.
[c]Assume immune if born before 1957.
[d]Routine usage in elderly controversial at this time.

incidence and prevalence of diseases that include poliomyelitis, rubella, rubeola, pertussis, diphtheria, and tetanus. However, recent data conclude that outbreaks of these illnesses still occur in populations that have resisted vaccination and that numerous adults may remain unvaccinated or undervaccinated against several of these diseases. Physicians who care for adults must assess vaccination needs on the basis of the age and prior vaccination status of the patient. Table 1.2 presents suggested vaccine approaches based on patient age and assumes the absence of special situations such as travel.

Under most circumstances, adults under the age of 24 should be able to document their vaccination status through school requirements, physician records, or military service. Immunity against diphtheria and tetanus should be updated every 10 years. Note that adults should not be routinely vaccinated against pertussis (whooping cough). If documentation of primary immunization cannot be obtained, then full immunization with the adult preparation (Td) should be undertaken with two doses given a month apart and followed by a third 6–12 months later.[12] Immunity against rubeola (measles) should be documented by either (1) immunization after 1956 given after 1 year of age, (2) physician documentation of clinical measles, or (3) serological testing. Vaccination with killed vaccine, used between 1963 and 1967, was ineffective. Immunity to rubella (German measles) should be documented in all women of childbearing age by either documented immunization after 1 year of age or serological testing. History of clinical disease should not be utilized because of the difficulty in making this diagnosis. Mumps vaccination is not routinely required, as most adults can be considered to be immune even without clinical disease.[5] However, when adults require either rubella or rubeola immunization, it is probably useful to administer the measles–mumps–rubella (MMR) trivalent vaccine.[5] Routine immunization against polio is generally not recommended unless there is high risk through either travel or occupational exposure.[13] In such circumstances, vaccination with the inactivated polio vaccine (IPV, Salk vaccine) is generally recommended rather than the oral form (OPV) because of decreased likelihood of adverse neuroparalytic reactions.[13]

Adults between 25 and 64 years of age should have documented immunity against diphtheria and tetanus and should be offered boosters at 10-year intervals.[4,5] Individuals for whom primary immunization cannot be documented should have it offered. Similarly, persons in this age group should have documented immunity to measles and rubella, either by proven immunization or by serological studies. For those persons who received measles immunization between 1963 and 1967, revaccination should be considered, as they may have received killed vaccine. The MMR vaccine should be utilized if persons are thought to be suceptible to more than one of these diseases. Persons in clinical situations that place them at risk for influenza should also be vaccinated annually against this viral disease. Examples include health care workers and military personnel.[5]

Persons over the age of 65 should receive Td boosters at 10-year intervals and should also be annually vaccinated against viral influenza. Usage of pneumococcal vaccine in this population is controversial. Further information concerning both influenza and pneumococcal vaccination is provided later in this chapter.

IMMUNIZATION IN SPECIAL CLINICAL SITUATIONS

Pregnancy

Pregnancy presents specific problems in immunization because of both real or hypothetical risks of selected vaccines to the fetus and changes in cell-mediated immunity in the mother. Ideally, childhood immunizations should be completed prior to pregnancy. Live virus vaccines such as rubella, rubeola, etc., should generally be avoided. Other vaccines must be used only when the risks of vaccination are smaller than the benefits of disease prevention. Diphtheria–tetanus immunization should be administered to all pregnant women who have not been previously immunized. This is especially true of persons likely to deliver a child in circumstances condusive to the development of neonatal tetanus.[12] Immunization against polio is generally not indicated unless travel to highly endemic areas is contemplated. In this situation, the inactivated form (IPV) should be utilized.[5,13] Vaccinations against measles, mumps, and rubella should be generally avoided during pregnancy because of the theoretical risks of live virus vaccines to the fetus. However, no clinical data exist that demonstrate that inadvertent vaccination during pregnancy poses documented risks to the fetus with any of these vaccines. Therefore, vaccine administration does not present an indication for therapeutic abortion.[14,15] Immunization with either pneumococcal or influenza vaccines is neither specifically indicated nor contraindicated in pregnancy. Hepatitis B vaccine may be used safely in pregnancy when clinically indicated[7] after appropriate exposures.

College Students and Military Recruits

These two groups share the likelihood of close living situations, where communicable diseases could rapidly spread to suceptible individuals. Military recruits are also at risk for infections acquired through foreign travel, a subject that is dealt with separately. Universal immunization against both measles and rubella should be documented either through prior vaccination history or serological positivity. As in other situations noted in young adults, MMR should be strongly considered if possibility of suceptibility to more than one virus is suspected. Diphtheria–tetanus (Td) vaccine should be administered as a booster if it has not been received within 10 years and if primary immunizations are up to date. Primary immunization should be administered if not given previously. Similarly, polio immunization should be given or updated as necessary in this cadre of individuals. In situations of outbreaks, it may be necessary to consider meningococcal or influenza immunization. These may be routinely administered to military recruits.

Health Care Personnel

For personnel in contact with hospitalized patients and outpatients, routine immunizations and boosters should be employed against poliomyelitis, rubella, measles, diphtheria, tetanus, and influenza.[5] For personnel at risk for hepatitis B, vaccination is strongly recommended.[5,8] Other needs must be individualized based on occupations and risks. Microbiology personnel may require immunization against cholera, plague, or tularemia. Veterinarians should be immunized against rabies, and possibly plague and tularemia.

Travelers

Persons traveling abroad face the possibility of exposure to a wide variety of infections not present in the United States. Methods to limit the likelihood of infection include (1) hygiene and sanitation precautions (evaluation of water and food supplies, mosquito netting, etc.), (2) prophylactic antibiotics, (3) immunoglobulins, (4) avoidance of high-risk areas, and (5) immunization.[16] With regard to the latter, choices must take into account the geographic area and

Table 1.3
Vaccines for International Travel

Probable benefit	Dubious benefit
Yellow fever[a]	Cholera
Typhoid	Typhus[c]
Hepatitis B	
Poliomyelitis	
Diphtheria–tetanus	
Japanese B encephalitis[b]	
Meningococcal	
Rabies	
Plague	

[a]Administered only through licensed centers in the United States.
[b]Investigational but available through selected sites.
[c]No longer produced in the United States.

duration of travel, the actual time to be spent in individual areas in a prolonged itinerary, risk of contact with vectors and infectious agents, prior immunization history, and allergies. Publications such as *Health Information for International Travel*[16] provide useful and relatively timely information for the practicing physician with regard to both general measures and risks and needs for specific immunizations by country of travel. Several commonly employed vaccines useful especially to travelers are now discussed and are listed in Table 1.3.

VACCINES OF ESPECIAL USE TO TRAVELERS

Typhoid Fever

Vaccination against typhoid fever is not required for international travel but is recommended if contact with the organism is likely. It is thought to be up to 70% effective when appropriately administered.[5,16] Travelers to third-world countries in Africa, South and Central America, and Asia should strongly consider vaccination if they depart from standard tourist routes and may have contact with contaminated food and water. Risk of disease may be greater for individuals who are immunosuppressed by steroids, acquired immune deficiency syndrome, or clinical situations that compromise the integrity of their gastric acid secretion. When feasible, a primary series of two 0.5-ml subcutaneous injections should be administered at least 4 weeks apart.[16] If time does not allow, similar doses can be given at weekly intervals. A booster is recommended at 3-year intervals. Side effects consist primarily of short-lived local soreness at the injection site and low-grade fever. No data are available concerning safety in pregnancy. Recent studies employing a new vaccine containing *Salmonella typhi* capsular polysaccharide (Vi antigen) demonstrated efficacy of about 75%.[17]

Yellow Fever

Yellow fever is endemic within parts of South America and Africa.[18] Selected countries require proof of vaccination prior to entry, and this vaccine is generally recommended for travelers entering endemic rural areas. This live virus vaccine must be administered through approved and licensed yellow fever vaccination centers. Locations are generally available through local public health facilities. A single 0.5-ml dose administered subcutaneously comprises primary immunization. Booster doses are sugged at 10-year intervals.[5,16,18] The vaccine is produced in chick embryos and is relatively contraindicated in persons with egg allergies. Use in pregnancy is not suggested unless value is thought to outweigh hypothetical risks. Reactions to yellow fever vaccine occur regularly and consist of mild constitutional complaints noted most commonly 3–10 days after vaccination.[18] With the possible exception of cholera, which should be administered at least 3 weeks after yellow fever vaccine, other immunobiologics can be given as necessary.[18]

Cholera

Although cholera exists in many underdeveloped countries, routine vaccination is neither required nor generally recommended.[5,16] Use should be reserved for tourists traveling to rural areas for prolonged periods, and even then cholera is an unusual circumstance.[19] The vaccine provides only 50% effectiveness and has a duration of action of less than 6 months.[5,16] A single 0.5-ml dose, given either subcutaneously or intramuscularly, satisfies international health requirements. Two injections given 1–4 weeks apart should be utilized for individuals at extremely high risk.[5,16] Boosters are necessary at 6-month intervals during the period of risk. Immunization results in local pain and modest constitutional symptoms for up to several days after vaccination. No data are available regarding use in pregnancy; generally it should be avoided. If administration of yellow fever vaccine is needed, the two should be given at least 3 weeks apart.

Japanese B Encephalitis

Japanese encephalitis is a mosquito-borne infection prevalent in parts of the Far East and associated with mortality rates of up to 20%.[16] Risk is greatest for long-term travelers to rural areas during appropriate seasons. Although vaccine is not produced in the United States, the Biken Laboratories product is available through the Centers for Disease Control and regional Japanese encephalitis vaccination centers. A two- or three-dose primary immunization series is recommended.[16] Boosters are necessary at 12–18 months and then at 4-year intervals if risks persist.[16] Persons with acute illnesses or underlying cardiopulmonary or malignant diseases and pregnant women should not be vaccinated.

Immune Serum Globulin

Immune serum globulin (ISG, γ-globulin) is not a vaccine but has a role to play in the prevention or amelioration of hepatitis A and selected other viral diseases.[5,8,16] With regard to travel, its major role is for prevention of hepatitis A, the risk of which varies with region of travel, length and location of stay, contact with inappropriately prepared food and water, and prior immunologic background. Risk is greatest in underdeveloped countries and in rural areas.[8,16] Dosage of this preparation varies with weight and estimated length of stay in areas of risk. Travel for periods of less than 3 months is managed with a dose of ISG of 2.0 ml for persons weighing greater than 100 lb. Longer travel periods mandate doses of 5.0 ml for a similarly sized individual.[7,15] No infectious diseases such as AIDS or hepatitis B have been noted to be transmitted by any immune globulin.[20] Side effects are minimal and usually consist of sore arm or buttock and mild constitutional symptoms. This product can be safely administered during pregnancy.

STRATEGIES FOR USE OF OTHER COMMONLY EMPLOYED VACCINES IN SPECIFIC CLINICAL SITUATIONS

Tetanus

Tetanus remains an important complication of wounds and trauma and may follow injuries that appear "incidental" or uncomplicated.[12,15] Documentation of tetanus immunization is important for all age groups, and active immunization with Td (tetanus and diphtheria toxoids, adsorbed for adult use) should be administered at 10-year intervals for all persons following primary immunization.[5,12] Following all injuries that have broken the skin or mucous membranes, assessment by the attending physician for risk of tetanus and immune status is mandatory. Management must take into account both of these factors. Table 1.4 summarizes recommendations for wound management. For individuals who have either never received primary immunization or whose status is unknown and who have neglected or significant wounds, the use of both Td (active immunization) and TIG (tetanus immune globulin) is strongly recommended.[5,12,15] The latter material is prepared from pooled human serum from individuals immune to this disease and renders passive immunity with little risk. It should be administered intramuscularly in doses of at least 250–500 units, although some investigators have recommended substantially higher doses.[21] Tetanus immune globulin is preferred over the previously employed horse antitoxin because of its enhanced safety.[21]

Table 1.4
Tetanus Prophylaxis for Wound Management in Adults[a]

History of tetanus immunization	Wound status			
	Clean, minor		All others	
	Td	TIG[b]	Td	TIG
Unknown, uncertain, 0–2 doses	Yes	No	Yes	Yes
3 doses	No[c]	No	No[c]	No

[a]Adopted from Centers for Disease Control[12] and Fedson.[15]
[b]Tetanus immune globulin, at least 250 units.
[c]No, if booster within past 10 years.

Rabies

Current data demonstrate that fewer than ten persons annually develop rabies.[22] Although human rabies remains an unusual (but highly lethal) infection in the United States, risk of this disease is potentially high because of the large numbers of animal reservoirs that exist and their possible contact with humans. Bats, skunks, raccoons, and other carnivorous wild animals are regularly noted to be infected, and rare cases have been noted in dogs and cats.[23] However, in the United States, rodents (squirrels, rabbits, gerbils, rats, mice, etc.) are almost never rabid. Bite wound injuries must be individually assessed for risk of rabies. Evaluation must include consideration of the species of biting animal, presence of rabies in the geographic region, circumstances of the bite, immunologic status of the person, allergy history, and the availability of the biting animal. Thorough cleansing and disinfection of the wound is always of primary importance. When rabies is a consideration, postexposure prophylaxis is indicated.[5,23] Approximately 25,000 persons per year receive such immunization.[23] Table 1.5 provides recommendations. When doubt exists concerning the presence of rabies in a geographic region or in a particular species of biting animal, local public health authorities should be promptly consulted. When rabies prophylaxis is indicated, both active and passive immunization should be administered. The only exception is the previously immunized individual (e.g., veterinarian) with a documented acceptable antibody titer. Such persons require only vaccine. Current recommendations call for use of human diploid cell rabies vaccine (HDCV) and human rabies immune globulin (RIG). Previously employed duck embryo vaccine (DEV) is no longer available in the United States. Antirabies serum (ARS) (equine) is manufactured from hyperimmune horses and is an alternative to RIG but should only be employed when RIG is not available.[23]

The HDCV is an inactivated vaccine produced from fixed rabies virus grown on human diploid cell culture.[23] It is administered in five 1-ml intramuscular doses, preferably in the deltoid region. First dose should be given as

Table 1.5
Rabies Postexposure Guide to Prophylaxis[a]

Species of animal	Condition of animal	Treatment
Dog, cat	Healthy and available for 10 days of observation	None (unless animal develops rabies)
	Rabid or suspected	RIG[b] plus HDCV[c]
	Escaped	Usually none, unless canine/feline rabies known in area (then RIG plus HDCV)
Skunks, raccoons, bats, foxes, other carnivores	Regard as rabid unless proven otherwise	RIG plus HDCV
Livestock, rodents, rabbits	Consult Health Dept., but rabies rare	None, unless special circumstances

[a]Adopted from Centers for Disease Control[23] and Anderson *et al.*[22]
[b]Rabies immune globulin, 20 IU/kg as single dose.
[c]Human diploid cell vaccine, five 1.0-ml doses.

soon as possible after the bite. Other doses are administered at intervals of 3, 7, 14, and 28 days.[23] Routine postvaccination serological testing is not indicated, although the Centers for Disease Control defines an acceptable postimmunization titer of 1 : 5 by rapid fluorescent focus inhibition test.[23] Human RIG is produced from plasma of hyperimmunized human donors that is concentrated by cold ethanol fractionization. Rabies neutralizing antibody content is standardized at 150 IU/ml, and it is supplied for adults in 10-ml vials containing a total of 1500 IU. It is administered only once as soon as possible after the bite. Dosage of 20 IU/kg is recommended, with half the dose infiltrated about the wound and the rest given intramuscularly. If RIG is not immediately available, it can be given up to 8 days after the bite.

Adverse effects from these products are common but do not routinely require discontinuation of therapy. The ARS (equine) is associated with serum sickness in 40% of recipients, which is the major reason why this preparation is now rarely employed. The HDCV is associated with local reactions in approximatly 20% of patients. A similar percentage demonstrate mild constitutional reactions such as low-grade fever, headache, and dizziness. These do not constitute reasons for discontinuation of therapy. Individuals who have been given preexposure prophylaxis (animal handlers, veterinarians, etc.) and then receive repeated boosters have been noted to develop an immune-complex-like illness characterized by pruritis, urticaria, and angioedema 2–21 days after the booster.[24] The rate is estimated at up to 6%, but this effect is generally mild and treated with antihistamines. No deaths have been reported. An unidentified component of the vaccine is suspected.

Rabies immune globulin has been associated with pain at the injection site and low-grade temperature elevations. Rarely, more significant allergic manifestations have been noted. Patients with a deficiency of IgA should receive this compound with care because of the possibility of sensitization against later IgA-containing blood products.[23]

Pneumococcal Vaccine

Streptococcus pneumoniae continues to represent the most common cause of treatable pneumonia in the adult and is associated with considerable morbidity and mortality.[25] Problems with management continue despite the availability of potent antimicrobial agents. Pneumococcal vaccines have been available for over 50 years and have been demonstrated to be effective in several groups of adults that include those who are otherwise healthy but are in high-risk employment (South African gold miners, military recruits) and postsplenectomy patients.[26] The vaccines have been considered to be safe and inexpensive. Routine immunization has been recommended in the United States for the elderly and those with underlying cardiopulmonary disease[27] and has been substantiated by retrospective data and mathematical models.[28] However, more recent prospective investigations have questioned this premise in older high-risk patients and have produced data demonstrating no advantage of the 14-valent vaccine when compared to placebo.[29,30] Those patients who received vaccine actually developed more pneumococcal lower respiratory events than the control group, and one study demonstrated an apparent failure to prevent bacteremic events.[30]

Vaccination is indicated for selected groups of individuals that include those who are postsplenectomy. A single 0.5-cc subcutaneous inoculation of the current 23-valent formulation should be given. For persons who have previously received the 14-valent preparation, repeat vaccination is generally not indicated, as incidence of local and systemic side effects appears to be enhanced. The decision to offer vaccination to older patients with underlying cardiopulmonary disease must be individualized. Although not statistically proven to be advantageous in this population, the vaccine remains safe and inexpensive and could offer some degree of protection in selected individuals.

Viral Influenza

Viral influenza is an important cause of morbidity and mortality in the United States and can be associated with either "A" or "B" strains. Changes in antigen structure occur regularly and are monitored by the Centers for Disease Control. Vaccine preparation attempts to anticipate the causative strains for the upcoming year. Influenza vaccine is indicated for those persons at risk for complications of viral influenza and those in whom morbidity (i.e., lost time from work) should be avoided.[31] The elderly, those with underlying cardiopulmonary disease, nursing home residents, etc., should be considered candidates for this immunization. Vaccine should be administered annually in late fall and can be given simultaneously with pneumococcal vaccine.[31] Protection is thought to occur in up to 80% of persons and is associated with the demonstration of protective antihemagglutinin titers. It is given as an annual 0.5-cc intramuscular injection as either the "whole" or "split" preparation. Because it is prepared in embryonated chicken eggs, it can cause hypersensitivity reactions in persons with immediate egg sensitivity.[31] Other complications are minor and consist of local tenderness and redness and mild constitutional symptoms lasting for up to 48 hr. There is no evidence of increased frequency of Guillain–Barré syndrome with current preparations. Although influenza vaccine was thought to be implicated as a cause of prolonged prothrombin time in a person simultaneously receiving coumadin, recent data conclude that no reproducible problems in this regard have been noted.[32]

Amantadine hydrochloride (Symmetrel®, Endo Laboratories) and rimantadine hydrochloride are antiviral medications with activity against influenza A but not influenza B.[31] Only the former is currently available in the United States. Amantadine is clinically useful both prophylactically and therapeutically. It is indicated during outbreaks of influenza A in nonimmunized populations (e.g., a nursing home with many nonvaccinated patients) or for "synergistic protection" in vaccinated patients deemed to be at risk for serious sequelae.[31] It can also be therapeutically useful for individuals with presumed influenza A if given during the first 48 hr of disease.[31] If used prophylactically, it must be administered daily for the period at risk, generally up to 12 weeks. For nonimmunized patients, during influenza A epidemics, amantadine can be given for the first 2 weeks after vaccination in order to offer immediate protection while awaiting protective antibody production by the host. For otherwise healthy, young individuals, daily dose is 200 mg daily, administered orally. Older patients, especially those with compromised renal function, should be given 100 mg daily.[5,31] Central nervous system side effects that include dizziness and irritability are regularly noted and require dosage reassessment or drug discontinuation. Seizures have occasionally been reported.

Hepatitis B

Hepatitis B constitutes a worldwide problem with both serious morbidity and mortality. In the United States, up to 0.5% of the population will experience infection with this virus, often asymptomatically.[8] Approximately 1% die acutely of this infection, while 5–10% develop chronic complications that include carriage of the virus and occasional cirrhosis. Chronic carriers may be infectious to others and form an inportant reservoir of infection. Selected groups of persons are at increased risk for infection with hepatitis B. These include male homosexuals, intravenous drug addicts, and health care workers who come into contact with blood from unknown sources.[33] Both active and passive immunization is available to deal with infection with hepatitis B. Table 1.6 summarizes strategies to utilize these products following percutaneous exposure.

Hepatitis B vaccine was licensed in 1981, and a "second-generation" product has recently become available. The initial vaccine, offering active protection

Table 1.6
Hepatitis B Prophylaxis following Percutaneous Exposure[a]

Source	Exposed person: Nonvaccinated	Exposed person: Vaccinated
HBsAg(+)	1. HBIG[b] × 1 stat 2. Hepatitis vaccine series	1. Test exposed person for anti-HBsAg 2. If inadequate antibody: HBIG × 1 stat; hepatitis vaccine booster
Known source High risk	1. Hepatitis vaccine series 2. Test source for HBsAg; give HBIG × 1 if positive	1. Test exposed person for HBsAb 2. Test source only if exposed is HBsAb(−) (nonresponder) 3. If source HBsAg(+): HBIG × 1; hepatitis vaccine booster
Low risk, HBsAg(+)	1. Hepatitis vaccine series	1. Nothing
Unknown source	1. Hepatitis vaccine series	1. Nothing

[a]Adopted from Centers for Disease Control.[8]
[b]HBIG in dose of 0.06 ml/kg i.m.; for adults 10 mg/i.m. per dose.

in up to 96% of vaccinated patients without significant underlying disease,[34] was administered in three intramuscular injections of 20 μg each at 0-, 1-, and 6-month intervals. Preparation steps preclude infection of the lots. However, poor acceptance among health care workers was frequently reported, presumably because of the fear of AIDS and other diseases, since the vaccine was manufactured from plasma of patients with high titers of hepatitis B antigen, often male homosexuals, who were felt to be at risk for AIDS. Other data demonstrated that criteria such as obesity and buttock site of injection could adversely impact on the likelihood of satisfactory antibody response.[9]

A newer product, Hepatitis B Vaccine (Recombinant), has been made available both to meet continued global needs for this product and to provide an acceptable alternative mode of production should plasma supplies decrease. It is free of associated blood or blood products. A portion of the hepatitis B genome, coded for HbsAg, is cloned into Bakers' yeast (*Saccharomyces cerevisiae*), and the vaccine is produced from cultures of this yeast.[35] This product offers an alternative to the original hepatitis B vaccine, is administered in a similar fashion, and appears to be equally effective. Three 1-cc vaccinations of 10 μg each are recommended, at 0-, 1-, and 6-month intervals. A pediatric formulation of 0.5 cc containing 5 μg is also available. Intramuscular administeration is advised, typically into the deltoid region, although the anterolateral thigh can be utilized in infants. Subcutaneous injection may be given in patients at risk for bleeding diatheses from intramuscular injection. There is more limited clinical experience with the new vaccine at the present time, and no definitive advantages. Length of protection of the recombinant product is not known; however, repeated booster injections are not currently recommended.

Hepatitis B immune globulin (HBIG) provides passive protection for time periods of up to 4 months and is indicated in selected postexposure settings.[8] It is the immune globulin of choice when definite exposure to hepatitis B virus has occurred. Unlike immune serum globulin (anti-HBs titers of at least 1 : 100), HBIG contains titers of at least 1 : 100,000 by radioimmunoassay.[8] The HBIG can be administered concomitantly with hepatitis B vaccine[36]; the combination is generally recommended as the most cost-effective approach to postexposure prophylaxis.[8] When administered in conjunction with hepatitis B vaccine, a single dose of HBIG of 0.06 ml/kg i.m. within 14 days is indicated. Efficacy is related to the proximity of HBIG administration to the initiating event, and it should be given as soon as possible after percutaneous exposures.[7]

CONCLUSIONS

Immunization for adults represents an important but underutilized strategy for disease prevention. The practicing clinician must become increasingly aware of the availability, indications, and implications of vaccination as an alternative to treatment of active infection. The future will see the development of new vaccines for various forms of diarrhea, varicella, and other diseases that will further impact on infectious diseases in the adult.

REFERENCES

1. Williams JS, Sanders CR: Cost-effectiveness and cost–benefit analysis of vaccines. *J Infect Dis* 1981; 144:486–493.
2. Koplan JP, Schoenbaum SC, Weinstein ME, *et al:* Pertussis vaccine—an analysis of benefits, risks and costs. *N Engl J Med* 1979; 301:906–911.
3. Centers for Disease Control: Summary of the Second National Community Forum on Adult Immunization. *Morbid Mortal Week Rep* 1987; 36:677–680.
4. Centers for Disease Control: General recommendations on immunization. *Ann Intern Med* 1983; 98(part I):615–622.
5. Committee on Immunizations, Council of Medical Societies, American College of Physicians: *Guide for Adult Immunization.* American College of Physicians, 1985.
6. Centers for Disease Control: Postexposure prophylaxis on hepatitis B. *Morbid Mortal Week Rep* 1984; 33:285–290.
7. Centers for Disease Control: Rabies prevention—United States, 1984. *Morbid Mortal Week Rep* 1984; 33:393–402.
8. Centers for Disease Control: Recommendations for protection against viral hepatitis. *Morbid Mortal Week Rep* 1985; 34:313–335.
9. Centers for Disease Control: Suboptimal response to hepatitis B vaccine given by injection into the buttock. *Morbid Mortal Week Rep* 1985; 34:105–113.
10. Hinman AR, Bart KJ, Orenstein WA: Immunization. In: Mandel GL, Douglas RG, Jr, Bennett JE, eds. *Principles and Practice of Infectious Disease,* ed 2. New York, John Wiley & Sons, 1986:1688–1698.

11. Felsenfeld O, Wolf RH, Gyr K, *et al:* Simultaneous vaccination against cholera and yellow fever. *Lancet* 1973; 1:457–458.
12. Centers for Disease Control: Diphtheria, tetanus and pertussis: Guidelines for vaccine prophylaxis and other preventive measures. *Morbid Mortal Week Rep* 1985; 34:405–426.
13. Immunization Practices Advisory Committees, Centers for Disease Control: Poliomyelitis prevention. *Ann Intern Med* 1982; 96:630–634.
14. Centers for Disease Control: Rubella vaccination during pregnancy—United States, 1971–1983. *Morbid Mortal Week Rep* 1984; 33:365–373.
15. Fedson DS: Adult immunization: Protocols and problems. *Hosp Pract* 1986; 21:143–158.
16. Centers for Disease Control: *Health Information for International Travel, 1986.* HHS Publication No. (CDC)86:8280, Washington, US Government Printing Office, 1986.
17. Acharya IL, Lowe CU, Thapa R, *et al:* Prevention of typhoid fever in Nepal with the Vi capsular polysaccharide of *Salmonella typhi. N Engl J Med* 1987; 317:1101–1104.
18. Centers for Disease Control: Yellow fever vaccine. *Morbid Mortal Week Rep* 1984; 32:679–688.
19. Snyder JD, Blake PA: Is cholera a problem for US travelers? *JAMA* 1982; 247:2268–2269.
20. Centers for Disease Control: Lack of transmission of human immunodeficiency virus through Rh_o (D) immune globulin (human). *Morbid Mortal Week Rep* 1987; 36:728–729.
21. Martin RR: *Clostridium tetani* (tetanus). In: Mandell GL, Douglas RG Jr, Bennett JE, eds. *Principles and Practice of Infectious Disease,* ed 2. New York, John Wiley & Sons, 1985:1355–1359.
22. Anderson LF, Nicholson KG, Tauxe RV, *et al:* Human rabies in the United States, 1960–1979: Epidemiology, diagnosis and prevention. *Ann Intern Med* 1984; 100:728–735.
23. Centers for Disease Control: Rabies prevention—United States, 1984. *Morbid Mortal Week Rep* 1984; 33:393–407.
24. Centers for Disease Control: Systemic allergic reactions following immunization with human diploid cell rabies vaccine. *Morbid Mortal Week Rep* 1984; 33:185–187.
25. Van Metre TE: Pneumococcal pneumonia treated with antibiotics: The prognostic significance of certain clinical findings. *N Engl J Med* 1954; 251:1048–1052.
26. Smit P, Oberholzer D, Hayden-Smith S, *et al:* Protective efficacy of pneumococcal polysaccharide vaccines. *JAMA* 1977; 238:2613–2616.
27. *Medical Letter:* Pneumococcal vaccine. *Med Lett* 1978; 20:13–14.
28. Bolan G, Broome CV, Facklam RR, *et al:* Pneumococcal vaccine efficacy in selected populations in the United States. *Ann Intern Med* 1986; 104:1–6.
29. Simberkoff MS, Cross AP, Al-Ibrahim M, *et al:* Efficacy of pneumococcal vaccine in high-risk patients. Results of a Veterans Administration cooperative study. *N Engl J Med* 1986; 315:318–327.
30. Forrester HL, Jahnigen DW, LaForce FM: Inefficacy of pneumococcal vaccine in a high risk population. *Am J Med* 1987; 83:425–430.
31. Centers for Disease Control: Prevention and control of influenza. Recommendations of the Immunization Practices Advisory Committee. *Ann Intern Med* 1987; 107:521–525.
32. Lipsky BA, Pecoraro RE, Roben NJ, *et al:* Influenza vaccination and warfarin anticoagulation. *Ann Intern Med* 1984; 100:835–837.
33. Dienstag JL, Ryan DM: Occupational exposure to hepatitis B virus personnel: Infection or immunization? *Am J Epidemiol* 1982; 115:26–39.
34. Szmuness W, Stevens CE, Harley EJ, *et al:* Hepatitis B vaccine. Demonstration of efficacy in a controlled clinical trial in a high-risk population in the United States. *N Engl J Med* 1980; 303:833–841.
35. Merck Sharp & Dohme: *Hepatitis B Vaccine* [*Recombinant, MSD*] *package insert.* West Point, PA, Merck Sharp & Dohme, undated.
36. Zachoval R, Jilg W, Corbeer B, *et al:* Passive/active immunization against hepatitis B. *J Infect Dis* 1984; 150:112–117.

2

Infectious Disease Problems for the Traveler

Richard B. Brown

INTRODUCTION

Travel has become far more routine than has historically been appreciated. Estimates indicate that up to eight million Americans travel to underdeveloped countries annually.[1] It is now common for people of all ages and backgrounds to travel regularly to domestic and foreign locations. In doing so, individuals must confront many issues and health risks not present in their home environs, and they often seek attention for many of these matters. Indeed, recent studies suggest that depending on itinerary, 15–75% of travelers may develop illness during or after foreign travel.[2] Advice and information for travelers can come from many sources that include the library, physicians, friends, and travel agents. Considerations that need to be addressed can include many that are "noninfectious," such as insurance coverage in foreign lands, availability of prescription medications, special needs of impaired travelers, remedies for motion sickness, etc. Table 2.1 depicts many of the important noninfectious disease issues that all travelers should consider prior to embarking on substantial travel.

Physicians who deal with travelers soon learn that many questions or problems do not fall within their usual knowledge base and that much new knowledge must be acquired in order for the clinician to deal optimally with this cadre of patient. Additionally, acquisition and dispensation of this information can be time consuming and not a "cost-effective" use of the clinician's time. Knowledge about vaccinations, infectious disease problems on a global scale, availability of prescription medications in overseas markets, etc. are common problems that must be addressed and answered. Some physicians have concluded that the field should actually be considered a separate specialty named "emporiatrics," defined as the science of the health of travelers.[3]

Table 2.1
Noninfectious Considerations for Travelers

Health insurance
Availability of prescription medications
First-aid kit
Insect repellants, mosquito netting
Jet lag
Locating a doctor abroad
Chronic lung disease and altitudes
Getting home if injured or ill
Traveling with children
Motion sickness

TRIP PREPARATION AND TRAVEL: INFECTIOUS DISEASE IMPLICATIONS

Persons preparing for travel abroad must allow sufficient time so that travel needs can be met. At least one and preferably 2–3 months should be allotted for adequate planning. It is important that adequate time be available for immunizations and that they be administered in an appropriate sequence. Details regarding selected immunizations are provided later in this chapter. Vaccine recipients must be aware of both the limitations of vaccination and the potential side effects. Patients taking long-term antibiotics, such as for chronic urinary tract or bronchial infections, or those on long-term prophylaxis for rheumatic fever should bring adequate supplies of medication with them. It is usually prudent to carry a signed letter from the physician indicating the name, dose, frequency of administration, and indication for selected antimicrobial agents. Agents to treat common complaints such as diarrhea and headache should be carried with the traveler in most instances rather than be purchased abroad. Products available in some areas may be quite different from those that the Western traveler is used to, and quality may vary quite dramatically from that typical in the United States and other developed countries. A travel packet should also include nonprescription medications such as disinfectants and topical antibacterial medications for dealing with minor injuries.

Depending on location and type of journey, other priorities may include insect repellants and materials to decontaminate water and food. Insects such as mosquitoes are a major source of spread of infections in underdeveloped countries, and the prevention of bites is more important than either medical prophylaxis or treatment of resultant disease. In areas where mosquito bites are anticipated, quality mosquito netting is indispensable, and a good insect repellant containing DEET (N,N-diethyl-*meta*-toluamide) in a concentration of about 30% should be utilized.[4] Although intake of regional foods and beverages may be considered a major source of travel enjoyment, it may also result in major health risks that range from hepatitis to gastroenteritis. Information regarding safety of foods and liquids must be given to the traveler going to underdeveloped areas having health and sanitation standards lower than those in the United States and similar countries.

In areas with poor sanitation standards or when chlorinated or filtered tap water is unavailable, only carbonated beverages, those made with boiled water, and beer and wine should be considered safe. Freezing does not afford protection, and the traveler should remember that ice cubes are potential sources of contamination and can transmit the same diseases as water.[2] In areas where these products are unavailable, water can be treated either by boiling (1 min for each 1000 feet above sea level) or by the addition of tincture of iodine (2%) at five drops per liter or tetraglycine hypoperiodide (Globaline, Potable-Agus) tablets according to manufacturer's directions.[4] Cloudy water should first be filtered to remove sediment, if possible. Swimming in contaminated water is also potentially dangerous and can result in either oral ingestion of infected liquid or percutaneous transmission of diseases such as schistosomiasis. In general, ocean water is safer than either fresh or brackish water. Pools should be chlorinated. The traveler is encouraged to check with local residents and health authorities with regard to the safety of water for swimming.

Foods from areas with poor sanitation standards should be considered contaminated. Raw fruits and vegetables should be avoided unless they can be peeled. Meats should be eaten hot and well-done. Unpasteurized milk and milk products should be avoided. Do not partake of foods that have been unrefrigerated for prolonged time periods. Seafood may be especially dangerous because of both infectious agents and toxins. Uncooked clams and oysters should generally be avoided because of risk of concentrated infectious agents such as hepatitis A virus. Avoid internal organs where toxins can be concentrated.

Sexually transmitted diseases can prove potentially troublesome to the unsuspecting traveler. Condoms should be employed if sexual activity with unknown partners is contemplated. Both hepatitis B and highly resistant strains of *Neisseria gonorrhoeae* have been sexually transmitted in selected areas of the world including many countries in Africa and Southeast Asia.[5] In an analogous vein, needles used for blood drawing or blood donation must be sterile and preferably disposable. Blood and blood products can carry unacceptably high risks of disease transmission in countries that do not screen for hepatitis and AIDS (acquired immune deficiency syndrome).

IMMUNIZATION (VACCINATION) FOR TRAVELERS

Individuals traveling to many parts of the world are candidates for immunization as a means of preventing transmission of selected infectious diseases. In general, all persons with itineraries outside of the United States or western

Table 2.2
Vaccination and Prophylaxis Recommendations for Travelers

A.	Recommended for all travelers
	Diphtheria, tetanus
	Poliomyelitis
	Measles, mumps, rubella
B.	Recommended, based on travel itinerary
	Typhoid fever
	Yellow fever
	Malaria
	Immune globulin (ISG)
	Japanese encephalitis
	Travelers' diarrhea
C.	Recommended in special situations only
	Plague
	Rabies
	Meningococcal disease
	Hepatitis B
	Cholera
	Other

Europe should seek counseling regarding the need for vaccination. Table 2.2 summarizes general vaccination recommendations. Immunization may be needed either to prevent diseases present in selected countries or to allow passage into countries in accordance with their own health policies. For these reasons, it is vital that such information be available for the traveler prior to departure. The typical clinician is unlikely to have this type of information immediately available. However, several publications both provide and regularly update these data.[4,6] Additionally, most larger cities contain either specialists in infectious diseases or ''travelers clinics'' where both information and services may be available for variable fees. Virtually all vaccines can be dispensed by the interested clinican with the exception of yellow fever vaccine, which requires licensure and is not typically dispensed by private physicians.[7]

Persons considering travel to areas requiring immunization should allot sufficient time for this procedure. Vaccines that include hepatitis B, cholera, and typhoid fever require two or more injections that should be given at least several weeks apart. The traveler should thus seek attention more than a month prior to departure. In addition to immunizations to prevent unusual illnesses capable of being acquired abroad, the traveler must also ensure that immunizations for poliomyelitis, tetanus, and diphtheria are updated.

An International Certificate of Vaccination should be obtained by all travelers and is available from designated yellow fever centers, travelers clinics, and other centers or physicians interested in travel. Sections are available for documenting a personal health history, prescription medications utilized by the traveler, and complete immunization history. It is mandatory that this certificate be utilized and appropriately stamped when either cholera or yellow fever vaccine is needed.

A wide variety of vaccines are potentially available for use in travelers and are summarized in Table 2.2. They can be broadly divided into those that are an extention of childhood vaccinations, those that can be commonly employed in the prevention of infectious diseases in selected parts of the world, and those that should be utilized only in special circumstances.

VACCINES THAT ARE AN EXTENSION OF CHILDHOOD IMMUNIZATIONS

Tetanus, Diphtheria, and Poliomyelitis

Regardless of travel status, tetanus immunization should be updated every 10 years in persons who have had a primary immunization series.[8] Recent studies demonstrate that up to 11% of adults under the age of 40 and approximately 50% of the elderly lack protection.[9] Most health authorities now recommend that updating tetanus (and diphtheria) immunization each decade be made part of standard health care practices in the United States. Travel may provide a reasonable "excuse" to reinitiate this immunization. Adults who have not received primary immunization should be given a series of three injections of Td (tetanus and diphtheria toxoids, adsorbed for adult use), with the first two doses administered 6–8 weeks apart and the third 6–12 months later.[8] Local reactions that include redness, induration, and pain are common, as are mild constitutional problems. More severe illness such as anaphylaxis or neurological complications are extremely rare.[10] The only contraindication is a history of severe neurological or hypersensitivity reaction to this material.

Diphtheria and tetanus vaccines (Td) should be coadministered once each decade for persons who have received primary immunizations, regardless of plans for travel. In the United States occasional outbreaks of diphtheria continue to occur, primarily in selected areas where immunizations have not be utiilized.[8]

Poliomyelitis is a minor health problem in the United States because of widespread use of vaccines. However, worldwide, this illness continues to be a major health problem, with over 24,000 cases of paralytic disease noted in 1984.[11] Southeast Asia and the western Pacific region accounted for 63% and 19% of cases, respectively.[11] Travelers to all areas of the world with the exception of the United States, Canada, western or eastern Europe, New Zealand, Australia, and Japan should be adequately vaccinated. As with diphtheria and tetanus, travel may prove to be an excellent time to update this immunization even if one is not traveling to an endemic or epidemic area. Adults who have completed a primary immunization series should receive an additional dose of vaccine prior to travel.[12] For those who were vaccinated with oral polio vaccine (OPV), an additional dose of OPV is indicated. For persons in whom inactivated polio vaccine (IPV) was utilized, either OPV or IPV can be administered. Adults traveling to areas with risk and who have not been vaccinated should receive a primary immunization series with IPV because of the slightly lower risk of paralytic side effects.[6] If time permits, two doses administered at 1- to 2-month intervals followed by a third dose 6–12 months later should be given. If less time is available, two doses of IPV given 4 weeks apart can be administered. If less than 4 weeks is available, a single dose of OPV is recommended. In all instances, completion of the series is necessary at a later date.

Measles, Mumps, and Rubella

Measles can be a severe disease with associated morbidity and mortality. Vaccination programs within the United States have greatly decreased the incidence of this disease; however, at least 20% of all cases as recently as 1985 were imported. Although no country requires proof of immunity to measles, travelers are strongly advised to be immune prior to travel.[6] Immunity can be inferred if persons were born prior to 1957, have had proven infection with measles virus, have been immunized, or have serological confirmation of immunity.[13] A single dose of either live attenuated measles vaccine or the combined measles, mumps, rubella (MMR) preparation should be employed. Side effects are common and consist of constitutional reactions that include fevers of up to 103°F.[13] Rare cases of encephalopathy have been noted. Pregnancy is considered a relative contraindication to immunization. Severe allergic reactions to egg should also be considered a contraindication to vaccination.[13] Persons who are also considered candidates for immune serum globulin (ISG, γ-globulin) should have measles vaccine given at least 2 weeks before or 3 months after ISG administration to prevent interference from passively acquired antibodies.

Documentation of immunity to mumps is not required for entry into any country. Most adults should be considered to be immune. Children, especially young boys, should be vaccinated, often with MMR.[14] Side effects are rare and usually mild. Because the vaccine is a live virus, it should not be employed during pregnancy. Because it is manufactured in chick embryos, persons with severe egg hypersensitivities should probably not be immunized. Use with ISG should follow guidelines given for measles vaccine.

Although proof of immunity to rubella is not required for entry into any country, vaccination or proof of immunity should be considered for international travelers. People should be considered immune only if born prior to 1957, have had prior vaccination after their first birthday, or have laboratory evidence of immunity.[15] Side effects can consist of mild constitutional problems, and arthritis and arthralgia are noted regularly in women. Vaccine should not be administered during pregnancy and should be used with caution in women of childbearing age. If it is administered to such individuals, steps should be taken to prevent pregnancy for at least three menstrual cycles.[15] As with other live vaccines, simultaneous use of ISG should be avoided.

VACCINES FOR SELECTED PARTS OF THE WORLD

Yellow Fever

Yellow fever is a severe viral disease present only in parts of Africa and Central and South America and transmitted by the bites of various mosquito vectors.[16] Preventive measures in endemic areas include the use of mosquito netting and insect repellants. Yellow fever vaccine is indicated for persons over the age of 6 months traveling to endemic areas. It is a live attenuated vaccine made from the 17D yellow fever virus strain and has been noted to be safe and effective.[17] Vaccine must be stored at temperatures between 41°F and −22°F and should preferably be frozen prior to reconstitution. Any unused reconstituted vaccine must be discarded within 1 hr of preparation, as it loses potency after that time. For purposes of international travel, yellow fever vaccine must be approved by the World Health Organization and dispensed by an approved yellow fever vaccine center, which are designated by State health departments.[17] Travelers must obtain an International Certificate of Vaccination, documenting appropriate receipt of the yellow fever vaccine. It must be signed by a duly licensed physician, and a Uniform Stamp must be utilized. The certificate does not become valid for 10 days after vaccination. A primary immunization of 0.5 ml of reconstituted vaccine is employed. Booster doses at 10-year intervals are currently recommended. Reactions are mild and typically consist of fever, myalgia, and local pain within 10 days of vaccination. Because this is a live attenuated vaccine, use in pregnancy is generally avoided, although this is not founded on a sound scientific basis. If travel by a pregnant woman to an endemic area cannot be postponed, than vaccination should certainly be contemplated. If travel requirements, rather than increased risk, are the only reason for vaccination, then a waiver from a physician should be obtained.

With the exception of cholera vaccine, all other vaccines (including ISG) can be given either with or after yellow fever vaccine. Cholera and yellow fever vaccines should either be coadministered or given at least 3 weeks apart.[17]

Typhoid Fever

Typhoid fever, caused by *Salmonella typhi,* is endemic in many areas of the world and is seen most commonly in tropical climates, especially in underdeveloped areas with poor sanitation standards and substandard water treatment facilities.[18] Measures aimed at avoiding contaminated food and water should be considered of primary importance and have been previously outlined. Vaccine usage should be considered for international travelers going to areas at risk but should not preclude the need to select food and water sources carefully. In general, this vaccine is not indicated for persons staying in major cities and eating in large tourist-oriented hotels. The currently available vaccine appears to be at least 70% effective in disease prevention.[19] Two 0.5-cc subcutaneous doses of vaccine administered at least 4 weeks apart are recommended. If insufficent time is available, then three doses given at weekly intervals provide an alternative. Booster doses are indicated at 3-year intervals. A more recently developed investigational vaccine, made from the Vi capsular polysaccharide of *S. typhi,* appears to be at least as effective.[20]

Vaccine-related reactions are common but usually mild. Local pain and constitutional complaints usually resolve in 48–72 hr. Although no specific problems have been identified in pregnancy, it may be best to avoid this vaccine on theoretical grounds. However, risks and benefits must be individually assessed.

Cholera

Cholera represents a severe gastrointestinal disease caused by *Vibrio cholerae* and is typically transmitted through ingestion of contaminated water or food.[21] The disease is endemic in large parts of the underdeveloped world. Despite this, disease acquired as a result of travel is extremely rare and is seldom noted in travelers.[22] Although a vaccine is available, it is generally not recommended for routine use unless proof of vaccination is required for entry into a specific country. Efficacy in field trials has been only about 50%.[23] Avoidance of high-risk water and food sources is, however, indicated. The vaccine should be considered only for individuals traveling into extremely high-risk areas and who will be far from immediate medical attention or who suffer from impaired gastrointestinal defense mechanisms. A single 0.5-cc subcutaneous or intramuscular dose will satisfy entry requirements into all countries.[6] For individuals felt to require the vaccine for prophylactic reasons, a primary series consisting of two 0.5-cc doses given 1 week to 1 month apart is recommended.[6] Boosters are needed at 6-month intervals. Reactions are unusual and are not severe.

Patients who receive cholera vaccine should receive documentation in an International Certificate of Vaccination signed by a licensed physician. It is not valid until 6 days after vaccination.

VACCINES FOR SPECIAL CIRCUMSTANCES

A diverse variety of vaccines are potentially available for use in specific instances of unique risk. Persons should be carefully questioned about their need for these based on potential for occupational exposure and/or travel to hyperendemic areas. Not all available vaccines are discussed at this time.

Rabies

Preexposure rabies vaccination should be considered for persons traveling to endemic areas that include Southeast Asia, Africa, and Central or South America, especially if persons are likely to be outside of usual tourist areas for prolonged periods.[24] It should also be considered for individuals in extremely rural areas where access to postexposure vaccination might be delayed. Persons who are bitten while traveling should seek immediate medical attention regardless of the biting species, as in many parts of the world animals including dogs and cats may harbor rabies.

Preexposure prophylaxis consists of three intramuscular doses of human diploid cell vaccine (HDCV) of 1 cc each on days 0, 7, and 21 or 28.[24] Boosters are given at 2-year intervals. Preexposure prophylaxis does not obviate the need for postexposure management; however, it greatly simplifies it by doing away with the need of rabies immune globulin (RIG) and decreases the number of postexposure shots of HDCV that are necessary. For persons who have received preexposure prophylaxis and are subsequently bitten, postexposure management consists of the administration of an additional 1-cc dose as soon as possible and an additional dose at 3 days. Alternatively, a lyophilized HDCV vaccine has been developed that can be reconstituted in the syringe (Merieux Institute).[25] Three 0.1-cc doses administered intradermally on days 0, 7, and either 21 or 28 can be employed. This alternative vaccine route and dose must not be employed for postexposure prophylaxis. Chloroquine phosphate may interfere with production of antirabies antibodies, but this can be decreased by employing the intramuscular route and dose of administration.

Postexposure prophylaxis is indicated for persons who have incurred rabies-prone injuries. Compulsive cleansing of the injury area is of paramount importance and should not be overlooked because vaccination is available. Postexposure prophylaxis for persons not previously vaccinated includes use of both HDCV and RIG. The former is given as five 1-cc intramuscular doses on days 0, 3, 7, 14, and 28.[24] The RIG is administered as 20 IU/kg, with half infiltrated at the injury site and the rest given intramuscularly.

Plague

Vaccination against plague is not required for entry into any country but should be considered in unusual circumstances. Plague is endemic in many countries of Southeast Asia, Africa, and Central or South America and is noted primarily in rural areas.[6] Persons traveling to such sites, especially for activities that place them in direct contact with potentially infected rodents or fleas, should consider vaccination. Primary immunization consists of three injections. The first and second are administered at least 4 weeks apart and are 0.5 ml each. The third should be given 1–3 months after the second and is 0.2 ml. Two booster doses of 0.2 ml each should be given 6 months apart, and further booster doses of 0.2 ml can be given at yearly intervals if risk of infection persists.

Side effects are generally mild and consist of local reactions. More significant constitutional symptoms and signs may be noted with repeated immunizations. Occasional sterile abscesses have been noted.[6]

Meningococcal Infection

Vaccination against meningococci is not a requirement for international travel but should occasionally be considered for itineraries that include endemic areas. These currently include sub-Sahara Africa and parts of Nepal, India, and Brazil. A quadrivalent vaccine consisting of types A, C, Y, and W-135 is generally recommended and is administered subcutaneously. A single dose is indicated and is thought to provide immunity for at least 3 years.[6] Adverse effects are infrequent and are usually localized to the injection site.

Japanese Encephalitis

This form of viral encephalitis is endemic in parts of Asia that include Korea, Bangladesh, Nepal, Burma, Japan, and China. The disease is most common in late summer and autumn. Transmission is through a mosquito vector, and travelers to endemic areas must take protective action against mosquitoes. Persons traveling to rural areas, especially for long periods, should consider vaccination against Japanese encephalitis. The vaccine is not produced in the United States but has been available through the Centers for Disease Control and is distributed through regional centers. Location of distribution centers has historically been available through the CDC, Fort Collins (telephone number 303-221-6429). However, recently the supply has become restricted, and it may not be available.

MANAGEMENT OF OTHER INFECTIOUS DISEASES

Hepatitis A

Hepatitis A is a common health problem in developing countries and is transmitted by the fecal–oral route. Boiling of water, adequate chlorination, proper cooking of foods, and other measures previously outlined will help to prevent disease transmission and acquisition.[6] Likelihood of disease varies with location and extent of travel. Tourist areas and major hotels in most countries are considered safe, but travel to rural areas with poor sanitation standards places the traveler at risk. Immune globulin should be administered to persons felt to be at risk for hepatitis A.[6,26] A dose of 0.02 ml/kg is indicated for travel of less than 3 months' duration, and 0.06 mg/kg should be utilized for travel of up to 5 months.[26] Repeated doses will be needed for persons with more prolonged stays in areas at risk.

Various forms of immune globulins are safe and have not been noted to transmit any infectious disease, including AIDS.[27] This agent can be safely utilized during pregnancy. In instances where it is to be employed in conjuction with vaccines, it should probably not be given concomitantly with live viral vaccines but rather at least several weeks afterwards to prevent interference with antibody production.

Hepatitis B

Risk of hepatitis B in international travel is low, and proof of immunization is not required for entry into any country. Transmission is either through contaminated blood products or sexual activity. The disease is prevalent in parts of Southeast Asia, Africa, and Central and South America, and risk assessment depends on length of travel and likelihood of contact with contaminated blood or body secretions from the local population. Primary vaccination consists of three 1-ml intramuscular doses of either hepatitis B immune globulin (HBIG) or the newer genetically engineered product.[6] Doses are administered at 0, 1, and 6 months. It is considered safe and has not been associated with the transmission of other infectious diseases.[28] Hepatitis B vaccine can be safely administered during pregnancy.

Non-A, Non-B Hepatitis

This form of hepatitis has been noted in underdeveloped countries that include parts of North Africa and Southeast Asia. Transmission can occur through contact with infected water or food. In actuality, most persons traveling to areas where this illness is endemic will have received ISG prophylaxis for hepatitis A. However, the protective value of ISG for non-A, non-B hepatitis is unknown, and protection should not be assumed.

Malaria

Malaria is a common worldwide disease that results in substantial morbidity and mortality. Worldwide, it is estimated that up to 11 million cases occur annually[29]; between 1978 and 1982, approximately 5200 cases of malaria were imported into the United States.[30] During 1986, 1091 cases were reported in this country, an increase of 4% over the previous year.[31] Only 36 persons acquired their infection within continental borders. Disease is spread through the bite of infected female anopheles mosquitoes. These creatures are active primarily after

Table 2.3
Regimens for Malaria Prophylaxis[a]

A. All patients traveling to areas with malaria
   Chloroquine
B. Travel to areas of Africa with chloroquine-resistant *P. falciparum*
   Chloroquine plus either:
   1. Pyrimethamine–sulfadoxine (Fansidar): Take only if symptoms of malaria develop and patient is away from immediate medical attention (less than 3-week exposure) or
   2. Pyrimethamine–sulfadoxine (Fansidar): weekly (longer than 3-week exposure) or
   3. Proguanil 200 mg/day[b]
C. Travel to areas of Southeast Asia and South America with combined Chloroquine and Fansidar-resistant *P. falciparum*
   Chloroquine plus:
   Doxycycline 100 mg/day beginning 2–4 days prior to departure

[a]See Health Advice for International Travel,[46] Medical Letter,[47] and text for specific regimens.
[b]Not available in the United States.

dusk, and highest risk occurs during the evening and night. Disease occurs in many parts of the world, including Central and South America, sub-Sahara Africa, Southeast Asia, and Oceania.[29] Risk of disease acquisition is highest in travelers to sub-Sahara Africa, and between 1982 and 1984 over 250 cases of disease caused by *Plasmodium falciparum* were noted from this area.[32] This comprises over 70% of the total cases reported worldwide in Americans.

Prevention of malaria is of paramount importance to all persons traveling to endemic areas. Mosquito netting, staying indoors during high-risk time periods, and the use of insect repellants should be routinely considered. Patients should be advised of typical presenting symptoms and signs and should contact a health care facility if problems arise. No consistent illness should be automatically ascribed to "flu" without an appropriate assessment for malaria.

Malaria chemoprophylaxis should be routinely employed for travelers to endemic areas. Choice of prophylaxis will vary with the type of malaria likely to be implicated. Table 2.3 depicts recommended prophylaxis regimens. Choice depends both on the likelihood of encountering chloroquine-resistant strains of *P. falciparum* and on the length of travel to endemic areas. Chloroquine-resistant strains have been noted primarily in East and Central Africa, Central and South America, and selected areas within Southeast Asia.[6] More recent data now demonstrate chloroquine-resistant *P. falciparum* in West Africa (Nigeria) as well.[33]

For prophylaxis against *P. ovale, P. malariae, P. vivax,* and sensitive strains of *P. falciparum,* chloroquine remains the agent of choice.[6] Dosage of 500 mg weekly should be employed and should be initiated 2 weeks prior to travel to ensure against adverse reactions and to achieve adequate tissue concentrations. The traveler should be encouraged to take medication on the same day each week and to continue for 6 weeks after return from endemic areas. The chemoprophylactic regimen for persons traveling to areas where the possibility of resistant *P. falciparum* exists will vary with the duration of exposure and is constantly being revised. Because of the possibility of infection with *P. vivax,* chloroquine should always be included in the regimen. Fansidar, a fixed combination of sulfadoxine and pyrimethamine, has been considered the agent of choice for chloroquine-resistant *P. falciparum* but does not provide adequate coverage for *P. vivax.* Additionally, therapeutic failures have been noted in patients receiving both Fansidar and chloroquine.[34] However, recent demonstration of a significant number of dermatological adverse reactions to this agent has caused a reassessment of the use of this compound. By 1985, ten cases of severe skin reactions (four fatal) that included Stevens–Johnson syndrome and toxic epidermal necrolysis had been described.[35] For travel to endemic areas that will last less than 3 weeks, chloroquine, 500 mg, should be taken weekly, and the traveler should also be provided with a single empiric dose of Fansidar to be taken at the onset of symptoms consistant with malaria.[6] Alternatively, proguanil 200 mg/day can be utilized in lieu of Fansidar. It must be purchased outside of the United States. Fansidar should still be carried for presumptive treatment.[46] For travel to Southeast Asia, where chloroquine and Fansidar resistance has been encountered, doxycycline 100 mg/day plus chloroquine should be considered[46] and used for 4 weeks after return.

Travelers' Diarrhea

Diarrhea associated with travel is well appreciated and occurs regularly. It has often been labeled with the name of the area visited and carries such connotations as "Delhi belly," the "Trotskys," or "Montezuma's revenge." Diarrhea occurs in 1–94% of travelers, and estimates are that up to 12 million persons annually develop diarrhea during travel.[36] This represents the single largest health problem noted during travel. Risks for the development of diarrhea depend on the travel destination, length of stay, and products ingested. Selected areas of the world that include many parts of Central and South America, Africa, and Southeast Asia carry risks that approach 50%, whereas others such as the United States, Western Europe, and Canada carry risks closer to 2–5%.[37]

Bacterial agents account for up to 80% of all cases of diarrhea noted in travelers.[38] Depending on the population and the location of the investigation, enterotoxigenic *E. coli* is most common and can be noted in 40–60% of cases.[39] Other bacterial pathogens that can be regularly encountered include strains of *Salmonella* and *Shigella, Campylobacter,* and *Aeromonas.* Other organisms oc-

Table 2.4
Causes of Travelers' Diarrhea[a]

Organism	Frequency (%)
E. coli (enterotoxigenic)	40–70
Shigella	18–25
Campylobacter jejuni	3–17
Salmonella	3–7
Aeromonas hydrophilia	1–5
Rotavirus	0–10
Giardia lamblia	1–4
Multiple agents	5–15
Unknown	15–25

[a]Adopted from Ericsson and DuPont.[37]

casionally noted include *Giardia, Cryptosporidium,* and rotavirus. In all investigations, 25–40% of cases of diarrhea are unassociated with any demonstrable infectious agent.[39,40] Table 2.4 summarizes data on the likely causes of travelers' diarrhea.

In most instances the infectious agent is ingested with contaminated food or water. The traveler must remember that ice remains an important vehicle for the spread of many forms of infectious diarrhea and that bacteria may exist for prolonged periods within this substance.[41] Less common is person-to-person spread. Vegetables may be the most common source of disease, and likelihood of diarrhea development may also depend on the location of ingestion, with meals eaten in the homes of local families appearing to carry highest risk.[37] It is unclear, however, whether judicious avoidance of contaminated foods or water will decrease the probability of acquiring travelers' diarrhea.

Clinical presentation is usually that of a self-limited rather mild illness characterized by three to five loose, watery stools per day, often associated with abdominal cramping and low-grade constitutional complaints.[37,42] Disease lasts an average of 5 days. However, up to 20% of cases will note substantial inconvenience from the disease and may be bedridden for at least part of the illness. Less commonly, travelers' diarrhea presents as either a choleralike syndrome or as dysentery, and in these instances pathogens such as *V. cholera* or *Shigella* and *Campylobacter* species should be suspected. However, neither specific symptoms nor signs are sensitive or specific enough for diagnosis.

Management strategies for dealing with traveler's diarrhea include both prophylaxis and treatment of symptomatic illness. The former can be accomplished with a variety of preparations that include doxycycline, trimethoprim–sulfamethoxazole, and bismuth subsalicylate (Pepto-Bismol®).[37,38,42] Regimens for both prophylaxis and treatment are summarized in Table 2.5. Problems with prophylactic regimens include (1) rash and other allergic phenomena, (2) possibility of photosensitization, and (3) risk of development of resistant fecal flora. Current recommendations are that not all people receive prophylaxis and that this

Table 2.5
Prevention and Treatment of Travelers' Diarrhea[a]

Medication	Dose
Prevention	
Doxycycline	100 mg/day
Bismuth subsalicylate	60 ml q.i.d
Trimethoprim–sulfamethoxazole	160 mg, 800 mg/day
Trimethoprim	200 mg/day
Treatment	
Loperamide	4 mg followed by 2 mg after each stool to maximum of 16 mg/day
Bismuth subsalicylate	1 oz q.$\frac{1}{2}$ hr to total of 8 oz
Trimethoprim–sulfamethoxazole	160 mg, 800 mg q. $\frac{1}{2}$ 12 hr for 3–5 days
Trimethoprim	200 mg q. 12 hr for 3–5 days
Ciprofloxacin	250–500 mg q. 12 hr for 3–5 days

[a]Adopted from Ericsson and DuPont.[37]

management strategy be reserved for selected individuals who cannot risk diarrhea while traveling.[37,38,42]

Therapy of travelers' diarrhea includes adequate hydration and possibly the use of symptomatic medications as discussed in Chapter 13. Patients with three to five loose stools per day, in the absence of major constitutional symptomatology, can benefit from either loperamide or bismuth subsalicylate.[37] Antibiotics have been successfully employed but should probably be reserved for those with at least moderately severe illness.[37,38] This is typified by the passage of at least six loose stools per day, when other symptoms are severe, or when bloody stools are noted. Medications successfully utilized include trimethoprim, trimethoprim–sulfamethoxazole, and doxycycline. Suggested regimens are provided in Table 2.5. Studies with these medications demonstrate improvement rates in excess of 80% at 48 hr compared with less than 15% in the placebo-treated group.[37] Therapy for 3–5 days is usually sufficient. More recent studies have demonstrated the efficacy of ciprofloxacin in travelers' diarrhea and show it to be as effective as trimethoprim–sulfamethoxazole.[43] This agent has as a major advantage clinical and *in vitro* efficacy against *Campylobacter* species, a group usually resistant to other antibiotics commonly employed for this condition.[44] However, the quinolones (of which ciprofloxacin is representative) have several drawbacks. First, they are relatively contraindicated in children because of the potential for developmental problems in cartilage. Secondly, they are associated with adverse drug interactions, which include theophylline, and thirdly, they can be associated with CNS toxicities that can include seizures, depression, and anxiety.[45] Thus, the decision to employ ciprofloxacin should take into account the travel agenda (and implied risk for infection with *Campylobacter* species), patient allergies, and concomitant administration of other medications.

Management of the Returning Traveler

Although most travelers arrive home physically fit, occasional individuals develop medical problems that must be assessed on return. The clinician must remember to question about recent travel as part of the evaluation of the patient with disease, and if travel has occurred, to obtain a complete itinerary. Infectious diarrhea and malaria are two common illnesses that can present after return from travel and that must be assessed in a timely fashion. Stools for ova and parasite determination and bacterial culture may be needed for the former, and the latter can usually be documented by blood smears obtained during symptomatic periods. Failure to consider and appropriately manage malaria can lead to death, and ineffective diagnosis and management of infectious diarrhea could cause sustained morbidity, occasional mortality, and the possibility of intrafamilial spread. Febrile patients without diarrhea in whom malaria cannot be documented should also be evaluated for typhoid fever and brucellosis, among other possibilities.

REFERENCES

1. Jong EC: Medical approach to the traveling patient. In: Jong EC, ed. *The Travel and Tropical Medicine Manual.* Philadelphia, WB Saunders, 1987:3–7.
2. Jones TC: Health advice and immunizations for travelers. In: Remington JS, Swartz, MN, eds. *Current Clinical Topics in Infectious Diseases,* Vol 6. New York, McGraw-Hill, 1985:40–65.
3. Mann JM: Emporiatric policy and practice: Protecting the health of Americans abroad. *JAMA* 1983; 249:3323–3325.
4. Denny SC, ed: *Travel Health Information Service,* Vol 1 (Sect A): *Medical Reference Guide.* Milwaukee, Shoreland Medical Marketing, 1986.
5. Hook, EW III, Holmes KK: Gonococcal infections. *Ann Intern Med* 1985; 102:229–243.
6. US Department of Health and Human Services: *Health Information for International Travel.* Atlanta, Centers for Disease Control, Division of Quarantine, 1987.
7. Centers for Disease Control: Yellow fever vaccine. *Morbid Mortal Week Rep* 1984; 32:679–688.
8. Centers for Disease Control: Diphtheria, tetanus, and pertussis: Guidelines for vaccine prophylaxis and other preventive measures. *Morbid Mortal Week Rep* 1985; 34:405–426.
9. Centers for Disease Control: Summary of the Second National Community Forum on Adult Immunization. *Morbid Mortal Week Rep* 1987; 36:677–680.
10. Jacobs RL, Lowe RS, Lanier BQ: Adverse reactions to tetanus toxoid. *JAMA* 1982; 247:40–42.
11. Denny SC, ed: *Travel Health Information Service,* Vol 1 (Sect C), *Medical Reference Guide.* Milwaukee, Shoreland Medical Marketing, 1986:C9.1–C9.4.
12. Immunization Practices Advisory Committee, Centers for Disease Control: Poliomyelitis prevention. *Ann Intern Med* 1982; 96:630–634.
13. Centers for Disease Control: Measles prevention. *Morbid Mortal Week Rep* 1987; 36:409–425.
14. Centers for Disease Control: Mumps vaccine. *Morbid Mortal Week Rep* 1982; 31:617–625.
15. Centers for Disease Control: Rubella prevention. *Morbid Mortal Week Rep* 1984; 33:301–318.

16. Centers for Disease Control: Summary of a symposium on yellow fever. *J Infect Dis* 1981; 144:87–91.
17. Centers for Disease Control: Yellow fever vaccine. *Morbid Mortal Week Rep* 1984; 32:679–688.
18. Butler T, Mahmoud AAAF, Warren KS: Algorithms in the diagnosis and management of exotic diseases. XXIII. Typhoid fever. *J Infect Dis* 1977; 135:1017–1020.
19. Centers for Disease Control: Typhoid vaccine. *Morbid Mortal Week Rep* 1978; 27:231–233.
20. Acharya IL, Lowe CU, Lthapa R, *et al:* Prevention of typhoid fever in Nepal with the Vi capsular polysaccharide of *Salmonella typhi. N Engl J Med* 1987; 317:1101–1104.
21. Carpenter CCJ, Mahmoud AAF, Warren KS: Algorithms in the diagnosis and management of exotic diseases. XXVI. Cholera. *J Infect Dis* 1977; 136:461–464.
22. Morgen H: Epidemiology of cholera in travelers and conclusions for vaccination recommendations. *Br Med J* 1983; 286:184–186.
23. Centers for Disease Control: Cholera vaccine. *Morbid Mortal Week Rep* 1978; 27:173–174.
24. Centers for Disease Control: Rabies prevention—United States, 1984. *Morbid Mortal Week Rep* 1984; 33:393–407.
25. Centers for Disease Control: Field evaluations of pre-exposure use of human diploid cell rabies vaccine. *Morbid Mortal Week Rep* 1983; 32:601–609.
26. Immunization Practices Advisory Committee: Immune globulins for protection against viral hepatitis. *Ann Intern Med* 1982; 96:193–197.
27. Centers for Disease Control: Lack of transmission of human immunodeficiency virus through $Rh_o(D)$ immune globulin (human). *Morbid Mortal Week Rep* 1987; 36:728–279.
28. Centers for Disease Control: Hepatitis B virus vaccine safety: Report of an inter-agency group. *Morbid Mortal Week Rep* 1982; 31:465–467.
29. Ruebush TK II, Breman JG, Kaiser RL, *et al:* Selective primary health care. XXIV. Malaria. *Rev Infect Dis* 1987; 8:454–466.
30. Lobel HO, Campbell CC: Trends in imported malaria, United States. *Morbid Mortal Week Rep* 1983; 32(suppl 3SS):15SS–18SS. 1983
31. Centers for Disease Control: *Malaria Surveillance Annual Summary 1986, Issued October 1987.* Atlanta, Centers for Disease Control, 1987.
32. US Department of Health and Human Services: *Health Information for International Travel, 1986.* Atlanta, Centers for Disease Control, Division of Quarantine, 1986.
33. Centers for Disease Control: Chloroquine-resistant *Plasmodium falciparum* malaria in West Africa. *Morbid Mortal Week Rep* 1987; 36:13–14.
34. Miller KD, Lobel HO, Pappaioanou M, *et al:* Failures of combined chloroquine and Fansidar prophylaxis in American travelers to East Africa. *J Infect Dis* 1986; 154:689–691.
35. Centers for Disease Control: Adverse reactions to Fansidar and updated recommendations for its use in the prevention of malaria. *Morbid Mortal Week Rep* 1985; 33:713–714.
36. Steffen R, van der Linde F, Gyr K, *et al:* Epidemiology of diarrhea in travelers. *JAMA* 1983; 249:1176–1180.
37. Ericsson CD, DuPont HL: Travelers' diarrhea: Recent Developments. In: Remington JS, Swartz MN, eds. *Current Clinical Topics in Infectious Diseases,* Vol 6. New York, McGraw-Hill, 1985:66–84.
38. DuPont HL, Ericsson CD, Johnson PC: Chemotherapy and chemoprophylaxis of travelers' diarrhea. *Ann Intern Med* 1985; 102:260–261.
39. Sack RB: Traveler's diarrhea. *Hosp Ther* 1987; 12:81–88.
40. Rohde JE: Selective primary health care: Strategies of control of disease in the developing world. XV. Acute diarrhea. *Rev Infect Dis* 1984; 6:840–854.
41. Dickens DL, DuPont HL, Johnson PC: Survival of bacterial enteropathogens in the ice of popular drinks. *JAMA* 1985; 253:3141–3143.
42. Consensus Development Conference: *Traveler's Diarrhea.* Bethesda, National Institutes of Health, Public Health Service, 1985.

43. Ericsson CD, Johnson PC, DuPont HL, *et al:* Ciprofloxacin or trimethoprim–sulfamethoxazole as initial therapy for travelers' diarrhea. *Ann Intern Med* 1987; 106:216–220.
44. Wolfson JS, Hooper DC: The fluoroquinolones: Structures, mechanisms of action, resistance, and spectra of activity *in vitro*. *Antimicrob Agents Chemother* 1985; 28:581–586.
45. Fass RJ: Efficacy and safety of oral ciprofloxacin. *Hosp Formul* 1987; 22(suppl A):16–20.
46. Hill DR, Pearson RD: Health advice for international travel. *Ann Intern Med* 1988; 108:839–852.
47. Medical Letter: Advice for travelers. *Med Lett* 1987; 29:53–56.

3

Intestinal and Lymphatic Infectious Disorders in the Male Homosexual

Richard A. Gleckman

INTRODUCTION

This chapter reviews two unique disorders experienced by homosexual men. These entities have been referred to as the "gay bowel syndrome" and the "diffuse (persistent) lymphadenopathy syndrome." This section of the text does not focus on the clinical features of the male homosexual who has developed AIDS (see Chapter 4). However, all homosexual men, regardless of their "presenting" or "chief complaint," deserve a thorough medical history and physical examination, and this process can often raise the physician's consciousness that the patient has AIDS or the AIDS-related complex.[1] Tables 3.1 and 3.2 list those findings that should suggest AIDS-associated conditions.

Ten years ago the term "gay bowel syndrome" was coined to denote the vast array of infectious and traumatic disorders that involve the rectum and colon of male homosexuals.[2] Previously it had been reported that a number of viral (hepatitis A, hepatitis B, herpes simplex, condyloma acuminatum), bacterial (*Neisseria gonorrhoeae, Treponema pallidum, Shigella* spp.), parasitic (*Entamoeba histolytica, Giardia lamblia*), and chlamydial (lymphogranuloma venereum) infections of the intestinal tract occurred among sexually active male homosexuals. The reader should appreciate, however, that homosexuality by itself is not a risk factor for the acquisition of intestinal infections, particularly for those men who only engage in "safe" sexual practices. Intestinal infections are proven to occur in those male homosexuals who have multiple anonymous sexual partners and participate in specific sexual practices, namely, passive anal

Table 3.1
Information from History That Suggests AIDS or the AIDS-Related Complex

1. Chronic ulcerating facial or perianal herpes simplex lesions
2. Incapacitating and protracted diarrhea caused by *Cryptosporidium, Isospora belli, Mycobacterium avium-intracellulare*, or cytomegalovirus
3. Central or peripheral nervous system alteration not attributable to syphilis or herpes simplex
4. *Salmonella* bacteremia, particularly recurrent
5. Significant weight loss
6. Prolonged unexplained fever, on occasion accompanied by night sweats and extreme fatigue

intercourse, anilingus, active finger/fist fornication, and fellatio of a fecally contaminated penis. Table 3.3 lists some of the infectious organisms that contribute to the "gay bowel syndrome" and the sexual practices involved in their transmission. A third factor responsible for the high prevalence of enteric infections in homosexual men is the frequent asymptomatic carriage of intestinal organisms.[3] Of additional importance is the observation that gay men often harbor **multiple** potential intestinal pathogens simultaneously.[4]

Various myths regarding male homosexuals continue to pervade some medical quarters. Contrary to the opinion held by some physicians, no appearance, occupation, or behavior denotes that a man is a sexually active homosexual. It should also be appreciated that prior or current marriage does not exclude the possibility that a man is a homosexual. Clinicians should be prepared to obtain a history of sexual orientation and explore sexual practices when a patient presents with complaints that might be associated with sexual activity.

A number of advantages accrue from correctly diagnosing intestinal infections in male homosexuals. Virtually all of the infections are amenable to therapy, and disabling symptoms can be alleviated.[5] Unrecognized or untreated, these intestinal infections can have serious sequelae (chronic malabsorption resulting from small intestinal infection with *G. lamblia,* liver abscess caused by invasive

Table 3.2
Manifestations on Physical Examination That Suggest AIDS or the AIDS-Related Complex

1.	Telangiectasia of upper chest	7.	Oral candidiasis
2.	Seborrheic dermatitis (extensive)	8.	Hairy leukoplakia
3.	Kaposi's sarcoma	9.	Squamous (oral) carcinoma
4.	Cotton-wool exudates	10.	Non-Hodgkin's (oral) lymphoma
5.	Retinitis of CMV	11.	Lymph nodes of increasing size
6.	Splenomegaly	12.	Persistent, diffuse lymphadenopathy

Table 3.3
Correlation of Infectious Organism and Sexual Practice

	Anilingus	
Passive anal intercourse	Rim	Passive
Neisseria gonorrhoeae	*Salmonella* spp.	Herpes simplex
Condyloma acuminatum	*Shigella* spp.	*Treponema pallidum*
Chlamydia sp.	*Campylobacter* spp.	*Neisseria meningitidis*
Herpes simplex	*E. histolytica*	
Treponema pallidum	*G. lamblia*	
	Enterobius vermicularis	

E. histolytica, rectal stricture produced by the host response to lymphogranuloma venereum, disseminated disease arising from gonococcal proctitis), and they can contribute to the reservoir of infection within the homosexual community.[6] In addition, if intestinal infections are incorrectly diagnosed (amebic colitis misdiagnosed as ulcerative colitis and treated with prednisone), grave consequences can ensue.

A clinical/anatomic classification has emerged that relates the patient's symptoms with localization of the infection and the putative infectious agent(s).[7,8] Patients with symptomatic proctitis (an inflammation limited to the distal 15 cm of the anorectum) demonstrate one or more of the following abnormalities: anorectal pain, pruritus, constipation, tenesmus (ineffectual effort to defecate), hematochezia (passage of bloody stools), and mucopurulent discharge. In homosexual men proctitis is most frequently caused by *Neisseria gonorrhoeae, Treponema pallidum,* herpes simplex, *Chlamydia trachomatis,* and condylomata acuminata (viral genital wart). Proctocolitis (inflammation proximal to the rectosigmoid junction) is clinically recognized by the presence of lower abdominal pain, malaise, diarrhea (which can contain blood and pus), and, on occasion, fever and myalgia. In gay men this symptom complex is usually attributed to *Shigella* spp., *Campylobacter* spp., *Chlamydia trachomatis* (LGV serotype), *E. histolytica,* and *C. difficile* (antibiotic-initiated pseudomembranous colitis). Enteritis (inflammation of the small intestine) has been identified by the following clinical features: nausea, bloating, abdominal pain, and noninflammatory diarrhea. The pathogen most often identified with this symptom complex is *G. lamblia,* although the disorder can be caused by the traditional bacterial pathogens (*Shigella* spp., *Campylobacter* spp.) associated with enterocolitis. Additional parasites (cryptosporidium, *Isospora belli*) and bacteria (*Mycobacterium avium-intracellulare*) produce enteritis in homosexual men with AIDS.[1]

No attempt is made to describe in detail the clinical features and therapy of all the infectious agents isolated from the intestinal tract of homosexual men, including such organisms as *Enterobius vermicularis* (pinworm), *Calymmatobacterium granulomatous* (cause of granuloma inguinuale), *Neisseria men-*

Table 3.4
Intestinal Disorders: Clinical/Laboratory Associations

Manifestation	Infectious agent(s)
Fever	HSV, LGV, *Shigella* spp., *Campylobacter* spp., *E. histolytica, Treponema pallidum, C. difficile*
Fever with inguinal adenopathy	HSV, LGV, *Treponema pallidum*
Rash	*Treponema pallidum*
Rectal mass	*Treponema pallidum*, LGV
Sacral neuralgia, urinary retention	HSV
Perianal ulcer	HSV, *Treponema pallidum*, calymmatobacterium granulomatous
Rectal ulcer	HSV, LGV, *Treponema pallidum, E. histolytica, Shigella* spp., *Salmonella* spp.
Hematochezia	HSV, LGV, *Treponema pallidum*
Prior antimicrobial therapy	*C. difficile*
Anorectal discharge	*Neisseria gonorrhoeae, Chlamydia trachomatis, Treponema pallidum, E. histolytica*, nontreponemal spirochete
Constipation	HSV, *Neisseria gonorrhoeae, Treponema pallidum*
Diarrhea with fecal leukocytes	*Shigella* spp., *Salmonella*, spp., *Campylobacter* spp., *C. difficile*
Granuloma on rectal biopsy	LGV
Markedly elevated serum alkaline phosphatase	*Treponema pallidum*
Polys on rectal swab	*Neisseria gonorrhoeae*, Herpes simplex, *C. trachomatis, Campylobacter* spp.
Histology resembling ulcerative colitis	LGV

ingitidis, Plesiomonas shigelloides, and nontreponemal spirochetes.[9–11] Comments will, however, be restricted to the unique manifestations of specific infections as well as their diagnosis and therapy. A proposed diagnostic evaluation (''workup'') will also be presented to serve as a guide for the clinician assessing the gay male with symptoms referable to the intestinal tract. Table 3.4 lists some clinical manifestations and those infectious organisms most frequently and uniquely associated with these clinical features.

SYPHILIS

Rectal syphilis can be asymptomatic, can cause intestinal symptoms (pain on defecation, tenesmus, rectal discharge, bloody diarrhea, hematochezia, constipation), or can be incidentally detected when the patient is being evaluated because of other findings, such as rash or inguinal adenopathy.[12,13] Anorectal syphilis can resemble an anal fissure, a herpetic ulcer, a wart, or a rectal malignancy.[14,15] The diagnosis of anal lesion syphilis is achieved by the detection of motile treponemes by dark-field examination. This test is not specific, however, for rectal lesions. Biopsies of the rectum should be processed by conventional histology as well as with silver staining or immunofluorescence. Serology will enhance the clinical impression of primary or secondary syphilis, but a negative serological test fails to exclude the possibility of primary syphilis.[16] It is important to remember that biological false-positive serological tests for syphilis are common for drug addicts.[17] Positive reagin tests (VDRL, RPR) detected in gay male addicts should be confirmed by specific treponemal tests such as the fluorescent treponemal antibody absorption (FTA-ABS).

NEISSERIA GONORRHOEAE

Gonococcal proctitis in the homosexual man can be a symptomatic or an asymptomatic disease.[18] The diagnosis is established by Gram stain and culture of rectal discharge or culture of a swab taken from the rectal mucosa, not the stool. In the symptomatic gay male with anorectal discharge caused by *Neisseria gonorrhoeae,* anoscopy should be performed to obtain "directed" cultures and to detect additional/alternative disorders, including intrarectal chancres, condylomata acuminata, and ulcers caused by herpes simplex and *E. histolytica.*[19]

HERPES

Although herpes proctitis can be an asymptomatic disorder, anorectal disease caused by herpes simplex is usually characterized by pain, tenesmus, constipation, inguinal adenopathy, and, often, fever.[20–22] Most patients will demonstrate perianal ulcers or vesicular/pustular lesions. When patients experience urinary difficulty or pain or paresthesias of the buttocks and upper thigh, the clinician should heighten his suspicion that herpes simplex is contributing to the patient's intestinal symptoms.[22,23] The diagnosis of anorectal herpes can be suspected from the appearance of the lesions and the patient's clinical features, but definitive diagnosis requires viral culture. The presence of intranuclear inclusion bodies on rectal biopsy also suggests the diagnosis of herpetic proctitis.

CHLAMYDIA TRACHOMATIS

Proctitis caused by *C. trachomatis* ranges from asymptomatic disease to symptomatic infection.[24,25] The latter is characterized by anorectal discharge and tenesmus.[26] Often fecal leukocytes are detected on swab of the rectal mucosa in both asymptomatic and symptomatic patients. The lymphogranuloma venereum (LGV) serotypes produce a more severe disease, a disorder that resembles herpes simplex proctitis.[27,28] Patients develop anal discharge, anorectal pain, tenesmus, abdominal pain, constipation, hematochezia, and, on occasion, fever with inguinal adenopathy. Histologically, the presence of crypt abscesses, granulomas, and giant cells resembles Crohn's disease. The Frei test, a measure of a delayed hypersensitivity skin reaction, is unreliable to establish the diagnosis of LGV.[29] Culture of *C. trachomatis* from the rectum is the definitive diagnostic procedure. Rapid diagnosis of rectal infection has been accomplished by the direct immunofluorescent staining technique applied to rectal secretions.[30]

ENTERIC BACTERIAL PATHOGENS

Shigella sp., *Aeromonas* sp., *Campylobacter fetus* subspecies *jejuni,* and newly recognized *Campylobacter* spp. (*cinaedi, fennelliae*) produce an enterocolitis syndrome in gay men who practice fellatio and anilinction that resembles the syndrome experienced by heterosexual men who acquire these pathogens by ingesting contaminated food or fluid.[31–34] Diagnosis of these organisms requires their recovery from rectal swabs or stool cultures.

ENTAMOEBA HISTOLYTICA

This intestinal protozoan can be excreted by asymptomatic gay men or can be associated with symptoms consistent with proctocolitis.[35–37] The groups of *E. histolytica* (referred to as zymodermes) most commonly recovered from the stools of male homosexuals are considered nonvirulent.[38] However, gay men have experienced invasive disease, both severe colitis and liver abscess, from this organism.[39] The diagnosis of intestinal amebiasis is confirmed by demonstrating the parasite in stool, wet mount of a rectal swab, or in a rectal biopsy.

GIARDIA LAMBLIA

Most male homosexuals who harbor *G. lamblia* are asymptomtic. The symptoms that can be produced by this intestinal parasite include abdominal bloating, cramps, flatulence, and nonbloody diarrhea.[40] Multiple stool examinations are often necessary to detect *G. lamblia,* and barium studies should not be performed prior to stool analysis. Alternatives to stool examination include duodenal aspiration and biopsy as well as the Entero-test (gelatin capsule containing a weighted nylon string). Serological detection of *G. lamblia* antigen in stool is currently being developed.[41]

Table 3.5
Treatment Regimens

Organism	Recommended	Alternative
Treponema pallidum	Benzathine penicillin, 2.4 million units i.m.	Tetracycline, 500 mg p.o. q.i.d for 15 days
Neisseria gonorrhoeae	Ceftriaxone, 125 mg i.m.	Spectinomycin, 2 g i.m.
Herpes simplex	400 mg acyclovir 5 times a day for 10 days	Sitz bath
Chlamydia trachomatis	Tetracycline, 500 mg p.o. q.i.d. for 7 days (for 21 days if LGV serovar)	Erythromycin base or stearate, 500 mg p.o. q.i.d for 7 days (for 21 days if LGV serovar)
Shigella spp.	Trimethoprim–sulfamethoxazole, one double-strength tablet b.i.d. for 7 days	Norfloxacin, 400 mg b.i.d.
Campylobacter spp.	Erythromycin, 500 mg p.o. q.i.d. for 7 days	
G. lamblia	Quinacrine, 100 mg p.o. t.i.d. for 7 days	Metronidazole, 250 mg p.o. t.i.d. for 7 days
E. histolytica	Metronidazole, 750 mg p.o. t.i.d. for 5–10 days, plus iodoquinol, 650 mg p.o. t.i.d. for 20 days	Paromomycin, 25–35 mg/kg per day in three divided oral doses

TREATMENT

Treatment recommendations for the intestinal infections experienced by homosexual men are listed in Table 3.5. Some guidelines, however, apply to each of these infections. All infections merit treatment; the frequent existence of polymicrobic infections should be appreciated; efforts should be made to make specific (laboratory-confirmed) diagnoses; patients should be advised to abstain from sexual activity (in its full dimensions) until treatment has been determined to be successful; efficacy of therapy must be established; and efforts should be made to identify, screen, and treat sexual partners, even if they are asymptomatic. In addition, advice should be offered regarding safe sexual practices for gay men (mutual masturbation; orogenital insertive/receptive and anogenital insertive/receptive only **when** a condom is used), and all sexually transmitted diseases identified should be reported to the public health workers to evaluate contacts.

Ceftriaxone may well be the drug of choice to treat homosexual men with rectal gonococcal infection. This third-generation cephalosporin is administered as a single intramuscular injection, thereby assuring compliance. It is an effective therapy for anorectal disease (when caused by either β-lactamase-producing or -nonproducing strains of *N. gonorrhoeae*) as well as for pharyngeal gonococcal infection. Spectinomycin should be prescribed for the penicillin-allergic patient with anorectal gonococcal infection, but this compound is not effective treatment for pharyngeal disease. Test of cure follow-up cultures should be obtained from the rectum 3–7 days after treatment.

With regard to the treatment of primary or secondary syphilis, it is important to appreciate that the recommended therapy (2.4 million units of penicillin G benzathine, i.m.) is not invariably successful and that patients should be asked to return for clinical and serological testing 3 and 6 months after administration of the antibiotic. Cured patients should have a fourfold decrease in VDRL titer (or RPR) by 3 months and an eightfold decrease by 6 months. Serological response in patients who have had previous syphilitic infection is less predictable, however.

When metronidazole is prescribed to gay men with amebiasis or giardiasis, these patients should be advised not to drink any alcohol, as a disulfiramlike reaction can develop. This untoward reaction is characterized by confusion, flushing, headache, nausea, vomiting, drowsiness, and a fall in blood pressure.

The evaluation of the homosexual man with symptoms referable to the intestinal tract is predicated on two concepts: identifying the precise etiologic organism(s) and recognizing that dual infections often exist. The workup consists of a thorough medical history (emphasizing past medical illnesses, specific sexual activities, illnesses among sexual contacts, use of antidiarrheal agents and antibiotics), a complete physical examination (supplemented by anoscopy), serological tests for hepatitis B and syphilis, sigmoidoscopy, and appropriate cultures (Gram stain and culture for *N. gonorrhoeae* if rectal exudate is present, rectal swab culture for *N. gonorrhea, Chlamydia trachomatis,* and herpes simplex if proctitis is present, stools for *E. histolytica* as well as stool cultures for *Shigella* sp., *Salmonella* sp., and *Campylobacter* sp. if proctocolitis is present, and a search for these organisms and *G. lamblia* if enteritis is the dominant clinical syndrome). A dark-field examination for *T. pallidum* is indicated on anorectal ulcers, and, if the patient has previously received antibiotic and has a clinical syndrome or consistent finding by sigmoidoscopy, a stool should be analyzed for the toxin of *C. difficile.* All the components of the evaluation (history, physical examination, anoscopy, sigmoidoscopy, cultures, and serology) will also serve to document cure of the intestinal infection(s).

The extent of the diagnostic evaluation will depend on a number of factors: the availability of the laboratory tests; the availability of sigmoidoscopy; the expense for the testing; and the ability of the patient to return for periodic office visits.

Table 3.6 indicates when the family physician should consider referring the patient to a specialist for further diagnostic evaluation.

Table 3.6
When to Refer to the Specialist

1. Resources are not available for "appropriate" cultures
2. Resources are not available for complete stool examination (bacteria, parasites)
3. Sigmoidoscopy not available
4. Studies are "negative," and symptoms persist
5. Accepted treatment regimen has been instituted, and symptoms persist
6. Further diagnostic tests are indicated (colonoscopy, barium enema, small bowel biopsy) to exclude intestinal giardiasis, inflammatory bowel disease, and intestinal neoplasm
7. Concern the patient has AIDS and there is a desire to exclude *Cryptosporidium* spp., *Isospora belli*, and *Mycobacterium avium-intracellulare*

DIFFUSE LYMPHADENOPATHY

Diseases associated with diffuse lymphadenopathy in gay men can be conveniently classified as infectious (infectious mononucleosis, cytomegalovirus, toxoplasmosis, hepatitis B, syphilis, tuberculosis, *Mycobacterium avium-intracellulare*), hypersensitivity (phenytoin), and neoplastic (Kaposi's sarcoma, Hodgkin's disease, non-Hodgkins's lymphoma). An alternative approach to the evaluation of the patient with diffuse adenopathy is to categorize the causes according to their therapeutic potential. Generalized adenopathy occurring as an expression of infectious mononucleosis, cytomegalovirus, and toxoplasmosis in the gay man requires no treatment. Diffuse adenopathy in the AIDS patient presenting as a manifestation of lymphoma, Kaposi's sarcoma, or *Mycobacterium avium-intracellulare* has a grave prognosis and is virtually recalcitrant to present drug therapy. However, secondary syphilis in the non-HIV-infected patient and extrapulmonary tuberculosis, even when the latter exists in the AIDS patient, are amenable to antimicrobial therapy. Preliminary data also indicate that patients with persistent diffuse adenopathy attributed to human immunodeficiency virus infection benefit from antiviral chemotherapy.[42]

Secondary syphilis in the gay male with adenopathy can be associated with cutaneous lesions (papular, macular, maculopapular), sore throat, deafness, tinnitus, and features of hepatitis.[43,44] The hallmark of syphilitic hepatitis is an elevated serum alkaline phosphatase that is out of proportion to the transaminase.[45,46]

Treatment of secondary syphilis with 2.4 million units of i.m. benzathine penicillin is usually curative. Tetracycline, administered as 500 mg p.o. q.i.d. for 15 days, is the alternative treatment for the penicillin-allergic patient. However, some homosexual men have failed to respond to this recommended treatment and developed neurological complications.

In HIV-infected homosexual patients with secondary syphilis, the serological test can be initially negative, and the standard treatment can fail.[47,48] These patients may require high-dose (aqueous penicillin 24 million units per day i.v. for 10 days) penicillin.[49] They also need clinical and laboratory follow-up.[50]

Generalized adenopathy can be a manifestation of extrapulmonary tuberculosis in gay men who are intravenous drug abusers with AIDS.[51] Tuberculous adenopathy often precedes the development of AIDS. The lymphadenopathy can be the exclusive or prominent feature of tuberculosis, or it can be one component of disseminated disease. The chest x ray is usually but not invariably abnormal and demonstrates infiltrates as well as paratracheal, hilar, and mediastinal adenopathy.

The tuberculin skin test is often falsely negative, particularly if the patient has AIDS. Respiratory secretions usually grow the organism, even when the chest x ray is "negative." Lymph node biopsies and bone marrow biopsy are helpful to establish the diagnosis. The tissues should be stained and cultured specifically for tuberculous organisms. Susceptibility tests should be performed on the organisms isolated.

For the gay man with coexistent tuberculosis and AIDS, a three-drug onset therapy is recommended.[52] Treatment should consist of INH (10–15 mg/kg per day but not to exceed 300 mg/day) plus rifampin (10–15 mg/kg per day but not to exceed 600 mg/day) plus either ethambutol (25 mg/kg per day) or pyrazinamide (20–30 mg/kg per day). The latter two drugs are prescribed for only the first 2 months of treatment.

Lymphadenopathy caused by *Mycobacterium avium* complex in the male homosexual is one component of disseminated infection. The disease is virtually restricted to those gay men with AIDS. These patients usually experience fever, malaise, weight loss, and, on occasion, abdominal pain and chronic diarrhea.[53] The recommended therapy for *Mycobacterium avium* complex in gay men with human immunodeficiency virus infection consists of a four-drug treatment that includes isoniazid, ethambutol, rifabutin (ansamycin), and clofazimine. The latter two drugs are experimental. Clinical and microbiological cure rarely occur, however.

Diffuse lymphadenopathy in the male homosexual can be a manifestation of the "persistent generalized lymphadenopathy" syndrome, a disorder that consists of palpable adenopathy, involving two more extrainguinal sites, that persists for at least 3 months. To fulfill the definition of the persistent generalized lymphadenopathy syndrome, the disease must be attributed exclusively to infection by the human immunodeficiency virus (HIV), the retrovirus that causes the acquired immunodeficiency syndrome (AIDS).[54] In addition to diffuse adenopathy, some patients experience constitutional symptoms, including fatigue, fever, weight loss, and night sweats, and/or focal abnormalities such as oral candidiasis, chronic sinus congestion, diarrhea, recurrent herpes zoster, hepatomegaly, and splenomegaly.[55,56]

The lymph nodes can resolve spontaneously, antedating AIDS, or can rapidly increase in size, correlating with the development of lymphoma or Kaposi's sarcoma. Histologically this is usually follicular hyperplasia, a microscopic appearance that resembles a viral or autoimmune process. On occasion, follicular involution is detected on the biopsy, a finding that more commonly evolves into lymphoma or Kaposi's sarcoma. The biopsy has served as a useful predictor of the patient's prognosis. Mediastinal adenopathy, detected by chest x ray or computed tomography, is not a component of the persistent generalized lymphadenopathy syndrome.[57] When mediastinal or abdominal adenopathy is identified in the gay man, the clinician should be concerned that the patient has AIDS complicated by a neoplasm or an opportunistic infection.

Patients with persistent generalized lymphadenopathy have antibody to HIV and often have viremia caused by this organism.[58,59] The indications for recommending lymph node biopsy are not precisely established. Some experts recommend that all patients have biopsies.[60,61] Other experts would restrict biopsy to the following: disproportionate increase in the size of one localized node group; hematological abnormalities and increased erythrocyte sedimentation rate (findings that suggest occult neoplasm or an infectious complication of AIDS); and documentation of follicular hyperplasia as a prelude for experimental protocol treatment.[62]

Morbidity attributed to lymph node biopsy has consisted of wound infections, infected lymphocele, prolonged pain with parasthesia, and unsightly scars. An alternative to surgical biopsy is fine-needle aspiration biopsy.[63] This latter technique requires considerable skill and experience and, on occasion, can be associated with false-negative results when hyperplasia is demonstrated.

Prospective studies consistently indicate that a decreased number of T helper lymphocytes is associated with the subsequent development of AIDS.[64–66] Additional factors predictive of AIDS have been the loss of adenopathy, the presence of oral candidiasis and/or constitutional symptoms, a history of sex with someone in whom AIDS developed, and decline in titer or disappearance of antibody to HIV core protein.[67]

Treatment with ribavirin in a daily oral dose of 800 mg presumably decreases the development of AIDS among patients with persistent generalized lymphadenopathy.[42]

When diffusely enlarged lymph nodes are detected in homosexual men with AIDS, and the histology confirms the presence of lymphoma or Kaposi's sarcoma, referral to an oncologist is indicated.[68–73] These malignancies have the histological characteristics of high-grade (aggressive) tumors, and they involve multiple intranodal sites. The aggressive nature of these tumors combined with the propensity of AIDS patients to experience life-threatening opportunistic infections explains the poor prognosis. However, on rare occasion, intensive cancer chemotherapy has resulted in complete remission.

REFERENCES

1. Rodgers VD, Kagnoff MF: Gastrointestinal manifestations of the acquired immunodeficiency syndrome. *West J Med* 1987; 146:57–67.
2. Kazal HL, Sohn N, Carrasco JI, *et al:* The gay bowel syndrome: Clinicopathologic correlation in 260 cases. *Ann Clin Lab Sci* 1976; 6:184–192.
3. Owen WF: Sexually transmitted diseases and traumatic problems in homosexual men. *Ann Intern Med* 1980; 92:805–808.
4. Phillips SC, Mildvan D, William DC, *et al:* Sexual transmission of enteric protozoa and helminths in a venereal-disease-clinic population. *N Engl J Med* 198; 305:603–606.
5. Baker RW, Peppercorn MA: Gastrointestinal ailments of homosexual men. *Medicine* 1982; 61:390–405.
6. William DC, Felman YM, Marr JS, *et al:* Sexually transmitted enteric pathogens in male homosexual population. *NY State J Med* 1977; 77:2050–2052.
7. Quinn TC, Corey L, Chaffee RG, *et al:* The etiology of anorectal infections in homosexual men. *Am J Med* 1981; 71:395–406.
8. Quinn TC, Stamm WE, Goodell SE, *et al:* The polymicrobial origin of intestinal infections in homosexual men. *N Engl J Med* 1983; 309:576–582.
9. Goldberg J, Bernstein R: Studies on granuloma inguinale: Two cases of perianal granuloma inguinale in male homosexuals. *Br J Vener Dis* 1964; 40:137–139.
10. Kaplan LR, Takeuchi A: Purulent rectal discharge associated with a nontreponemal spirochete. *JAMA* 1979; 241:52–53.
11. Surawicz CM, Roberts PL, Rompalo A, *et al:* Intestinal spirochetosis in homosexual men. *Am J Med* 1987; 82:587–592.
12. Akdamar K, Martin RJ, Ichinose H: Syphilitic proctitis. *Am J Dig Dis* 1977; 22:701–704.
13. Smith D: Infectious syphilis of the anal canal. *Dis Colon Rectum* 1963; 6:7–13.
14. Samenius B: Primary syphilis of the anorectal region. *Dis Colon Rectum* 1968; 11:462–466.
15. Quinn TC, Lukehart SA, Goodell S, *et al:* Rectal mass caused by *Treponema pallidum:* Confirmation by immunofluorescent staining. *Gastroenterology* 1982; 82:135–139.
16. Gluckman JB, Kleinman MS, May AG: Primary syphilis of rectum. *NY State J Med* 1974; 74:2210–2211.
17. Kaufman RE, Weiss S, Moore JD, *et al:* Biological false positive serological tests for syphilis among drug addicts. *Br J Vener Dis* 1974; 50:350–353.
18. Janda WM, Bohncroff M, Morello JA, *et al:* Prevalence and site-pathogen studies of *Neisseria meningitidis* and *N. gonorrhoeae* in homosexual men. *JAMA* 1980; 244:2060–2064.
19. William DC, Felman YM, Riccardi NB: The utility of anoscopy in the rapid diagnosis of symptomatic anorectal gonorrhea in men. *Sex Transm Dis* 1980; 8:16–19.
20. Goldmeier D: Proctitis and herpes simplex virus in homosexual men. *Br J Vener Dis* 1980; 56:111–114.
21. Jacobs E: Anal infections caused by herpes simplex virus. *Dis Colon Rectum* 1976; 19:151–157.
22. Goodell SE, Quinn TC, Mkrtichian E, *et al:* Herpes simplex virus proctitis in homosexual men. *N Engl J Med* 1983; 308:868–871.
23. Samarasinghe PL, Oates JK, MacLennan PB: Herpetic proctitis and sacral radiculomyelopathy—a hazard for homosexual men. *Br Med J* 1979; 2:365–366.
24. Goldmeier D, Darougar S: Isolation of *Chlamydia trachomatis* from throat and rectum of homosexual men. *Br J Vener Dis* 1977; 53:184–185.

25. Rompalo AM, Price CP, Roberts PL, *et al:* Potential value of rectal-screening cultures for *Chlamydia trachomatis* in homosexual men. *J Infect Dis* 1986; 153:888–892.
26. Quinn TC, Goodell SE, Mkrtichian E, *et al: Chlamydia-trachomatis* proctitis. *N Engl J Med* 1981; 305:195–200.
27. Grace AW: Anorectal lymphogranuloma venereum: *JAMA* 1943; 122:74–78.
28. Bolan RK, Sands M, Schachter J, *et al:* Lymphogranuloma venereum and acute ulcerative proctitis. *Am J Med* 1982; 72:703–706.
29. Schachter J, Smith DE, Dawson CR, *et al:* Lymphogranuloma venereum: Comparison of the Frei test, complement fixation test and isolation of the organism. *J Infect Dis* 1969; 120:372–375.
30. Rompalo AM, Suchland RJ, Price CB, *et al:* Rapid diagnosis of *Chlamydia trachomatis* rectal infection by direct immunofluorescence staining. *J Infect Dis* 1987; 155:1075–1076.
31. Bader M, Pedersen AHB, Williams R, *et al:* Venereal transmission of shigellosis in Seattle–King County. *Sex Transm Dis* 1977; 4:89–91.
32. Roberts IM, Parenti D, Albert MB: *Aeromonas hydrophila*-associated colitis in a male homosexual. *Arch Intern Med* 1987; 147:1502–1503.
33. Quinn TC, Goodell SE, Fennell C, *et al:* Infections with *Campylobacter jejuni* and *Campylobacter*-like organisms in homosexual men. *Ann Intern Med* 1984; 101:187–192.
34. Totten PA, Fennell CL, Tenover FC, *et al: Campylobacter cinaedi* (sp.nov.) and *Campylobacter fennelliae* (sp. nov.): Two new campylobacter species associated with enteric disease in homosexual men. *J Infect Dis* 1985; 151:131–139.
35. Jones EA, Mindel A, Sargeaunt P, *et al: Entamoeba histolytica* as a commensal intestinal parasite in homosexual men. *N Engl J Med* 1986; 315:353–356.
36. Burnham WR, Reeve RS, Finch RG: *Entamoeba histolytica* infection in male homosexuals. *Gut* 1980; 21:1097–1099.
37. Schmerin MJ, Gelston A, Jones TC: Amebiasis: An increasing problem among homosexuals in New York City. *JAMA* 1977; 238:1386–1387.
38. Goldmeier D, Sargeaunt PG, Price AB, *et al:* Is *Entamoeba histolytica* in homosexual men a pathogen? *Lancet* 1986; 1:641–644.
39. Ylvisaker JT, McDonald GB: Sexually acquired amebic colitis and liver abscess. *West J Med* 1980; 132:153–157.
40. Schmerin MJ, Jones TC, Klein H: Giardiasis: Association with homosexuality. *Ann Intern Med* 1978; 88:801–803.
41. Ungar BLP, Yolkin RH, Nash TE, *et al:* Enzyme-linked immunosorbent assay for the detection of *Giardia lamblia* in fecal specimens. *J Infect Dis* 1984; 149:90–97.
42. Hirsch MS, Kaplan JC: Treatment of human immunodeficiency virus infections. *Antimicrob Agents Chemother* 1987; 31:839–843.
43. Chapel TA: The signs and symptoms of secondary syphilis. *Sex Transm Dis* 1980; 7:161–164.
44. Willcox RR, Goodwin PG: Nerve deafness in early syphilis. *Br J Vener Dis* 1971; 47:401–406.
45. Baker AL, Kaplan MM, Wolfe HJ, *et al:* Liver disease associated with early syphilis. *N Engl J Med* 1971; 284:1422–1433.
46. Keisler DS, Starke W, Looney DJ, *et al:* Early syphilis with liver involvement. *JAMA* 1982; 247:1999–2000.
47. Hicks CB, Benson PM, Lupton GP, *et al:* Seronegative secondary syphilis in a patient infected with the human immunodeficiency virus (HIV) with Kaposi sarcoma. *Ann Intern Med* 1987; 107:492–495.
48. Markovitz DM, Beutner KR, Maggio RP, *et al:* Failure of recommended treatment for secondary syphilis. *JAMA* 1986; 255:1767–1768.
49. Tramont EC: Syphilis in the AIDS era. *N Engl J Med* 1987; 316:1600–1601.
50. Guinan ME: Treatment of primary and secondary syphilis: Defining failure at three and six-month follow-up. *JAMA* 1987; 257:359–360.
51. Sunderam G, McDonald RJ, Maniatis T, *et al:* Tuberculosis as a manifestation of the acquired immunodeficiency syndrome (AIDS). *JAMA* 1986; 256:362–366.

52. CDC: Diagnosis and management of mycobacterial infection and disease in persons with human immunodeficiency virus infection. *Ann Intern Med* 1987; 106:254–256.
53. Hawkins CC, Gold JWM, Whimbey E, *et al: Mycobacterium avium* complex infections in patients with the acquired immunodeficiency syndrome. *Ann Intern Med* 1986; 105:184–188.
54. Safai B, Sarngadharan MG, Groopman JE, *et al:* Seroepidemiological studies of human T-lymphotropic retrovirus type III in acquired immunodeficiency syndrome. *Lancet* 1984; 1:1438–1440.
55. Metroka CE, Rundles SC, Pollack MS, *et al:* Generalized lymphadenopathy in homosexual men. *Ann Intern Med* 1983; 99:585–591.
56. Wagh UM, Enlow RW, Spigland I, *et al:* Longitudinal study of persistent generalized lymphadenopathy in homosexual men: Relation to acquired immunodeficiency syndrome. *Lancet* 1984; 1:1033–1038.
57. Stern RG, Gamsu G, Golden JA, *et al:* Intrathoracic adenopathy: Differential feature of AIDS and diffuse lymphadenopathy syndrome. *Am J Roentgenol* 1984; 142:689–692.
58. Gallo RC, Salakuddin SZ, Popovic M: Frequent detection and isolation of cytopathic retroviruses (HTLV-III) from patients with AIDS and at risk for AIDS. *Science* 1984; 224:500–503.
59. Kaplan JE, Spira TJ, Feorino PM, *et al:* HTLV-III viremia in homosexual men with generalized lymphadenopathy. *N Engl J Med* 1985; 312:1572–1573.
60. Gold JWM, Weikel CS, Godbold J, *et al:* Unexplained persistent lymphadenopathy in homosexual men and the acquired immune deficiency syndrome. *Medicine* 1985; 64:203–213.
61. Benoth PM, Jenkins RL, Cady B, *et al:* Surgical approach to generalized lymphadenopathy in homosexual men. *J Surg Oncol* 1987; 36:231–234.
62. Abrams DI: Lymphadenopathy syndrome in male homosexuals. In: Gallin JD, Fauci AS, eds. *Advances in Host Defense Mechanisms,* Vol 5. New York, Raven Press, 1985:75–97.
63. Bottles K, McPhaul L, Voeberding P: Fine-needle aspiration biopsy of patients with the acquired immunodeficiency syndrome (AIDS): Experience in an outpatient clinic. *Ann Intern Med* 1988; 108:42–45.
64. Kaplan JE, Spira TJ, Fishbein DB, *et al:* Lymphadenopathy syndrome in homosexual men. *JAMA* 1987; 257:335–337.
65. Goedert JJ, Biggar RJ, Melbye M, *et al:* Effect of T4 count and cofactors on the incidence of AIDS in homosexual men infected with human immunodeficiency virus. *JAMA* 1987; 257:331–334.
66. Polk BF, Fox R, Brookmeyer R, *et al:* Predictors of the acquired immunodeficiency syndrome developing in a cohort of seropositive homosexual men. *N Engl J Med* 1987; 316:61–66.
67. Carne CA, Weller IVD, Loveday C, *et al:* From persistent generalised lymphadenopathy to AIDS: Who will progress? *Br Med J* 1987; 294:868–869.
68. Ziegler JL, Drew WL, Miner RC, *et al:* Outbreak of Burkitt's-like lymphoma in homosexual men. *Lancet* 1982; 2:631–633.
69. Levine AM, Meyer PR, Begandy MK, *et al:* Development of B-cell lymphoma in homosexual men. *Ann Intern Med* 1984; 100:7–13.
70. Ziegler JL, Beckstead JA, Volberding PA, *et al:* Non-Hodgkin's lymphoma in 90 homosexual men. *N Engl J Med* 1984; 311:565–570.
71. Levine AM, Gill PS, Meyer PR, *et al:* Retrovirus and malignant lymphoma in homosexual men. *JAMA* 1985; 254:1921–1925.
72. Schoeppel SL, Hopp RT, Dorfman RF, *et al:* Hodgkin's disease in homosexual men with generalized lymphadenopathy. *Ann Intern Med* 1985; 102:68–70.
73. Finkbeiner WE, Egbert BM, Groundwater JR, *et al:* Kaposi's sarcoma in young homosexual men. *Arch Pathol Lab Med* 1982; 106:261–264.

4

Outpatient Management of Acquired Immunodeficiency Syndrome

Richard B. Brown

INTRODUCTION

The acquired immunodeficiency syndrome (AIDS) is a recently recognized viral disease that represents one of the major health care problems of the 1980s. "Full-blown" AIDS requires the presence of opportunistic infection or specific malignancy in an individual made at risk by virtue of infection with the human immunodeficiency virus (HIV).[1] Recently, this definition has been expanded to include wasting disease and dementia. Several other diseases may also be included if accompanied by evidence of HIV positivity.[2] These include extrapulmonary tuberculosis and recurrent nontyphoidal *Salmonella* bacteremia. AIDS-related complex (ARC) is noted by the presence of weight loss, persistent lymphadenopathy, fever, and other constitutional complaints in the absence of the infections, malignancies, or other parameters that define AIDS.[3] Asymptomatic infection with HIV can also be demonstrated serologically by testing for the presence of either antibodies to the virus or actual viral antigen.[4]

Over 55,000 cases of AIDS have been diagnosed in the United States with well over 25,000 deaths.[5] This illness has also been reported from over 110 foreign countries. Recent calculations indicate that over 250,000 cases may be diagnosed in the United States by the end of 1991 and that more than 170,000 deaths will be noted by that time.[6] It is estimated that five to ten cases of ARC exist for each case of AIDS and that currently at least 1,500,000 persons in our country are felt to harbor HIV asymptomatically.[7] What percentage of these individuals will ultimately emerge with AIDS or other forms of symptomatic

Table 4.1
Outpatient Management of
AIDS-Related Diseases

Counseling and options regarding HIV testing
Evaluation of the "worried well"
Assessment of symptoms in nondiagnosed persons
Psychological counseling
Periodic follow-up of patients with AIDS/ARC
Treatment of *Pneumocystis carinii* pneumonia (non-critically ill)
Prophylaxis of *Pneumocystis carinii* pneumonia
Management of diarrhea
Chemotheraphy of Kaposi's sarcoma, other malignancies
Management of skin lesions, rashes

disease is unclear. However, best estimates are that up to 50% can develop AIDS within 5 years.[8]

The health care implications for HIV-related illness are astounding. Recent estimates suggest that each patient with AIDS costs as much as $140,000.00.[9] Much of this cost is related to that of hospitalization for care related to either diagnosis or treatment of opportunistic infection or malignancy in patients with "full-blown" AIDS. Because of the large health care expenditures required for each patient with symptomatic HIV infection and the documented massive increases in the numbers of such individuals, health care planners have been and will continue to be forced to utilize outpatient strategies in creative ways. Table 4.1 depicts several of the clinical situations in which patients with AIDS-related illness may be managed in the outpatient setting. Additionally, patients with asymptomatic HIV-related disease and the "worried well" who deem themselves to be at risk for this illness also require access to clinicians for reassurance and/or periodic evaluation.

MANAGEMENT OF ISSUES RELATED TO HIV TESTING

An increasing number of patients will seek medical guidance regarding HIV testing. The availability of an "AIDS test" is now public knowledge; however, the pros and cons of testing, recommendations regarding who should be tested, and counseling regarding results require significant and enlightened medical input. Presently, several statements can be made concerning testing: (1) all positive screening tests should be confirmed with a back-up "gold standard" test such as Western blot; (2) testing should not be routinely administered to all individuals who request it; (3) patients who fall into acknowledged "high-risk" categories should be offered testing; (4) testing should not be administered without the informed consent of the patient; (5) results should be confidential; (6) testing should be accompanied by appropriate counseling; and (7) contact follow-up should be performed as allowed by law on patients who test positive.[10]

Prior to the initiation of testing, the clinician should assess the reasons for testing, the risk category of the patient, and how the results would be utilized. Patients who fall into high-risk categories should be offered testing, since positive tests are more likely to be "true positives," and subsequent counseling efforts may help control the spread of disease. Low-risk patients are statistically far less likely to test positive, and those that do have a higher likelihood to be "false positives," which can impact adversely on their lives and those of their families. Individuals who test positive (after confirmatory testing) should be counseled about alterations in life style. This should include, but not be limited to, concepts of "safer sex," risks of sharing intraveneous needles and paraphernalia, and risks from donating blood or blood products.

EVALUATION FOR SUSPECTED AIDS-RELATED DISEASE

The presentation of patients with suspected AIDS-related illness is diverse and requires a high index of suspicion on the part of health care personnel. In many instances initial contact with a suspect for AIDS-related illness will be in the office of the clinician. Such physicians must be capable of rendering competent, sensitive, and compassionate care to all individuals who present with AIDS-related problems. Table 4.2 depicts many of the more common presentations. The practicing physician must become comfortable in assessing likelihood of AIDS-related disease on the basis of risk factors.

Despite the fact that an increasing number of patients are being noted outside of high-risk groups, at least 85–90% of individuals may still be identified within such groupings.[5] For this reason, clinicians must become comfortable in assessing patients' sexual orientation and use of illicit substances. With regard to the former, best estimates are that up to one third of males will have had at least one homosexual experience leading to orgasm between 16 and 55 years of age,[11] and that labeling patients as either "homosexual" or "heterosexual" may be misleading.[11] Sexual orientation may not be fixed but rather may change in relation to environmental or other situations. Thus, the clinician who is assessing a specific patient should not assume that male homosexuals have not had heterosexual contacts or that the middle-aged married male with several adolescent children has not had an occasional and possibly recent homosexual exposure. Additionally, physicians must discuss the possibility of sexual exposure to individuals who may be in high-risk categories. Finally, physicians must develop strategies to investigate actual types of sexual activities that may be engaged in by selected patients. Sexual activities such as anal intercourse are far more likely

Table 4.2
Common Presentations of AIDS-Related Diseases

Constitutional	
	Weight loss
	Fever, chills
	Night sweats
	Anorexia, malaise
	Mononucleosislike syndrome
	Anemia
Pulmonary	
	Shortness of breath
	Cough (productive or nonproductive)
Other organ systems	
	Diarrhea, often severe and chronic
	Skin lesions, rashes
	Headache, stiff neck
	Swollen glands, often multiple areas
	Oral or vaginal thrush, often chronic or recurrent
	Peripheral neuropathy
	Progressive dementia

to be associated with the spread of HIV than others such as mutual masturbation.[12]

Clinical presentation of acute HIV infection as a mononucleosis syndrome has been noted in an increasing number of patients.[13] Recent onset of fever, lymphadenopathy, and malaise is commonly seen in this group, and the clinical expression of this illness is usually self-limited. HIV positivity may be noted if checked, and the disease should be suspected in patients whose history places them at risk for AIDS-related disease. If strong clinical suspicion persists despite a negative test, and if other diagnosis cannot be made, repeat testing should be performed in 3–6 months. These patients will be serologically negative for acute mononucleosis caused by Epstein–Barr virus and cytomegalovirus, and this author feels that HIV testing should be routinely offered to those individuals in high-risk groups, especially if other diagnoses cannot be readily documented. Failure to document HIV-related disease in this clinical context may result in spread to sexual partners, offspring, and others at risk from the index case. Additionally, disease may progress to either ARC or AIDS over variable time periods. A variety of acute neurological diseases that include Guillain–Barré syndrome have also been demonstrated in association with acute HIV infection.[14]

Chronic lymphadenopathy with or without associated fever and weight loss is another common presentation of AIDS-related disease to the practitioner.[15] In many instances it represents a nonspecific manifestation of HIV infection rather than a marker of specific opportunistic infection and may thus be noted in

Table 4.3
Differential Diagnosis of Lymphadenopathy in Patients Suspected of AIDS/ARC

Epstein–Barr virus mononucleosis
Cytomegalovirus
Toxoplasmosis
Syphilis
Hodgkin's disease, other lymphomas
Metastatic solid tumors
Hepatitis B
Disseminated fungal infections
Disseminated mycobacterial infections
Angioblastic lymphadenopathy

patients with infections that do not directly involve the lymphatic system. Although biopsies may occasionally demonstrate a specific etiologic diagnosis, more commonly findings consist only of benign reactive hyperplasia. Patients with far advanced AIDS may acually demonstrate involution of the nodes with associated lymphocyte depletion. This may be a sign of impending opportunistic infection. Differential diagnosis of lymphadenopathy in this patient population is provided in Table 4.3; HIV infection should be in the differential diagnosis of such patients, and an assessment of risk factors should ensue. The presence of such factors will trigger appropriate serological testing. In addition, testing for hepatitis B, syphilis, CMV, Epstein–Barr virus, and possibly toxoplasmosis infections should also be considered.

Approximately 33% of patients who present with lymphadenopathy will have noted a recent ''viral'' syndrome, and the others note prior illness.[15] About one third are asymptomatic, whereas the remainder note a wide variety of diverse complaints. Physical examination will usually reveal widespread nodal involvement, with an average of ten groups of glands involved.

Asymptomatic HIV-positive patients require counseling and should be followed at regular intervals for evidence of disease progression. The role of specific antiviral therapy with agents such as azidothymidine (AZT) is currently unclear. Clinical trials have recently been initiated in an attempt to answer this question.

HEALTH MAINTENANCE OF THE PATIENT WITH ARC OR AIDS

Patients with symptomatic ARC or AIDS should be regularly assessed by the clinician, do not represent an unusual health risk to medical personnel, and can be evaluated in the office during regular working hours. The rate of progression of AIDS or ARC varies considerably among individuals. Evaluation should include relevant interim history, physical examination with especial assessment of vital signs, weight, skin, lymphatics, and lungs, and appropriate laboratory tests. In general, patients seen in the office do not require extensive infection control precautions.[16] Physicians and other paramedical personnel should routinely wear gloves when examining weeping lesions or mucosal surfaces. Masks, goggles, gowns, and other protective gear should be reserved for specific procedures where splatters or splashes may be anticipated.

Patients with early ARC or AIDS (e.g., just after recovery from first-bout *Pneumocystis carinii* pneumonia) should be encouraged to adopt a life style that ensures good nourishment, adequate rest, and vitamin supplementation.[17] Elimination of stress, drugs, and alcohol should also be encouraged. Complete blood count and differential should be performed monthly even in the absence of specific complaints or antiviral therapy. Periodic evaluation of T4/T8 ratio and absolute T4 count should also be performed, as these may be prognostic indicators of AIDS.[18,19] Individuals with T4 counts of less than 200/mm^3 are more likely to develop AIDS in the near future and may be candidates for antiviral chemotherapy. All individuals with AIDS or ARC should have a base-line chest PA and lateral x ray to be used in case of the future onset of pulmonary symptoms. Other tests should be performed based on specific symptoms or signs demonstrated on history and physical examination. Patients who are noted to be febrile in the office should routinely have blood cultures performed as part of the evaluation, and the laboratory should be notified of the need to assess for mycobacteria and fungi in addition to routine bacterial pathogens.[16] If no source for fever can be documented, then strong consideration can be given to a trial of salicylates or nonsteroidal antiinflammatory agents in an attempt to obtain symptomatic relief.

Patients with late-stage ARC or AIDS should have efforts aimed at maintaining comfort and dignity. Physicians must routinely address issues such as indications for hospitalization, admission to intensive care units, and resuscitation status with the patient prior to the time when the actual needs arise.[16] In most circumstances these subjects are best discussed in the office setting during a routine visit. The clinician should also attempt to ensure that a will has been prepared and that the personal affairs of the patient are in order. Personal comfort should be ensured through the use of pain medications appropriate for the needs of the patient. In late stages of AIDS or ARC, this may well requite the regular use of opiates. Many companies that specialize in home health care are now providing parenteral pain medication.

Availability of Azidothymidine

Azidothymidine has recently been demonstrated to be useful in the treatment of HIV infection itself.[20,21] Although it has historically been available only through the Burroughs-Wellcome Company (hotline telephone number

800-843-9388), it can now be dispensed directly by the private clinician. The drug can then be ordered by any pharmacy and dispensed directly to the patient. Prior to initiating treatment, the physician is wise to inform the patient about costs, which can be prohibitive, and the patient should inquire at several pharmacies regarding their costs for this product. Currently, charges are estimated to be at least $8000.00 annually, which may not be covered by insurance.

Available data demonstrate significantly enhanced survival in patients with AIDS treated with AZT following first-bout *Pneumocystis carinii* pneumonia or far-advanced ARC,[21] and this remains the primary indication for this product. Numerous other investigations are currently proceeding to ascertain optimal dosage and alternative indications for use. These could include asymptomatic HIV-positive patients, patients with early symptomatic ARC, and those with Kaposi's sarcoma.

Typical adult dose of AZT is two tablets (100 mg each) orally every 4 hr (AZT product information, Burroughs-Wellcome Inc.). Minor side effects that include nausea and vomiting are often encountered but are uncommonly associated with the need to discontinue the product.[22] The major side effect of AZT is bone marrow suppression, noted in approximately 25% of patients.[22] However, it must be remembered that most patients with symptomatic AIDS-related diseases may present both anemic and neutropenic, and this must be taken into consideration when assessing the results of medical treatment. Progressive anemia is the most commonly noted hematological side effect of AZT, but thrombocytopenia and neutropenia also can be seen.[22] These problems are most commonly encountered during the second or third month of drug treatment, and careful assessment for this must be given during therapy. Most patients can be successfully managed with short-term discontinuation of treatment and reinitiation with a dose of one tablet (100 mg) every 4 hr. Occasional patients will fail to tolerate even this dosage, and up to 21% may require periodic transfusions to maintain satisfactory hemoglobin concentrations.[21] Problems with neutropenia are even more worrisome, can be noted in approximately 16% of patients, and may occasionally force discontinuation of the agent.[22] Severe pancytopenia, which may not be reversible, has recently been reported.[23] In the near future the problem of hematological complications will become even more muddled by the impending availability of agents such as gancyclovir (for management of infections caused by cytomegalovirus), which are also capable of causing bone marrow suppression. The author has also recently encountered a case of severe toxic hepatitis associated with the use of AZT in a patient with AIDS and chronic hepatitis B carriage. Another individual with Stevens–Johnson syndrome attributable to AZT has also been seen.

Management of *Pneumocystis carinii* Pneumonia

Pneumonias caused by the protozoan *Pneumocystis carinii* are the manifestation of AIDS in approximately 65% of patients and are a significant reason for both hospitalization and mortality.[24–26] Many efforts have centered on approaches to prevent second occurrences of *Pneumocystis carinii* pneumonia. The role of AZT in the management of AIDS-related disease may actually impact on the frequency of recurrence of *Pneumocystis carinii* pneumonia, but this has not been fully explored and is not discussed further at this time. Historically, either parenterally administered trimethoprim–sulfamethoxazole (TMP/SMX) or pentamidine isethionate has been employed for treatment of pulmonary infections with this protozoan.[27,28] The former has been given in doses of 20 mg/kg per day of trimethoprim in 3–4 divided doses, whereas the latter is typically administered at 4 mg/kg per day either intramuscularly or intravenously.[27,28] With regard to therapeutic efficacy, results have usually demonstrated equal outcomes. Satisfactory responses have been noted in up to 80% of patients treated with either agent with first bouts of this disease.[28–30] A recent investigation has also noted good therapeutic efficacy in "mild" *Pneumocystis carinii* pneumonia with the smaller dose of 3 mg/kg of pentamidine isethionate.[31]

For patients who tolerate TMP/SMX, outpatient therapy to complete a 3-week course is indicated. Many physicians are loathe to administer pentamidine out of hospital because of the risk of severe and possibly irreversible hypotension. However, hospital-related clinics and physicians' offices can provide useful alternatives to inpatient care with this agent, and it has been successfully employed out of hospital. Prolonged therapy with reduced doses (e.g., 160 mg TMP/800 mg SMX b.i.d.) of TMP/SMX have been tried as a prophylactic measure.[29] But adverse effects have been noted in close to 50% of patients. Although such numbers may be acceptable for in-hospital therapy of life-threatening illness, they are generally considered to be excessive for prevention of recurrences.[29] Furthermore, pentamidine has historically required parenteral administration, making long-term prophylaxis cumbersome. Although TMP/SMX may be employed orally, over 60% of patients with AIDS may manifest severe bone marrow or dermatological toxicity after prolonged use.[32] Thus, alternative strategies have been sought to prevent recurrences of this common form of pneumonia in this patient population.

Table 4.4 lists some of the recent novel approaches to the prophylaxis and treatment of *Pneumocystis carinii* pneumonia. Several recent preliminary communications and pilot studies have utilized aerosolized pentamidine.[31,33–36] The rationale for this is that disease with this protozoan is mostly respiratory and typically centered within the alveoli. Preliminary investigations have utilized variable amounts of pentamidine, ranging from 4 mg/kg per day for therapy of documented disease to 600 mg biweekly for prophylaxis. Results in small series to date indicate that such preventative treatment lowers recurrences to about 10% of that seen in historical controls and that outcomes of treatment are good, although earlier relapses may be noted.[31] Pentamidine adminstered by aerosolization is not readily absorbed and thus spares the host from many of the untoward effects of this product. Additionally, it appears to be concentrated in

Table 4.4
Prophylaxis of *Pneumocystis carinii* Pneumonia

Agent and route	Dose
Pyrimethamine–sulfadoxine (Fansidar), p.o.	One tablet weekly
Pentamidine isethionate, i.v./i.m.	4 mg/kg biweekly
Pentamidine isethionate, aerosolized	300–600 mg biweekly
Diaminodiphenylsulfone (dapsone), p.o.	50 mg daily
Trimethoprim–sulfamethoxazole (Bactrim, Septra), p.o.	One DS b.i.d.

respiratory secretions to a greater extent than is i.v. drug and is well tolerated with few adverse reactions.[31]

Although bronchospasm has been anticipated, it appears to be an infrequent complication but should be anticipated in patients who have a previous history of this problem. Several unanswered questions remain. Optimal dose and interval between treatments is not known. Similarly, it is not yet clear what constitutes the best particle size for aerosolization. Preliminary data suggest that particles of 1–3 μm should be sought and that this may require special forms of aerosolization such as the Wright-type nebulizer.[36]

Diaminodiphenylsulfone (dapsone) has also been employed for both the treatment and prevention of pneumonia with *Pneumocystis carinii*.[37] Although doses are not yet standardized, several investigators have employed doses of 50 mg p.o. daily for prophylaxis for extended time periods with apparent success and with limited toxicity. They recommend that persons be screened for glucose-6-phosphate dehydrogenase deficiency prior to initiation of treatment with this agent. Noteworthy is the fact that new studies appear to demonstrate that significant allergy to one sulfa preparation (e.g., trimethoprim–sulfamethoxazole) does not preclude therapy with another (e.g., dapsone).[38] However, care must be taken to exclude patients who have had immediate reactions or who require treatment with the alternative agent within 3 months.[38] The fixed combination of pyrimethamine and sulfadoxine (Fansidar®) has also been employed for *Pneumocystis carinii* pneumonia prophylaxis.[29] Dosage of half to one tablet weekly or biweekly for indefinite periods has been utilized with early apparent success, and it appears that this regimen can be safely employed despite allergy to TMP/SMX.[29,38]

Assessment and Management of Diarrhea

At least 50% of patients with AIDS or ARC will develop diarrhea, and it may either be the presenting complaint that leads to the diagnosis of AIDS or become manifest at any time thereafter.[39,40] It may be more common in homosexual patients than in those who abuse intravenous drugs.[41] This problem may

Table 4.5
Common Etiologies for Diarrhea in AIDS

A.	Bacterial
	Salmonella (often bacteremic)
	Shigella
	Campylobacter
	C. difficile (antibiotic-associated)
B.	Protozoal
	Cryptosporidia
	Isospora
	Entamoeba histolytica
C.	Other infectious
	Mycobacterium Avium-intracellulare
	Cytomegalovirus
	Herpes simplex
	Candida albicans
D.	Noninfectious
	AIDS enteropathy
	Kaposi's sarcoma
	Non-Hodgkin's lymphoma

become disabling, prolonged, and frustrating for both patient and clinician. In most instances the initial assessment and management of this problem may occur in the office. However, hospitalization, at least on a limited basis, may be required on occasion for invasive studies such as intestinal biopsy or colonoscopy and for initial clinical management. The patient who presents with complaints of diarrhea should have a thorough history and physical examination performed in order to document potential involvement of other organ systems. Routine assessment should include stools for fecal leukocytes, ova, and parasites and culture and sensitivity. Depending on the results of these studies, it may be necessary to proceed with more invasive procedures that could include sigmoidoscopy, colonoscopy with biopsy, or upper gastrointestinal endoscopy with biopsy. Special smears and cultures for acid-fast bacilli and fungi may also be needed.

Table 4.5 depicts the most common causes of diarrhea in patients with AIDS-related diseases. Although many potentially treatable infectious causes are included, it must be noted that others that include Kaposi's sarcoma, diarrhea of unexplained etiology ("AIDS enteropathy"), and untreatable pathogens may also be regularly encountered. Recent data suggest that a specific infectious diagnosis may be made in 50–60% of patients with diarrhea and that stool examination for ova and parasites is the single most useful procedure.[42] However, complete assessment that also includes stools for fecal leukocytes and culture and sensitivity should routinely be performed because multiple pathogens may be identified in up to 25% of cases.[42] Blood cultures may be positive in over

25% of instances and should be obtained routinely in patients who present with fever and diarrhea.[43–46] Assessment should center on the diagnosis of treatable causes that include primarily selected bacterial and parasitic pathogens.

Salmonella gastrointestinal infections have been increasingly recognized in patients with AIDS, are at least 100 times more common in this population than in the general population, and may be associated with bacteremia.[43,44] This species may account for 5–10% of all infectious diarrheas in patients with AIDS. In patients who have diarrhea caused by this pathogen, the disease may be unusually severe, recurrent, and virtually impossible to eradicate.[43] *S. enteritidis* has been most commonly implicated. Diagnosis is easily confirmed by stool and blood cultures, and antibiotic therapy should be directed by the suceptibility patterns of the isolate.

In general, appropriate antimicrobial agents are efficacious in this illness, and it is one of relatively few gastrointestinal diseases in patients with AIDS for which therapy appears reproducibly worthwhile.[43,45] Although complete cure is unlikely, long-term suppression may be achieved. Ampicillin, TMP/SMX, and chloramphenicol have all been utilized; however, the former agent is probably preferred because of the least likelihood of toxicity. Quinolones such as ciprofloxacin may provide an additional means of therapy, but their efficacy in this disease and this population has not yet been established. However, it is the author's opinion that one of these agents should be utilized for chronic treatment of *Salmonella* gastroenteritis if ampicillin cannot be utilized because of organism resistance, patient intolerance, or allergy. Ciprofloxacin, 250–500 mg p.o. b.i.d. would be reasonable treatment once suceptibility to this agent is established and offers the advantage of activity against other enteric pathogens such as *Campylobacter* and *Shigella* species. Patients with recurrent *Salmonella* gastroenteritis or bacteremia require indefinite therapy and will usually relapse if treatment is halted.[43–45] Recently, severe bacteremic infections with strains of *Shigella* have also been noted.[46] Bacteremic infection with this species is distinctly uncommon, and diagnosis should prompt both an assessment for immunodeficiency and initiation of appropriate antibiotic therapy.

Cryptosporidia and *Isospora* are important causes of profuse, watery diarrhea in patients with AIDS and may be intractible.[40,41,47,48] These protozoa account for 10–21% of diarrhea in patients with AIDS.[36,38] Although the former protozoan has also been noted to cause diarrhea in immunocompetent individuals, the disease is significantly more severe and long-lived in patients with AIDS.[49] Weight loss, anorexia, and wasting often supervene and can be associated with death. Involvement of the entire gastrointestinal tract, including the biliary tract, has been noted at autopsy. Diagnosis rests on demonstrating the organism within the stool or gastrointestinal tract. Special methods of stool staining are necessary for the organism to be documented. Perhaps the easiest is the modified Kinyoun acid-fast stain.[50] Therapy is generally supportive; specific treatment has generally been unrewarding. Spiramycin, an agent available in

Canada, has been used successfully[51–53] but is not generally felt to be reproducibly useful. Dosage has been approximately 3 g/day, orally, in divided doses. Other agents that have been employed with little clinical benefit include trimethoprim–sulfamethoxazole, clindamycin, quinine, and indomethacin.

Gastrointestinal infection with *Mycobacterium avium-intracellulare* (MAI) has frequently been noted late in the course of AIDS, often in association with disseminated infection that includes high-grade bacillemia.[39–41,54] Debilitating diarrhea is common, and therapy is unrewarding. The MAI can be suspected from acid-fast positive smears of stool, and cultures will ultimately define this specific pathogen. Clinical presentation often consists of abdominal pain, diarrhea, and hepatosplenomegaly. Lymphadenopathy may also be noted on CT scan. Small bowel biopsy will demonstrate changes similar to those seen in Whipple's disease, with foamy macrophages and PAS-positive material noted. Presumably because of poor host immune response, granulomata are rarely noted. Therapy has been unrewarding and probably is not indicated except on an investigational basis. Multiple-drug regimens that often include the experimental drugs ansamycin and clofazamine have been utilized. However, any improvement rarely lasts for more than several months, and toxicity can be substantial.

Other Gastrointestinal Infections

Other infectious etiologies for gastrointestinal complaints in patients with AIDS include cytomegalovirus (CMV), herpes simplex, and *Candida albicans*.[39–41,55,56] Infections with CMV are common in patients with AIDS. Gastrointestinal infection with this virus has been noted in up to 90% of autopsies of persons dying with AIDS, with involvment noted at any level of the GI tract.[39,40,55] In patients with AIDS and diarrhea, infection with CMV is noted in up to 10% of cases.[39] Often, it can be isolated in conjunction with other enteric pathogens. Clinical manifestations include toxic megacolon, hemorrhage from ulceration, and granulomatous hepatitis. The most characteristic lesion associated with CMV is an ulcer, typically located within the cecum. A syndrome mimicking inflammatory bowel disease has also been reported, and perforation associated with this virus has been reported.[57] Diagnosis rests on demonstrating characteristic inclusion bodies within intestinal biopsies and isolating the virus. No acceptable therapy is currently available, and treatment is generally supportive. Gancyclovir, an experimental analogue of acyclovir, has been shown to have some efficacy in infections caused by CMV, primarily retinitis. However, it must be given for prolonged periods, has substantial bone marrow toxicity, and is only available as an intravenous preparation.

Herpes simplex infection of the gastrointestinal tract should be suspected in patients with AIDS who demonstrate unexplained ulcerative lesions. Involvement is primarily of the anus, rectum, mouth, and esophagus.[39,40,56] Painful ulcers are most commonly noted. Diagnosis is established by demonstrating multinucleated giant cells on Tzanck preparation and by isolating the virus. Therapy has been successfully employed with acyclovir in doses of 5–10 mg/kg per day in divided doses. Severe cases may require initial therapy with the intravenous preparation of this agent, and response is usually good. However, relapses are common, and either prolonged or intermittent treatment regimens may be necessary.

Infections with *C. ablicans* usually involve the mouth and esophagus, with relative sparing of the lower gastrointestinal tract.[39,40,58] Oral thrush is common and can be associated with pain and anorexia. Esophagitis should be suspected in patients with severe dysphagia and may be unaccompanied by clinical evidence of oral disease. Diagnosis of oral thrush can be suspected on clinical grounds and confirmed by wet prep, Gram stain, or culture. Therapy with either clotrimazole troches (Mycelex®) or oral ketoconazole has generally been successful; however, relapses are common once treatment has been discontinued. Chronic suppression may be indicated. Esophageal disease is best documented by esophagoscopy, which allows both culture and biopsy. Other diseases that include CMV and Herpes simplex can simultaneously be ruled out. Barium swallow will usually be abnormal in patients with esophagitis of any etiology. Abnormalities include spasm, disordered motility, and cobblestoning. Successful therapy of esophageal candidiasis has included ketoconazole, low-dose amphotericin B, and even topical agents. No scientifically valid studies have been conducted among these modalities.

Unfortunately, some patients with AIDS and diarrhea will be noted to have enteropathy unassociated with any itentifiable pathogen.[59] Evaluation of such individuals reveals pathological changes with jejunum and colon that suggest a specific disease process as yet undetermined. Treatment is supportive.

EVALUATION OF FEVER IN THE PATIENT WITH AIDS/ARC

Many patients with AIDS-related disease will have fever, which may be of any magnitude and duration. A major problem for the clinician is to discriminate among fever that may be related to underlying HIV infection, that which is secondary to associated infection or malignancy, and that which is unrelated to the disease. Unfortunately, is is unlikely that assessment of fever curve, magnitude, longevity, or association with chills or sweats will provide useful information. Diagnosis of fever caused by underlying HIV infection requires ruling out other treatable and identifiable causes. Complete history and physical examination provide a starting point for further assessment. Possible clinical clues should be pursued by cultures, x rays, etc. Several sets of blood cultures should be obtained in all patients; the need for cultures from other sites rests on clinical suspicions. Blood cultures should be specifically evaluated for mycobacteria and fungi in addition to routine bacteria. For patients whose initial assessment fails to provide a reason for fever, bone marrow biopsy with smears and cultures for acid-fast bacilli, routine bacterial pathogens, and fungi should be obtained. If diagnosis is still uncertain, a careful trial of antiinflammatory nonsteroidal agents is warranted and may allow discrimination between infectious and noninfectious etiologies for fever. These medications should be administered on an around-the-clock basis rather than only when temperatures reach a certain level.

CONCLUSIONS

Within the next several years, AIDS-related diseases will impact on most physicians within the United States regardless of location and practice patterns. Many clinical problems related to this illness can and should be managed by the enlightened family practitioner or internist, and to the greatest extent possible care should be rendered in the office rather than hospital setting. In the upcoming years an increasing proportion of patients will be managed in areas removed from the high-incidence areas, and all clinicians must become increasingly comfortable in acquiring strategies to deal with this trend. An awareness of clinical presentations of AIDS and an approach to dealing with the common complaints of patients with this disease are mandatory if patients with this ever-increasing problem are to be managed in a humane and medically forthright manner.

REFERENCES

1. Jaffe HW, Bregman DJ, Selik RM: Acquired immune deficiency syndrome in the United States: The first 1,000 cases. *J Infect Dis* 1983; 148:339–345.
2. Centers for Disease Control: Revision of the CDC surveillance case definition for acquired immunodeficiency syndrome. *Morbid Mortal Week Rep* 1987; 36:3S–15S.
3. Swartz MN: Lymphadenitis and lymphangitis. In: Mandell GL, Douglas RG Jr, Bennett JE, eds. *Principles and Practice of Infectious Diseases,* ed 2. New York, John Wiley & Sons, 1985:618–624.
4. Allain JP, Laurian Y, Paul DA, *et al:* Long-term evaluation of the HIV antigen and antibodies to p24 and gp41 in patients with hemophilia. *N Engl J Med* 1987; 317:1114–1121.
5. Centers for Disease Control: Update: Acquired immunodeficiency syndrome and human immunodeficiency virus infection among health care workers. *Morbid Mortal Week Rep* 1988; 37:229–234.
6. Coolfont Report: A PHS plan for prevention and control of AIDS and the AIDS virus. *Public Health Rep* 1986; 101:341–348.
7. Centers for Disease Control: Public health guidelines for counseling and antibody testing to prevent HIV infection and AIDS. *Morbid Mortal Week Rep.* 1987; 36:509–515.
8. Goedert JJ, Biggar RJ, Weiss SH, et al: Three-year incidence of AIDS in five cohorts of HTLV-III-infected risk group members. *Science* 1986; 231:992–995.
9. Hardy AM, Rauch K, Echenberg D, *et al:* The economic impact of the first 10,000 cases of acquired immunodeficiency syndrome in the United States. *JAMA* 1986; 255:209–211.
10. Centers for Disease Control: Public Health Service guidelines for counseling and antibody testing to prevent HIV infection and AIDS. *Morbid Mortal Week Rep* 1987; 36:509–515.

11. Ross MW: Social and behavioral aspects of male homosexuality. *Med. Clin North Am* 1986; 70:537–547.
12. Curran JW, Morgan WM, Hardy AM, *et al:* The epidemiology of AIDS: Current status and future prospects. *Science* 1985; 229:1352–1358.
13. Selwyn PA: AIDS: What is now known, III. Clinical aspects. *Hosp. Pract* 19O6; 21:119–153.
14. Vendrell J, Geredia C, Pujol M, *et al:* Guillain–Barre syndrome associated with seroconversion for acute HTLV-III. *Neurology (NY)* 1987; 37:544.
15. Abrams DI: Lymphadenopathy related to the acquired immunodeficiency syndrome in homosexual men. *Med Clin North Am* 1986; 70:693–706.
16. Centers for Disease Control: Summary: Recommendations for preventing transmission of infection with human T-lymphotrophic virus type III/lymphadenopathy-associated virus in the workplace. *Morbid Mortal Week Rep* 1985; 34:681–695.
17. Abrams DI, Dilley JW, Maxey LM, *et al:* Routine care and psychosocial support of the patient with the acquired immunodeficiency syndrome. *Med Clin North Am* 1986; 70:707–720.
18. Kaslow RA, Phair JP, Friedman HB, *et al:* Infection with the human immunodeficiency virus: Clinical manifestations and the relationship to immune deficiency. *Ann Intern Med* 1987; 107:474–480.
19. Goedert JJ, Biggar RJ, Melbye M, *et al:* Effect of T4 count and cofactors on the incidence of AIDS in homosexual men infected with the human immunodeficiency virus. *JAMA* 1987; 257:331–334.
20. Chaisson RE, Allain JP, Leuther M, *et al:* Decline in serum HIV p 24 antigen (Ag) in patients treated with AZT. In: *International Conference on AIDS,* 1987
21. Fischl MA, Richman DD, Grieco MH, *et al:* The efficacy of azidothymidine (AZT) in the treatment of patients with AIDS and AIDS-related complex. *N Engl J Med* 1987; 317:185–191.
22. Richman DD, Fischl MA, Grieco MH, *et al:* The toxicity of azidothymidine (AZT) in the treatment of patients with AIDS and AIDS-related complex. *N Engl J Med* 1987; 317:192–197.
23. Gill PS, Rarick M, Brynes RK, *et al:* Azidothymidine associated with bone marrow failure in the acquired immunodeficiency syndrome (AIDS). *Ann Intern Med* 1987; 107:502–502.
24. Kovacs JA, Hiemenz JW, Macher AM, *et al: Pneumocystis carinii* pneumonia: A comparison between patients with the acquired immunodeficiency syndrome and patients with other immunodeficiencies. *Ann Intern Med* 1984; 100:663–671.
25. Fauci AS, Macher AM, Longo DL, *et al:* Acquired immunodeficiency syndrome: Epidemiologic, clinical, immunologic, and therapeutic considerations. *Ann Intern Med* 1984; 100:92–106.
26. Lerner CW, Tapper ML: Opportunistic infections complicating acquired immune deficiency syndrome. *Medicine* 1984; 63:155–164.
27. Sands M, Kron MA, Brown RB: Pentamitine: A review. *Rev Infect Dis* 1985; 7:625–634.
28. Wharton JM, Coleman DL, Wofsy CB, *et al:* Trimethoprim–sulfamethoxazole or pentamidine for *Pneumocystis carinii* pneumonia in the acquired immunodeficiency syndrome. *Ann Intern Med* 1986; 105:37–44.
29. Young LS: Management of opportunistic infections complicating the acquired immunodeficiency syndrome. *Med Clin North Am* 1986; 70:677–692.
30. Mills J: *Pneumocystis carinii* and *Toxoplasma gondii* infections in patients with AIDS. *Rev Infect Dis* 1986; 8:1001–1011.
31. Conte JE, Hollander H, Golden JA: Inhaled or reduced-dose intravenous pentamidine for *Pneumocystis carinii* pneumonia. *Ann Intern Med* 1987; 107:495–498.
32. Gordin FM, Simon GL, Wofsy CB, *et al:* Adverse reactions to trimethoprim–sulfamethoxazole in patients with the acquired immunodeficiency syndrome. *Ann Intern Med* 1984; 100:495–499.
33. *Medical World News.* June 8, 1987.
34. Debs RJ, Blumenfeld W, Brunette EN, *et al:* Successful treatment with aerosolized pentamidine of *Pneumocystis carinii* pneumonia in rats. *Antimicrob Agents Chemother* 1987; 31:37–41.

35. Montgomery AB, Debs RC, Corkery LK, *et al:* Concentration of pentamidine in bronchoalveolar lavage fluid after aerosol and intravenous administration. *Am Rev Respir Dis* 1987; 135:A167.
36. Bernard EM, Pagel L, Schmitt HJ, *et al.* Clinical trials with aerosol pentamidine for prevention of *Pneumocystis carinii* pneumonia. *Clin Res* 1987; 35:468A.
37. Leoung GS, Mills J, Hopewell PC, *et al:* Dapsone–trimethoprim for *Pneumocystis carinii* pneumonia in the acquired immunodeficiency syndrome. *Ann Intern Med* 1986; 105:45–48.
38. Medina I, Wofsy FD: Cross-allergy to sulfonamides/sulfones (sulfa) and folic acid antagonists in AIDS. In: *3rd International Conference on AIDS,* Washington 1987
39. Dworkin B, Wormser GP, Rosenthal WS, *et al:* Gastrointestinal manifestations of the acquired immunodeficiency syndrome: A review of 22 cases. *Am J Gastroenterol* 1985; 80:774–778.
40. Gelb A, Miller S: AIDS and gastroenterology. *Am J Gastroenterol* 1986; 81:619–622.
41. Laurence J: Gastrointestinal infections in AIDS patients. *Infect Surg* 1986; 5:651–658.
42. Antony MA, Brandt LJ, Klein RS, *et al:* Infectious causes of diarrhea in patients with AIDS. In: *3rd International Conference on AIDS,* Washington 1987
43. Jacobs JL, Gold JwM, Murray HW, *et al: Salmonella* infections in patients with the acquired immunodeficiency syndrome. *Ann Intern Med* 1985; 102:186–188.
44. Nadelman RB, Mathur-Wagh U, Yancovitz SR, *et al: Salmonella* bacteremia associated with the acquired immunodeficiency syndrome (AIDS). *Arch Intern Med* 1985; 145:1968–1971.
45. Profeta S, Forrester C, Eng RHK, *et al: Salmonella* infections in patients with acquired immunodeficiency syndrome. *Arch Intern Med* 1985; 145:670–672.
46. Baskin DH, Lax JD, Barenberg D: *Shigella* bacteremia in patients with the acquired immune deficiency syndrome. *Am J Gastroenterol* 1987; 82:338–341.
47. Soave R, Danner RL, Honig CL, *et al:* Cryptosporidiosis in homosexual men. *Ann Intern Med* 1984; 100:504–511.
48. Pitlik SD, Fainstein V, Garza D, *et al:* Human cryptosporidiosis: Spectrum of disease. *Arch Intern Med* 1983; 143:2269–2275.
49. Current WL, Reese NC, Ernst JV, *et al:* Human cryptosporidsiosis in immunocompetent and immunodeficient persons. *N Engl J Med* 1983; 308:1252–1257.
50. Ma P, Soave R: Three-step stool examination for cryptosporidiosis in 10 homosexual men with protracted watery diarrhea. *J Infect Dis* 1983; 147:824–828.
51. Soave R, Armstrong D: Cryptosporidium and cryptosporidiosis. *Rev Infect Dis* 1986; 8:1012–1023.
52. Centers for Disease Control: Update: Treatment of cryptosporidiosis in patients with acquired immunodeficiency syndrome (AIDS). *Morbid Mortal Week Rep* 1984; 33:117–119.
53. Portnoy D, Whiteside ME, Buckley E III, *et al:* Treatment of intestinal cryptospridiosis with spiramycin. *Ann Intern Med* 1984; 101:202–204.
54. Greene JB, Sidhu GS, Lewin S, *et al: Mycobacterium avium-intracellulare:* A cause of disseminated life-threatening infection in homosexuals and drug abusers. *Ann Intern Med* 1982; 97:539–546.
55. Levinson W, Bennetts RW: Cytomegalovirus colitis in acquired immunodeficiency syndrome—a chronic disease with varying manifestations. *Am J Gastroenterol* 1985; 80:445–447.
56. Kalb RE, Grossman ME: Chronic perianal herpes simplex in immunocompormised hosts. *Am J Med* 1986; 80:486–490.
57. Frank D, Raicht RF: Intestinal perforation associated with cytomegalovirus infection in patients with acquired immunodeficiency syndrome. *Am J Gastroenterol* 1984; 79:201–205.
58. Klein RS, Harris CA, Small CB, *et al:* Oral candidiasis in high-risk patients as the initial manifestation of the acquired immunodeficiency syndrome. *N Engl J Med* 1984; 311:354–358.
59. Kotler DP, Gaetz HP, Lange M, *et al:* Enteropathy associated with the acquired immunodeficiency syndrome. *Ann Intern Med* 1984; 101:421–428.

5

Sinusitis and Pharyngitis

Richard A. Gleckman

SINUSITIS

Acute Bacterial Sinusitis

Acute sinusitis can be arbitrarily defined as an infection of the sinuses in which the signs and symptoms have been present for less than a month. Usually multiple sinuses are infected simultaneously. Isolated maxillary sinusitis necessitates a search for an infected tooth.

Acute sinusitis usually follows in the wake of a preceding viral infection that has caused destruction of mucosal surface cells, tissue edema, exudate formation, and occlusion of the ostium of the sinus. Ostial obstruction causes an anaerobic environment in the sinus, which in turn interferes with mucociliary clearance, bacterial phagocytosis, and bacterial killing. Ostial obstruction causes the release of proteolytic enzymes from granulocytes, and these enzymes cause damage to the mucosa of the sinus.[1] Acute sinusitis can also develop from barotrauma or secondary to an allergic disorder.

Clinical Manifestations

Symptoms of acute maxillary sinusitis include facial pain or pressure localized to the cheek or maxillary teeth that is aggravated by bending over, nasal congestion, purulent nasal discharge (both anterior and posterior), and often a foul taste. The discharge and associated swelling of the middle and inferior turbinates can cause anosmia or hyposmia. Fever occurs in approximately 50% of adults with acute sinusitis. Impressive temperature elevations, headaches, and ocular symptoms are not characteristic of uncomplicated acute bacterial maxillary sinusitis. Aching pain over the orbit or forehead suggests frontal sinusitis. Ethmoid sinusitis can produce pain in the temporal area, retroorbital area, upper nose, and mastoid area. Patients with acute sphenoid sinusitis have fever and a headache that interferes with sleep and is unrelieved by traditional analgesics. Location of the pain is variable: the discomfort can be most marked in the frontal, temporal, periorbital, or occipital region.

Physical examination elicits pain over the sinuses and reveals purulent discharge from erythematous turbinates. Transillumination of the maxillary and frontal sinuses can provide supportive information, particularly when dullness or opacification is detected.[2] However, the technique of transillumination requires skill, and the findings can be difficult to interpret in patients who have had previous episodes of disease or who have normal variations in bone thickness.

Radiographic Studies

Sinus x rays can help confirm the clinical suspicion of sinusitis, particularly when the sinus radiographs demonstrate air–fluid levels, complete antral opacity, or mucosal thickening. These latter abnormalities have been correlated with bacterial isolation following sinus aspiration.[2] On occasion, x rays of the maxillary sinus will be normal in the patient with acute maxillary sinusitis.[3,4] Sinus x rays, as well as the newer diagnostic techniques such as ultrasonography, sinoscopy, and computerized tomography, are currently considered too expensive for the routine evaluation of most outpatients with traditional manifestations of acute sinusitis.

Microbiology

Cultures of nasal discharges and exudates from nasal turbinates provide unreliable information regarding the etiology of acute bacterial sinusitis. Precise microbiology of acute sinusitis would require direct needle puncture and aspiration of the sinus or culture of the sinus mucosa itself. These procedures are restricted to the evaluation of the immunosuppressed host or the patient who has failed to respond to traditional forms of treatment. Studies of patients with acute maxillary sinusitis that employed the needle-puncture technique have revealed that most of these infections are caused by *Streptococcus pneumoniae, Haemophilus influenzae,* and *Staphylococcus aureus.*[5] Less frequently incriminated are *Branhamella catarrhalis* and anaerobes.[6] When maxillary sinusitis arises from dental sepsis, anaerobes are the etiologic agents, particularly *Bacteroides* spp. and streptococci. *Staphylococcus aureus,* aerobic streptococci (including *S. pneumoniae*), and anaerobic streptococci are the predominant organisms isolated from patients with acute sphenoid sinusitis. Comparable data are not available from patients with acute frontal or ethmoid sinusitis. However, the organisms isolated from patients with intracranial complications arising from acute ethmoid and frontal sinusitis have included aerobic, microaerophilic, and anaerobic streptococci as well as *S. aureus* and *S. epidermidis.*

When a patient with cystic fibrosis has acute bacterial sinusitis, the clinician should consider the possibility of disease caused by *Pseudomonas aeruginosa*. In the diabetic with acute sinusitis, particularly when ketoacidosis occurs, the physician should also be aware of the possibility of a fungal etiology, an entity described later.

Therapy

The lion's share of patients with acute bacterial sinusitis are treated in an outpatient setting. Hospital admission is restricted to compromised hosts, patients with severe disease, patients with acute sphenoid sinusitis, and patients with disease that extends beyond the sinuses.

The goals of therapy are to eradicate the existent infection, prevent spread of the infection, and provide symptomatic relief. It is assumed that early institution of appropriate treatment will prevent irreparable sinus damage and the development of chronic sinusitis. Traditional outpatient management consists of breathing through hot moist towels, applying a topical nasal vasoconstricting (decongestant) agent such as oxymetazoline (Afrin®) or xylometazoline (Otrivin®) as 0.05% t.i.d., and ingesting an oral antimicrobial agent. Although topical decongestants improve ostial drainage and provide symptomatic improvement, they also cause ciliostatis and decrease blood flow to the mucosa. The latter activity could impair antibiotic penetration.

Oral agents such as pseudoephedrine (Sudafed®) will cause a marked nasal decongestant effect.[7] However, oral decongestants do not significantly increase the size of the ostium in patients with acute sinusitis.[8] Use of oral antihistamine–vasoconstrictor combinations is probably counterproductive, since these preparations tend to thicken sinus exudates.

The role of the antibiotic in the treatment of acute bacterial sinusitis is to achieve sterilization of the sinus, accomplish rapid clinical cure, and prevent complications such as spread of the disease and the development of chronic sinusitis. No one antibiotic has emerged as the preferred agent for the therapy of acute bacterial sinusitis. Comparable results have occurred with all the compounds listed in Table 5.1. Antibiotic selection is often influenced by history of drug allergy, the spectrum of activity of the compound, and the cost. Table 5.2 lists the advantages and disadvantages of some agents.

Currently, no oral quinolone is FDA-approved for the treatment of acute bacterial sinusitis. These compounds do not possess impressive *in vitro* inhibitory activity for *Streptococcus pneumoniae*.

Following the introduction of therapy, progressive clinical improvement should be anticipated within a few days. Bacteriological cure of the sinusitis, as documented by repeat sinus aspiration, results when an appropriate antimicrobial is prescribed and compliance occurs.[2] Infection of the sinus will persist if the infecting organism is resistant *in vitro* to the therapy, the antibiotic is discon-

Table 5.1
Treatment of Acute Bacterial Sinusitis

Agent	Dose
Amoxicillin	500 mg t.i.d.
Ampicillin	500 mg q.i.d.
Cyclacillin	500 mg t.i.d.
Bacampacillin	800 mg b.i.d.
Trimethoprim–sulfamethoxazole	Two tablets b.i.d.
Minocycline	100 mg b.i.d.
Cefaclor	500 mg q.i.d.
Amoxicillin–clavulanic acid	500 mg/125 mg t.i.d.

tinued prematurely, or adequate drainage has not been accomplished.[4] The treatment course should be 10–14 days, as 20% of sinuses will retain the infecting organism after a week of treatment.[4]

Complete radiographic resolution of the sinusitis usually will not occur within 10 days of antibiotic therapy.[9] If sinus x rays reveal air–fluid levels or opacification after 10–14 days of antibiotic treatment, there should be consideration for referring the patient to an ENT specialist for sinus aspiration and lavage.[10]

Table 5.2
Advantages and Disadvantages of Antibiotic Agents

Agent	Advantages	Disadvantages
Ampicillin	Inexpensive; activity for pneumococci and most *H. influenzae*	Contraindicated in the penicillin-allergic patient; can cause skin rashes, diarrhea; resistant strains of *H. influenzae, B. catarrhalis*, and *S. aureus*
Minocycline	Infrequent dosing	Resistant strains of *H. influenzae, S. aureus*, and *S. pneumoniae*; more expensive than tetracycline
Cefaclor	Activity for pneumococci, virtually all *H. influenzae*, and *S. aureus*	Contraindicated in the penicillin-allergic patient; expensive
Trimethoprim–sulfamethoxazole	Infrequent dosing; activity for virtually all pneumococci, *H. influenzae*, and *S. aureus*	Adverse reactions (fever, rash, GI); interactions with drugs (warfarin, oral hypoglycemic agents, phenytoin)
Amoxicillin–clavulanic acid	Activity for virtually all pneumococci, *H. influenzae, S. aureus*, and *B. catarrhalis*	Contraindicated in the penicillin-allergic patient; potential to cause diarrhea; expensive; clinical activity for disease caused by *S. aureus* not proved

Concerns

Follow-up of the patient is the key to successful management of acute sinusitis. Patients should be advised to contact their physician if any signs or symptoms of uncontrolled infection occur. Immediate hospitalization, an emergency consultation, or both should be considered if the patient complains of severe headache, headache unrelieved by mild analgesics, persistent or high fever, lethargy, visual impairment, or orbital or forehead swelling. Vomiting, aphasia, paresis, seizures, or altered mental status demand immediate hospitalization.

Spread of infection, particularly from the ethmoid, frontal, and sphenoid sinuses, can lead to osteomyelitis, orbital cellulitis, orbital abscess, cavernous sinus thrombophlebitis, cerebral epidural abscess, subdural empyema, brain abscess, meningitis, and cerebral venous infarction. These life-threatening complications require rapid neurological and neuroradiologic evaluation.

Acute Fungal Infection in the Diabetic

There is a unique, rapidly progressive, and life-endangering fungal infection of the sinus and orbit that develops in diabetics with ketoacidosis.[11] Rarely this disease occurs as a subacute process in a well-controlled diabetic or as an acute process in an immunocompromised nondiabetic host. The disease is caused by fungi of the order Mucorales, fungi with a predilection to invade blood vessels.

Initial manifestations consist of facial pain, eye pain, and, on occasion, blood-tinged nasal discharge. Additional features can include fever, lethargy, headache, proptosis, periorbital edema, visual blurring, increased lacrimation, tenderness over the maxillary sinus, and facial cellulitis.

X rays reveal nodular thickening of the soft-tissue lining of the paranasal sinuses and spotty destruction of the bony walls. Air–fluid levels are not present. The diagnosis is suggested by an awareness of this unique, aggressive form of acute infectious sinusitis in the diabetic with ketoacidosis and is established by histological examination and culture of biopsied infected tissue. Therapy consists of control of ketoacidosis, infusion of amphotericin B, and extensive debridement. This form of sinusitis is frequently fatal. Survivors often require extensive reconstructive surgery.

Chronic Maxillary Sinusitis

Patients with signs and symptoms consistent with chronic maxillary sinusitis merit diagnostic tests and appropriate referral. In addition to sinus x rays to help confirm the clinical diagnosis and exclude alternative noninfectious diseases (granulomatous, neoplastic), a dental consultation is appropriate. Approximately 20% of these patients will have dysfunction or infection of the masticatory system (such as periodontitis or periapical infection).[12] This probably explains why some studies have indicated an important role for anaerobes.[13] Additional investigations underscore the polymicrobic nature of chronic maxillary sinusitis and implicate the importance of *Haemophilus influenzae*.[14] In addition to sinus and dental x rays as well as dental consultation, most patients with documented chronic maxillary sinusitis should be referred to the ENT specialist for consideration of an antimicrobial program plus the performance of a drainage procedure (either lavage or more definitive surgical intervention).

PHARYNGITIS

Patients who acutely develop a severe sore throat may elect to consult a physician to obtain relief of their discomfort. There are some clinicians who arrange to have the patient evaluated initially by a nurse or a physician's assistant. It is important to note that well-trained physician-extenders, acting under careful supervision and in accordance with a predefined protocol, can often effectively assess (''screen'') patients, perform appropriate cultures, and determine when a physician referral is indicated.[15]

Viruses (rhinovirus, adenovirus, herpes simplex, influenza, Epstein–Barr, Coxsackie), bacteria (*Neisseria gonorrhoeae, C. diphtheriae, C. haemolyticum, Francisella tularensis*), and mycoplasma have been implicated in pharyngitis.[16] A sore throat can be a prominent feature of secondary syphilis, Vincent's angina, Lyme disease, epiglottitis, and retropharyngeal space infections. Streptococcal pharyngitis, however, is of greatest concern to practitioners because group A β-hemolytic streptococci cause most acute bacterial pharyngitis, are readily identified, are capable of initiating both nonsuppurative (acute rheumatic fever, acute glomerulonephritis) and suppurative sequelae, and, most importantly, are amenable to antimicrobial therapy.

Streptococcal pharyngitis has a peak incidence in late winter and early spring. The organism is transmitted by large airborne droplets through direct person-to-person spread. Rare epidemics are attributed to ingestion of contaminated food. Infected school children are the primary source of streptococcal pharyngitis that occurs in family units.

The classical description of streptococcal pharyngitis consists of the acute onset of sore throat accompanied by fever, malaise, headache, and dysphagia. Examination reveals pronounced inflammation of the pharynx, edema of the uvula, a discrete yellow exudate, and tender submandibular nodes. A leukocytosis is the anticipated laboratory finding. Those strains that produce an erythrogenic toxin produce the erythematous rash of scarlet fever. The experienced clinician appreciates, however, that there is considerable variability associated with the clinical manifestations of a streptococcal pharyngitis and that comparable signs and symptoms can develop when a pharyngitis is caused by alternative infectious organisms.[17]

The presence of conjunctivitis, nasal discharge, hoarseness, cough, and diarrhea is suggestive of a nonstreptococcal pharyngitis. Detection of vesicles or ulcers in the pharynx usually indicates disease caused by herpes simplex or Coxsackie virus. The patient with cough and muscle aches may well have influenza. Diffuse adenopathy and splenomegaly are most consistent with infectious mononucleosis.

Recovery of group A β-hemolytic streptococci from the pharynx of the patient with a sore throat has been statistically associated with three abnormalities: a fever >101°F, tonsillar exudate, and tender anterior cervical adenitis. This observation has formed the foundation for a probability-based management protocol that is designed to encourage the discriminating use of throat cultures and antibiotics for patients with sore throats.[18] It is apparent, however, that physicians who are guided by the presence or absence of specific physical findings to estimate the probability of streptococcal pharyngitis will often err, particularly when there is a low prevalence of the disease.[19]

A confirmed diagnosis of streptococcal pharyngitis requires a compatible clinical syndrome **plus** the detection of a significant rise in antibody titer to the extracellular hemolysin known as streptolysin O. This definition has been established to differentiate the acutely infected patient from the patient without a bona fide streptococcal infection whose pharynx contains group A streptococci, a condition referred to as the carrier state. A consensus has emerged that the chronic carrier does not require identification because the chronic carrier is unlikely to transmit the *Streptococcus* or to develop rheumatic fever.

Because the rise in ASO titer develops weeks after the onset of the acute streptococcal pharyngitis, and because early antibiotic therapy aborts this immune response, clinicians have sought practical alternatives to establish the diagnosis of streptococcal pharyngitis. Although it does not confirm infection, traditionally the throat culture has served as a means to determine the presence or absence of group A streptococci. It has been appreciated for years that there are a number of variables that influence the recovery of group A streptococci from the pharynx of infected patients.[20] These include the following: faulty collection (failure to sample thoroughly); the use of multiple specimen swabs; the interval between the onset of symptoms and collection of the specimen; previous antibiotic treatment; and expertise in preparing, incubating, and interpreting cultures. There are three problems with throat cultures: they can not distinguish the acutely infected patient from the carrier; there is a 10% false-negative rate in detection of group A streptococci; and the process requires overnight incubation. However, this technique remains the "gold standard" to confirm or exclude the presence of group A β-hemolytic streptococci.

Recently, a number of rapid direct antigen tests have become available and provide an alternative to throat cultures.[20] These tests can be interpreted in 10–

30 min, and they provide excellent specificity. However, these systems may fail to identify small numbers of group A β-hemolytic streptococci. Contrary to popular opinion, the recovery of small numbers of group A β-hemolytic streptococci can occur in infected patients, and these small numbers should not be summarily discarded and attributed to the carrier state.

There are a number of approaches physicians have taken when challenged by the patient with acute sore throat. Some clinicians culture each patient and await the results. This approach can be justified because the majority of patients will not have streptococcal pharyngitis, and a delay of as many as 9 days will not enhance the risk of rheumatic fever. In addition, this approach will reduce needless antibiotic costs and drug allergies. There are physicians who elect to perform no cultures but prefer to institute treatment immediately for those patients who have a "classical" streptococcal sore throat. They defend this position by noting that it reduces the laboratory cost and expedites the return to school or work for the patient. Other practitioners advocate an individualized approach and culture and immediately treat selected patients. I would suggest that the clinician swab the patient's throat with two swabs simultaneously and then perform the rapid antigen detection test. If the antigen detection test is positive, the second swab can be discarded, and antimicrobial treatment initiated. If the rapid antigen detection test is negative, the second swab should be cultured.

Streptococcal pharyngitis is usually a self-limited disease lasting for less than 5 days. There are four reasons to identify rapidly and treat the patient with acute streptococcal pharyngitis, however. Therapy initiated within 48 hr of the onset of symptoms can expedite the rate of resolution of fever and symptoms. Antibiotic treatment can prevent interpersonal dissemination and the development of suppurative complications (suppurative cervical adenitis, peritonsillar abscess, retropharyngeal abscess).[21] Treatment with penicillin can prevent the development of acute rheumatic fever. No evidence exists that antibiotic therapy prevents poststreptococcal acute glomerulonephritis, however.[22]

An acceptable antibiotic regimen for streptococcal pharyngitis is benzathine penicillin G, 1.2 million units administered once i.m.[23] This therapy assures compliance. However, it causes pain and is more sensitizing than oral treatment. Intramuscular therapy should be restricted to patients with a previous history of rheumatic fever and patients with an anticipated poor compliance with oral regimens. The preferred treatment of streptococcal pharyngitis is oral penicillin V potassium, administered as 250 mg four times a day for 10 days.[23] Penicillin is inexpensive, produces few untoward reactions, possesses inhibitory activity for all group A β-hemolytic streptococci, and has achieved an unsurpassed record of therapeutic efficacy. For the patient who is allergic to penicillin, the recommended treatment is erythromycin prescribed as 250 mg orally every 6 hr for 10 days. The erythromycin should be given with food to enhance absorption and tolerance. Oral cephalosporins are contraindicated for the patient who has sustained an immediate or accelerated hypersensitivity event from a penicillin. Sulfonamides, tetracycline, and trimethoprim–sulfamethoxazole are ineffective for the treatment of streptococcal pharyngitis. Ancillary treatment consists of warm saline gargles, rest, aspirin, liquids, and lozenges.

There is no reason to culture or treat asymptomatic family contacts unless a member has had rheumatic fever. Evaluation and treatment should be restricted to symptomatic members of the household.

A consensus of opinion has emerged that there is no reason to reculture patients at the end of a course of therapy and retreat those individuals with a positive culture. Perhaps an exception to this guideline is the patient who has had prior rheumatic fever. This consensus position has been reached for the following reasons: physicians will not be able to differentiate the initial streptococcal strain from colonization by a new strain; rheumatic fever is now a rare disease in most areas of the United States; most persistent streptococci represent a carrier state and not organisms that have become resistant to penicillin; and eradication of the carrier state is difficult to achieve.

Streptococci of Lancefield groups B, C, and G can cause exudative pharyngitis associated with fever and cervical adenopathy.[24] Disease caused by groups C and G can be accompanied by a rise in ASO titer, and, in fact, poststreptococcal glomerulonephritis has followed in the wake of group-C-related pharyngitis. No evidence exists, however, that these streptococcal groups can initiate rheumatic fever or that antibiotic therapy modifies either the severity or duration of the pharyngitis ascribed to these organisms.

Gonococcal pharyngeal infections are usually asymptomatic.[25] On occasion, patients experience a sore throat, which can be associated with pharyngeal erythema and exudate. Pharyngeal gonococcal infections are identified most often in homosexual men and less frequently in heterosexual women. The infection appears to be most frequently acquired by fellatio. There is a risk of transmission of pharyngeal gonococcal infection to the pharynx or urethra of an uninfected sexual partner. Of greater importance, however, is the fact that pharyngeal gonococcal infection can serve as the focus for disseminated gonococcal infection in the patient.[25]

It appears that for most patients there is spontaneous resolution of pharyngeal gonorrhea. However, because this disorder can produce local symptoms, can be a source of transmission, and can result in disseminated disease, antimicrobial therapy is indicated. Patients should also have a serological test for syphilis.

Because of its efficacy, the concern for the increasing gonococcal resistance to penicillin, and patient acceptability, ceftriaxone (125 mg i.m.) could be considered the preferred treatment. The penicillin-allergic patient should receive nine tablets of trimethoprim–sulfamethoxazole (720 mg/3600 mg) per day in one daily dose for 5 days. Inadequate numbers of patients with pharyngeal gonorrhea have been treated with norfloxacin to recommend this oral treatment.

An effort should be made to obtain a follow-up culture approximately 5–7 days after the completion of drug therapy and to contact, examine, and culture recent (within the past 30 days) sex partners.

The bacterium known as *Corynebacterium hemolyticum* is a rare, potentially treatable form of pharyngitis for teenagers and young adults.[26] The organism, a gram-positive rod, can cause a peritonsillar abscess as well as a pharyngeal or tonsillar membrane that resembles the exudate traditionally associated with diphtheria. In addition to pharyngitis, some patients experience fever, cervical adenopathy, and nonproductive cough. The distinctive clinical manifestation is the red (scarlatiniform) rash that develops in approximately 50% of the patients. The rash usually is confined to the extremities and trunk, occurs early in the course of the illness, and can desquamate. The combination of a pharyngitis and a red rash is not diagnostic of *Corynebacterium hemolyticum*-related illness, however, as these two findings can occur in streptococcal pharyngitis, toxic shock syndrome, secondary syphilis, Lyme disease, and infectious mononucleosis patients who have received ampicillin.

A presumptive diagnosis of pharyngitis caused by *Corynebacterium hemolyticum* can be made by the presence of gram-positive rods associated with polys on a Gram-stained smear of pharyngeal exudate. The definitive diagnosis requires recovery of the organism from pharyngeal culture, as this bacterium is not part of the normal flora.

The disease can resolve spontaneously. The suggestion has been made that patients experiencing persistent symptoms be treated with either 1.2 million units of benzathine penicillin G administered i.m. or 250 mg of oral erythromycin prescribed four times a day for 10 days.

Yersinia enterocolitica is a gram-negative bacillus that is capable of producing a wide range of infections. This organism is most frequently identified with a severe enterocolitis and, on occasion, Reiter's syndrome. *Yersinia enterocolitica* can cause a pharyngitis syndrome (even exudate) in patients with the enterocolitis syndrome (varying elements of fever, headache, nausea, vomiting, diarrhea, abdominal pain), or it can be responsible for sporadic cases of pharyngitis with accompanying cervical lymphadenopathy.[27] Patients with *Yersinia enterocolitica*-related pharyngitis fail to respond to penicillin. The optimum antibiotic therapy for this disease remains unknown. *In vitro* susceptibility testing indicates that tetracycline and trimethoprim–sulfamethoxazole inhibit the growth of this bacillus. Whether these compounds or the new quinolone drugs would hasten the resolution of this disease remains to be determined.

Similar to the pharyngitis associated with *Yersinia enterocolitica,* the pharyngitis caused by *Francisella tularensis* can represent the primary illness or be a component of ulceroglandular or typhoidal tularemia.[28] The pharynx can appear normal or demonstrate erythema, exudate, petechiae, ulcers, or "diphtherialike" membranes. Fever and cervical lymphadenopathy are frequent concomitant findings. *Francisella tularensis*-related pharyngitis is also a cause of penicillin-unresponsive pharyngitis. The bacterium will not be isolated (''culture-negative'') on the conventional blood agar designed to recover the group A β-hemolytic streptococcus. The organism constitutes a hazard for the microbiologist (through the development of aerosols or penetration of the skin), and laboratories do not usually have the ideal media available to grow this fastidious bacterium. The diagnosis is usually considered because of epidemiologic information (history of tick bite, ingestion or handling of animals, particularly muskrats and rabbits) and supportive clinical manifestations (cutaneous ulcers, lymphadenopathy, pneumonia). In the management of acutely ill patients, clinicians should not rely on the results of the initial serological test, as ''diagnostic agglutinin titers'' ($>1:160$) are not usually detected within the first week of exposure. Streptomycin remains the drug of choice, and it should be administered as 500 mg intramuscularly b.i.d. for 10–14 days.

A study published in 1983 attracted considerable attention because the authors suggested that *Chlamydia trachomatis* was responsible for pharyngitis in adults.[29] Subsequent investigations have provided inconclusive evidence.[30,31] Thus, the role of *Chlamydia trachomatis* as a cause of acute pharyngitis in adults remains to be established.

There are three life-threatening infections of the head and neck in which soreness of the throat is a prominent early complaint. These infections are epiglottitis, retropharyngeal phlegmon or abscess, and suppurative thrombophlebitis of the internal jugular vein (''postanginal sepsis''). In contemporary medicine epiglottitis is one of the more frequent infections of the neck to require hospitalization. The other two infections are distinctly unusual today.

Epiglottitis is an acute infectious disease that involves the supraglottic structures. Most patients are febrile and initially present with a sore throat. There then ensues the rapid progression of acute painful dysphagia and respiratory distress (upper airway obstruction). Of note are the fact that there is neither edema nor erythema of the oropharynx, and the patient's pain is disproportionate to the visible signs of pharyngitis. Lateral neck x rays reveal an edematous epiglottis and edema of the prevertebral soft tissue. Indirect laryngoscopy provides visual documentation of the process. Once the diagnosis of epiglottitis is considered, the focus of therapy is to maintain an airway (endotracheal intubation if necessary), obtain cultures (blood and, if possible, the epiglottis), and initiate antibiotic therapy. A number of bacteria have been incriminated in this infection, including *Streptococcus pneumoniae,* streptococci, staphylococci, and *Haemophilus parainfluenzae,* although this disease is most often caused by *Haemophilus influenzae,* frequently β-lactamase-producing strains. I would consider ceftriaxone, administered as 1–2 g i.v. ql2h, as the preferred initial antibiotic selection. For the penicillin/cephalosporin-allergic patient, I would commence treatment with chloramphenicol, 1 g i.v. q6h. Patients usually improve within 48 hr of the onset of antibiotic, and supportive therapy and antibiotic therapy should be continued for 7–10 days.

Retropharyngeal abscess is a rare life-threatening disorder in adults that usually results from trauma (penetration of the pharynx by a bone or endoscope) but can occur spontaneously or secondary to a continguous infection of the pharynx or nose. Patients usually experience fever and sore throat associated with considerable difficulty swallowing. On occasion, bulging of the posterior pharynx is noted. Routine x rays of the neck invariably demonstrate retropharyngeal swelling, and computed tomography has emerged as the most sensitive and specific radiographic study to identify the abscess. These infections are caused predominantly by aerobic streptococci, bacteroides, and peptostreptococci. Retropharyngeal abscesses endanger life because they can drain spontaneously and pose the threat of aspiration, they can penetrate the lateral pharyngeal space and threaten the great vessels, and they can dissect into the mediastinum. Therapy consists of controlled surgical drainage and antibiotics. Until definitive identification and susceptibility reports are available, the clinician should consider initiating therapy with chloramphenicol, 1 g i.v. every 6 hr, or clindamycin, 600 mg i.v. every 8 hr.

The term used for infection that begins in the throat and dissects into the parapharyngeal space, causing septic jugular thrombophlebitis, is ''postanginal sepsis''.[32] The disease is characterized by hectic fever, bacteremia, septic pulmonary infarcts, hematogenous dissemination (often involving the joints), and mediastinal suppuration. Of critical importance is the fact that throat discomfort, the patient's initial manifestation, can resolve spontaneously and completely, and the pharynx can appear absolutely normal when the second or systemic phase of the disease is ushered in. In fact, there can be a latent or asymptomatic period of 1–2 weeks between the original soreness of the throat and the subsequent appearance of the systemic (high fever, chills, sweating, prostration) and metastatic events. The most valuable clinical features to search for include tenderness at the angle of the jaw of the involved side (that can be accompanied by slight swelling) and tender induration along the anterior border of the sternocleidomastoid muscle. This life-endangering infection is usually caused by upper respiratory tract anaerobes (*Fusobacterium necrophorum, Peptostreptococcus* sp.) and much less frequently by *Streptococcus pyogenes*.

Treatment consists of the administration of antibiotics that possess inhibitory activity for the incriminated anaerobes (chloramphenicol, metronidazole, or clindamycin), drainage of metastatic abscesses and empyema, and, if computed tomography indicates a parapharyngeal space abscess, surgical exploration of the parapharyngeal space. The role for anticoagulation has not been defined. Patients have been successfully treated without this maneuver.

REFERENCES

1. Lundberg C, Engquist S: Pathogenesis of maxillary sinusitis. *Scand J Infect Dis* [*suppl*] 1983; 39:53–55.

2. Gwaltney JM, Sydnor A, Sande M: Etiology and microbiology treatment of acute sinusitis. *Ann Otol Rhinol Laryngol [suppl 84]* 1981; 90:68–71.
3. McNeill RA: Comparison of the findings on transillumination, X-ray and lavage of the maxillary sinus. *J Laryngol Otol* 1963; 77:1009–1013.
4. Hamory BH, Sande MA, Sydnor A Jr, *et al:* Etiology and antimicrobial therapy of acute maxillary sinusitis. *J Infect Dis* 1979; 139:197–202.
5. Scheld WM, Sydnor A Jr, Farr B, *et al:* Comparison of cyclacillin and amoxicillin for therapy of acute maxillary sinusitis. *Antimicrob Agents Chemother* 1986; 30:350–353.
6. Evans FO Jr, Sydnor JB, Moore WEC, *et al:* Sinusitis of the maxillary antrum. *N Engl J. Med* 1975; 293:735–739.
7. Roth RP, Cantekin EI, Bluestone CD, *et al:* Nasal decongestant activity of pseudoephedrine. *Ann Otol* 1977; 86:235–242.
8. Aust R, Drettner B, Falck B: Studies of the effect of peroral fenylpropanolamin on the functional size of the human maxillary ostium. *Acta Otolaryngol* 1979; 88:455–458.
9. Mattuccci KF, Levin WJ, Habib MA: Acute bacterial sinusitis. *Arch Otolaryngol Head Neck Surg* 1986; 112:73–76.
10. Gray WC, Blanchard CL: Sinusitis and its complications. *Am Fam Physician* 1987; 35:232–243.
11. Rangel-Guerra R, Martinez HR, Saenz C: Mucormycosis. *Arch Neurol* 1985; 42:578–581.
12. Lindahl L, Melen I, Ekedahl C, *et al:* Chronic maxillary sinusitis. *Acta Otolaryngol* 1982; 93:147–150.
13. Su WY, Lin C, Hung SY, *et al:* Bacteriological study in chronic maxillary sinusitis. *Laryngoscope* 1983; 93:931–934.
14. Karma P, Jokippi L, Sipila P, *et al:* Bacteria in chronic maxillary sinusitis. *Arch Otolaryngol* 1979; 105:386–390.
15. Greenfield S, Bragg FE, McCraith DL, *et al:* Upper-respiratory tract complaint protocol for physician-extenders. *Arch Intern Med* 1974; 133:294–299.
16. Mandel JH: Pharyngeal infections. Postgrad Med 1985; 77:187–199.
17. Schachtel BP, Fillingim JM, Beiter DJ, *et al:* Subjective and objective features of sore throat. *Arch Intern Med* 1984; 144:497–500.
18. Walsh BT, Bookheim WW, Johnson RC, *et al:* Recognition of streptococcal pharyngitis in adults. *Arch Intern Med* 1975; 135:1493–1497.
19. Roses RM, Cebul RD, Collins M, *et al:* The accuracy of experienced physicians' probability estimates for patients with sore throats. *JAMA* 1985; 254:925–929.
20. Kellogg JA, Manzella JP: Detection of group A streptococci in the laboratory or physician's office. *JAMA* 1986; 255:2638–2642.
21. Bennike T, Brochner-Mortensen K, Kjaer E, *et al:* Penicillin therapy in acute tonsillitis, phlegmonous tonsillitis and ulcerative tonsillitis. *Acta Med Scand* 1951; 139:253–274.
22. Weinstein L, LeFrock J: Does antimicrobial therapy of streptococcal pharyngitis or pyoderma alter the risk of glomerulonephritis? *J Infect Dis* 1971; 124:229–231.
23. Bass JW: Treatment of streptococcal pharyngitis revisited. *JAMA* 1986; 256:740–743.
24. McCue JD: Group G streptococcal pharyngitis. *JAMA* 1982; 248:1333–1336.
25. Weisner PJ, Tronca E, Bonin P, *et al:* Clinical spectrum of pharyngeal gonococcal infection. *N Engl J Med* 1973; 288:181–185.
26. Miller RA, Brancato F, Holmes KK: *Corynebacterium hemolyticum* as a cause of pharyngitis and scarlatiniform rash in young adults. *Ann Intern Med* 1986; 105:867–872.
27. Jacket CO, David BR, Carter GP, *et al: Yersinia enterocolitica* pharyngitis. *Ann Intern Med* 1983; 99:40–42.
28. Evans ME, Gregory DW, Schaffner W, *et al:* Tularemia: A 30-year experience with 88 cases. *Medicine* 1985; 64:251–269.
29. Komaroff AL, Aronson MD, Pass TM, *et al:* Serologic evidence of chlamydial and mycoplasmal pharyngitis in adults. *Science* 1983; 222:927–928.

30. Gerber MA, Ryan RW, Tilton RC, *et al:* Role of *Chlamydia trachomatis* in acute pharyngitis in young adults. *J Clin Microbiol* 1984; 20:993–994.
31. McDonald CJ, Tierney WM, Hui SL, *et al:* A controlled trial of erythromycin in adults with nonstreptococccal pharyngitis. *J Infect Dis* 1985; 152:1093–1094.
32. Seidenfeld SM, Sutkev WL, Luby JP: *Fusobacterium necrophorum* septicemia following oropharyngeal infection. *JAMA* 1982; 248:1348–1350.

6

Infectious Bronchitis

Richard A. Gleckman

INTRODUCTION

It has been estimated that approximately 18 million episodes of bronchitis are treated in an ambulatory care setting in the United States each year.[1] These inflammatory events produce troublesome symptoms, often result in absenteeism from work, and, on occasion, threaten the life of the patient. With the introduction of new culture and serological techniques, the infectious organisms contributing to actue bronchitis and the exacerbation of chronic bronchitis are being more completely defined. This chapter reviews contemporary concepts pertaining to the pathogenesis, microbiology, clinical features, differential diagnosis, therapy, and prevention of bronchitis in adults.

ACUTE BRONCHITIS

Acute bronchitis is an inflammatory disorder of the bronchi that occurs most commonly during the winter. The disease is usually preceded by or associated with coryza, pharyngitis, and headache and is frequently caused by viruses, particularly rhinovirus, coronavirus, adenovirus, and influenza virus, less commonly by *Mycoplasma pneumoniae,* and rarely by bacterial pathogens including *Legionella* sp. and *Bordetella pertussis*. Both *Legionella pneumophila* and *Legionella feeleii* produce a self-limiting influenzalike illness known as Pontiac fever.

Pontiac fever occurs in epidemic form in individuals exposed to droplet nuclei of aerosols of contaminated water.[2] The disease is ushered in acutely, and the clinical manifestations consist of shaking chills, headache, myalgias, sore throat, and a nonproductive cough. Patients demonstrate a leukocytosis, but the chest x ray does not reveal an infiltrate. Pontiac fever is a self-limiting disorder, and secondary spread does not occur among family members.

Recently, a new respiratory pathogen capable of causing both acute bronchitis and pneumonia in adults has been identified.[3] The pathogen is a new strain of *Chlamydia psittaci* known as the TWAR agent. Currently, the ability to detect this organism, by culture or serological tests, remains restricted to a very small number of reference laboratories.

The hallmark of acute bronchitis is cough, and approximately one half of the patients with acute bronchitis produce sputum. As a general rule, when acute bronchitis is caused by rhinovirus or coronavirus, patients remain afebrile. When the disease is caused by adenovirus, influenza, or *M. pneumoniae,* patients are often febrile. In evaluating a patient with acute bronchitis, there is no need to analyze the sputum or blood. Chest x rays are indicated only for those elderly patients with fever and/or rales.

Acute bronchitis is usually a self-limiting infection. Bronchitis caused by influenza, however, can be complicated by viral pneumonia or a secondary bacterial pneumonia, both life-endangering diseases.

During the last year, cases have been reported of patients who developed staphylococcal-induced toxic shock syndrome in the wake of influenza-B-related acute bronchitis.[4] This sequence of events was first described by Thucydides, Greek historian of the fifth century BC.

Antibiotics are not indicated for the management of acute bronchitis. A placebo-controlled study failed to identify any advantage with the use of an antibiotic.[5] Treatment is directed at controlling cough and fever. Codeine is the preferred antitussive medication. Glyceryl guaiacolate has no documented ability to reduce cough frequency.[6]

Physicians should consider prescribing amantadine hydrochloride, 100 mg orally twice daily, for patients with suspected influenza-A-related bronchitis. Amantadine shortens the duration and severity of the symptoms and has been found to be more effective than aspirin in relieving signs and symptoms. In addition, amantadine accelerates resolution of the altered function of the peripheral airways that occurs as a result of influenzal bronchitis. To be effective, amantadine must be prescribed within 48 hr of the onset of symptoms. Adverse reactions attributed to amantadine include anxiety, lethargy, and anorexia, and in those predisposed patients, this medication can induce a seizure. Amantadine should not be administered to patients who are pregnant, have a seizure disorder, are performing work requiring constant alertness, or are receiving chlopheniramine. The dose of amantadine must be reduced in the patient with renal insufficiency.[7]

There are data to indicate that ribavirin is an effective oral therapy for disease caused by influenza A and B. This compound is not currently FDA approved for this indication, however.

CHRONIC BRONCHITIS

Chronic bronchitis, a disease characterized by mucosal inflammation of the cartilaginous airways, represents a response to chronic bronchial irritation. Patients experience a chronic or recurrent productive cough. To satisfy the official definition, the productive cough should be present almost every day for a minimum of 3 months in 1 year and for not less than two successive years.[8] Approximately 7.5 million Americans have chronic bronchitis.

There are a number of alternative diseases that cause chronic cough and sputum production over a period of years. These diseases, such as cystic fibrosis, bronchietasis, and asthma, need to be excluded before the diagnosis of chronic bronchitis is accepted.

Among American women a disturbing trend has developed over the last 20 years. More women now are considered "heavy" smokers, and these women inhale deeply. In fact, there is 300% more bronchitis and emphysema among women who smoke, and lung cancer has become the leading cause of cancer death in women. In 1983 there were 41,000 new cases of lung cancer and 35,000 deaths from cancer among American women. The risk for fatal and nonfatal cardiac events is also enhanced for women who smoke.[9]

For patients with bronchitis, the prognosis is related to the degree of airflow obstruction and the age at which spirometric abnormalities are first identified.[8] Smoking cessation is the single most important therapeutic maneuver that can alter the course of chronic bronchitis with airflow obstruction.[10,11] Among the identifiable causes of chronic bronchitis are cigarette smoking, air pollution, and perhaps respiratory illness in early life.[12]

Physicians should encourage their patients to stop smoking. It is important, however, to appreciate that nicotine is six to eight times more addictive than alcohol and that patients are concerned with the withdrawal syndrome, which consists of increased appetite and decreased ability to concentrate.

An exacerbation of chronic bronchitis is considered to have occurred when the patient experiences a worsening cough accompanied by purulent or mucopurulent sputum. Inconsistent manifestations of the exacerbation consist of malaise. increasing dyspnea, fever, and leukocytosis.During the exacerbation there can be rhonchi, coarse rales, wheezes, or decreased breath sounds. There can be no abnormality detected. Since the abnormalities can be present when the patient's condition is stable, the detection of these ausculatory findings has no diagnostic value. Objective findings that develop with the exacerbation of chronic bronchitis include an elevated sedimentation rate, a decreased vital capacity, and a decreased forced expiratory volume in the first second. The exacerbation of chronic bronchitis has attracted considerable medical attention, because for the patient it often results in incapacitation, medical costs, lost work time, and, less commonly, hospitalization, respiratory failure, and even death.

A number of factors are considered to be able to precipitate an exacerbation of chronic bronchitis: infection, hypersensitivity with acute bronchospasm, and environmental irritants. With regard to the "infectious" exacerbation of chronic bronchitis, this is believed to develop because of the combined effects of retained secretions, diminished cough, decreased mucociliary activity, and unrestrained multiplication of respiratory pathogens.

Whether infection contributes to the onset or perpetuation of the exacerbation has been disputed for a number of years, since there are studies that both support and refute a role for viruses, *M. pneumoniae, Streptococcus pneumoniae, Haemophilus influenzae,* and *Branhamella catarrhalis.* In fact, the resolution of this issue has been hampered by the assumption that patients with chronic bronchitis invariably have bacteria colonizing their bronchi. A more recent investigation, however, indicates that patients with chronic bronchitis do not invariably have a tracheobronchial microflora but that colonizing of the bronchi occurs selectively in those patients who continue to smoke.[13]

There are three lines of evidence that indicate that specific bacterial respiratory pathogens, such as *H. influenzae* and *S. pneumoniae,* contribute to the infectious exacerbation of chronic bronchitis. When transtracheal aspiration is performed on patients experiencing an exacerbation, *S. pneumoniae* and *H. influenzae,* as well as α-hemolytic *Streptococcus* and *Neisseria* spp. (? *B. catarrhalis*), are the bacteria most commonly isolated.[14] *Branhamella catarrhalis,* a gram-negative diplococcus that resembles two other respiratory pathogens by Gram stain, namely, *Neisseria meningitidis* and *Acinetobacter* sp., has been incriminated as a cause of exacerbation of chronic bronchitis. Antibody develops in patients who manifest purulent bronchitis associated with the recovery of *H. influenzae.*[15] Antibiotic therapy has been documented to be effective treatment for a specific segment of patients with an exacerbation of chronic bronchitis.[16]

It has been suggested that the elaboration of an IgA protease enzyme by *H. influenzae* and *S. pneumoniae* inactivates secretory IgA in the bronchial epithelium, thereby permitting these respiratory pathogens to adhere to and invade the bronchial epithelium.[17] This mechanism would not explain the role of *B. catarrhalis,* however, since this bacterium does not produce IgA protease.[18] It has also been suggested that secretory IgA blocks the bactericidal and opsonizing effect of antibody to nontypable *H. influenzae,* thereby allowing for colonization and subsequent invasive bronchitis by this organism.[19]

Since 1974, an increasing number of *H. influenzae* strains, both typable and nontypable, have been noted to be resistant to ampicillin. The most common ampicillin-resistant mechanism is explained by the elaboration in the periplasmic space of a β-lactamase enzyme mediated by a plasmid. The β-lactamase hydrolyzes the amide bond of the β-lactam nucleus, thereby rendering ampicillin inactive. Some strains of type B *H. influenzae* are resistant to ampicillin because of altered penicillin-binding proteins in the bacterium's plasma membrane, and presumably others are resistant because of an alteration of the organisms's outer membrane proteins (porins) that regulate drug diffusion. Many strains of *B. catarrhalis* also elaborate an inactivating enzyme, but this is a chromosome-mediated β-lactamase.

In this era of cost containment, physicians have reconsidered the need to obtain a complete blood count, Gram stain of sputum, sputum culture, or blood culture when evaluating patients in an outpatient setting. Sputum culture adds to the costs and requires 48 hr for identification and susceptibility data. If sputum is not processed, however, there will be no recognition of β-lactamase-producing *H. influenzae* and *B. catarrhalis*. All patients with exacerbations of chronic bronchitis merit chest x rays to exclude coexisting pneumonia, tuberculosis, or pulmonary neoplasm. The presence or absence of fever or leukocytosis does not effectively differentiate an exacerbation from pneumonia.[20]

Traditionally, physicians have prescribed antibiotics for patients experiencing an exacerbation. Physicians are convinced that patients improve faster and are concerned that patients will develop respiratory failure. Physicians also feel that antibiotics can forestall progressive pulmonary deterioration. Since the introduction of the sulfonamides, the value of administering an antimicrobial agent for the patient with an exacerbation has been an unresolved issue. The previously published studies designed to assess the contribution of the antibiotic have had major methodological and statistical defects. Investigators have often evaluated nonhomogeneous groups, used variable adjunctive therapy, failed to randomize patient entry into the study or to use a double-blind technique, and have not monitored drug compliance. Other researchers have failed to identify the causative infectious agents, exclude patients with pneumonia, or use objective efficacy criteria in their study protocols. In addition, patient entry into the studies has been so limited that if a difference existed among patients receiving antibiotics, the merit of the drug could not be demonstrated statistically.[21]

A recent large study that enrolled 173 patients and evaluated 362 exacerbations appears to have resolved this issue.[16] This randomized placebo-controlled investigation demonstrated that antimicrobial agents, when prescribed for 10 days, were well tolerated and resulted in a more complete resolution of symptoms, less frequent clinical failures requiring intervention (new medication or the need for hospitalization), and achieved a more rapid increase in peak flow rates. Of note is the fact that the patients who benefited from the antibiotic were those individuals who had an exacerbation characterized by increasing dyspnea, sputum volume, and sputum purulence or at least two of these abnormalities. Antibiotics conferred no benefit when only one of these manifestations had occurred.

No study has identified the preferred antimicrobial agent.[22] Erythromycin, prescribed as 500 mg q.i.d., is an inexpensive and safe compound that would be an appropriate selection when the exacerbation is caused by *S. pneumoniae, B.*

catarrhalis, or *M. pneumoniae.* This drug does not possess inhibitory activity for many strains of *H. influenzae,* and it interacts with theophylline, warfarin, carbamazepine, and cyclosporine.

Tetracycline, prescribed as 500 mg q.i.d., is inexpensive and has stood the test of time. There are pneumococci and *H. influenzae* strains that are resistant to tetracycline, however, and this drug can augment azotemia in patients with renal insufficiency. Alternatively, doxycycline, prescribed as 100 mg b.i.d., can be offered. This drug does not affect renal function. Ampicillin, prescribed as 500 mg q.i.d., and amoxicillin, prescribed as 500 mg t.i.d., inhibit the growth of *S. pneumoniae* and most *H. influenzae.* These antibiotics are contraindicated in the patient allergic to penicillin, can cause fever, skin rashes, and diarrhea, and fail to impede the growth of β-lactamase-producing *H. influenzae* and *B. catarrhalis.* Bacampicillin, prescribed as 800 mg b.i.d., is as effective as ampicillin, and it offers several advantages, such as twice-a-day dosage without regard to meals and fewer gastrointestinal side effects.[23] It is more expensive, however.

Trimethoprim–sulfamethoxazole possesses inhibitory activity for *S. pneumoniae* and most *H. influenzae,* including β-lactamase-producing strains. The combination agent can be prescribed as infrequently as twice a day. When prescribed in a dose of two tablets t.i.d. in a randomized blinded controlled study comparing trimethoprim–sulfamethoxazole to tetracycline, 500 mg q.i.d., deterioration in clinical status that required an alternative antibiotic occurred significantly more often in those patients receiving the tetracycline.[24] The disadvantages of this compound are its potential to cause fever and rash and its interaction with numerous other drugs, including warfarin, phenytoin, and oral hypoglycemic agents. Cefeclor possesses a spectrum of activity that includes *S. pneumoniae* and many *H. influenzae,* including β-lactamase-producing strains. This compound is expensive and contraindicated for the patient who has experienced an immediate or accelerated hypersensitivity reaction (anaphylaxis, laryngospasm, giant urticaria) from a penicillin antibiotic. The long-acting cefadroxil should not be considered as an alternative to cefaclor because the former compound does not possess inhibitory activity for *H. influenzae.*

The fixed-dose antimicrobial compound consisting of amoxicillin and clavulanic acid is known as Augmentin®. The clavulanic acid component binds irreversibly to the active sites of many β-lactamase enzymes capable of inactivating amoxicillin. Clavulanic acid functions as a true "suicide inhibitor," since it forms a complex with some β-lactamases, and the complex then decomposes. By removing some β-lactamase hydrolytic enzymes, this allows the amoxicillin component of the combination to exert its inhibitory activity on bacterial respiratory pathogens that are normally resistant to amoxicillin. In essence, the addition of clavulanic acid has extended the spectrum of amoxicillin to include β-lactamase producing strains of both *H. influenzae* and *B. catarrhalis.* The amoxicillin–clavulanic acid combination, however, is expensive, is contraindicated in the penicillin-allergic patient, and often causes diarrhea.

Physicians now have access to a new cephalosporin and a quinolone for treatment of the bacterial exacerbation of chronic bronchitis. The oral cephalosporin cefuroxime axetil possesses excellent inhibitory activity against virtually all strains of *H. influenzae,* and this compound can be administered infrequently.[25] Initial clinical studies with the quinolone ciprofloxacin for the treatment of the bacterial exacerbation of chronic bronchitis appear promising, but this compound is expensive, can interact with theophylline, and does not possess impressive *in vitro* inhibitory activity directed against *S. pneumoniae.*[26]

The conventional duration of antimicrobial therapy for the exacerbation is 10 to 14 days. Ancillary therapies consist of cessation of smoking, adequate hydration, and bronchodilators. No evidence exists, however, that hydration actually facilitates sputum production. Chest physiotherapy and expectorants have not produced consistent, significant improvement. In colder climates, humidification should be considered during the heating season.

Assessing the efficacy of therapy for the exacerbation of chronic bronchitis is crude. The patient should experience a sense of well-being and produce less sputum. There should be a change in the appearance of the sputum, from purulent to mucoid. Clinical improvement is recognized within 3 to 4 days of the onset of therapy, and complete resolution of the exacerbation occurs in approximately 11 days.[22] If clinical improvement does not ensue within 3 to 4 days of the onset of therapy, three concerns surface. Has the patient failed to comply with the therapeutic program? Has an inappropriate medication been prescribed? Should hospitalization be considered to offer an intense supervised therapy or to initiate steroid treatment? Although there are not rigid guidelines, most physicians would hospitalize the patient when the oxygen pressure at room air is <50 mm Hg and/or the carbon dioxide at room air is >50 mm Hg. For the hospitalized patient intravenous methylprednisolone improves airflow.[27] No benefit has been attributed to intravenous aminophylline, however.[28]

In addition to the conventional parameters to measure antimicrobial effectiveness, the suggestion has been made that another important dimension that merits consideration is the posttreatment infection-free period.[22] Unfortunately, this has not been precisely determined for many antimicrobial patients.

An unresolved issue is whether or not patients with chronic bronchitis should receive prophylactic antibiotic during the winter months. Limited data indicate that some patients who take prophylactic antibiotics experience fewer exacerbations and lose less work time. Certainly the data supporting the prophylactic value of influenza vaccine for patients with chronic bronchitis are compelling. The vaccine has been shown to be able to reducc the length of illness of influenza, the necessity for hospitalization, the development of pneumonia, and the number of deaths. For those patients with chronic bronchitis who fail to receive influenza immunization, amantadine should be administered continuously throughout influenza epidemics.

It is important to emphasize that recent influenza vaccines have not been associated with the development of the Guillain–Barré syndrome and that, contrary to initial reports, influenza vaccine does not inhibit the clearance of warfarin or theophylline.

Although patients with chronic bronchitis are considered prime candidates for immunization with the 23-valent pneumococcal vaccine, there currently exist no published data indicating its prophylactic value in this population.[29] When elderly patients with chronic bronchitis receive pneumococcal vaccine, they do not achieve persistent protective antibody concentrations, and their sera fail to develop adequate opsonizing capacity.

REFERENCES

1. Dixon RE: Economic costs of respiratory tract infections in the United States. *Am J Med* 1985; 78(suppl 6B):45–51.
2. Glick FH, Gregg MB, Berman B, *et al:* Pontiac fever. *Am J Epidemiol* 1978; 107:149–160.
3. Grayston JT, Kuo CC, Wang SP, *et al:* A new *Chlamydia psittaci* strain, TWAR, isolated in acute respiratory tract infections. *N Engl J Med* 1986; 315:161–168.
4. MacDonald KL, Osterholm MT, Hedberg CW, *et al:* Toxic shock syndrome: A newly recognized complication of influenza like illness. *JAMA* 1987; 257:1052–1058.
5. Stott NCH, West RR: Randomised controlled trial of antibiotics in patients with cough and purulent sputum. *Br Med J* 1976: 2:556–559.
6. Kuhn JJ, Hendley JO, Adams KF, *et al:* Antitussive effect of guaifenesin in young adults with natural colds. *Chest* 1982; 82:7–13.
7. Horadam VW, Sharp JG, Similack JD, *et al:* Pharmacokinetics of amantadine hydrochloride in subjects with normal and impaired renal function. *Ann Intern Med* 1981; 94:454–458.
8. American Thoracic Society: Definitions and classification of chronic bronchitis, asthma and pulmonary emphysema. *Am Rev Respir Dis* 1962; 85:762–768.
9. Willett EC, Green A, Stampfer MJ, *et al:* Relative and absolute excess risks of coronary heart disease among women who smoke cigarettes. *N Engl J Med* 1987; 317:1303–1309.
10. Peto R, Speiger FE, Cochrane AL, *et al:* The relevance in adults of airflow obstruction, but not of mucus hypersecretion, to mortality from chronic lung disease. *Am Rev Respir Dis* 1983; 128:491–500.
11. Camilli AE, Burrows B, Knudson RJ, *et al:* Longitudinal changes in forced expiratory volume in one second in adults. *Am Rev Respir Dis* 1987; 135:794–799.
12. Britten N, Davies JMC, Colley JRT: Early respiratory experience and subsequent cough and peak expiratory flow rate in 36 year old men and women. *Br Bed J* 1987; 294:1317–1320.
13. Irwin RS, Erickson AD, Pratter MR, *et al:* Prediction of tracheobronchial colonization in current cigarette smokers with chronic obstructive bronchitis. *J Infect Dis* 1982; 145:234–241.
14. Irwin RS, Corroa WM, Erickson AD, *et al:* Characterization by transtrachaeal aspiration of the tracheobronchial microflora during acute exacerbations of chronic obstructive bronchitis. *Am Rev Respir Dis* 1980; 121(suppl):150.
15. Musher DM, Kubitscheck KR, Crennan J, *et al:* Pneumonia and acute febrile tracheobronchitis due to *Haemophilus influenzae*. *Ann Intern Med* 1983; 99:444–450.
16. Anthonisen NR, Manfreda J, Warren CPW, *et al:* Antibiotic therapy in exacerbations of chronic obstructive pulmonary disease. *Ann Intern Med* 1987; 106:196–204.
17. Mulks MH, Kamfeld SJ, Plaut AG: Specific proteolysis of human IgA by *Streptococcus pneumoniae* and *Haemophilus influenzae*. *J Infect Dis* 1980; 141:450–456.

18. Mulks MH, Plaut AG: IgA protease production as a characteristic distinguishing pathogenic from harmless Neisseriaceae. *N Engl J Med* 1978; 299:973–976.
19. Musher DM, Goree A, Baughn RE, *et al:* Immunoglobulin A from bronchopulmonary secretions blocks bactericidal and opsonizing effects of antibody to nontypable *Haemophilus influenzae. Infect !mmun* 1984; 45:36–40.
20. Raheja AK, Weiss EB: The significance of fever in acute exacerbations of chronic obstructive airways disase. *Am Rev Respir Dis* 1981; 123(Suppl):71.
21. Nicotra MB, Rivera M, Awe RJ: Antibiotic therapy of acute exacerbations of chronic bronchitis. *Ann Intern Med* 1982; 97:18–21.
22. Chodosh S: Acute bacterial exacerbations in bronchitis and asthma. *Am J Med* 1987; 82(Suppl 4A):154–163.
23. Chodosh S: Bacampicillin in chronic bronchitis: Clinical experience. *Bull NY Acad Med* 1983; 59:505–514.
24. Pines A: Trimethoprim–sulfamethoxazole in the treatment and prevention of purulent exacerbations of chronic bronchitis. *J Infect Dis* 1973; 128(Suppl):706–709.
25. Cooper TJ, Ladusans E, Williams PEO, *et al:* A comparison of oral cefuroxime axetil and oral amoxycillin in lower respiratory tract infections. *J Antimibroc Chemother* 1985; 16:373–378.
26. Rubinstein E, Segev S: Drug interactions of ciproflozacin with other nonantibiotic agents. *Am J Med* 1987; 82(Suppl 4A):119–123.
27. Albert RK, Martin TR, Lavois SW: Controlled clinical trial of methylprednisolone in patients with chronic bronchitis and acute respiratory insufficiency. *Ann Intern Med* 1980; 92:753–758.
28. Rice KL, Leatherman, JW, Duane PG, *et al:* Aminophylline for acute exacerbations of chronic obstructive pulmonary disease. *Ann Intern Med* 1987; 107:305–309.
29. Leech JA, Gervais A, Rubin FL: Efficacy of pneumococcal vaccine in severe chronic obstructive pulmonary disease. *Can Med Assoc J* 1987; 136:361–365.

7

Management of Pneumonia in Outpatients

Richard B. Brown

INTRODUCTION

Pneumonia constitutes one of the most frequent and perplexing infections facing the primary care physician. In pediatric practice, this disease constitutes 13% of infections demonstrated during the first 2 years of life. Under the best of circumstances the diagnosis may be easily made, although the exact etiology may be difficult to prove. However, in patients with underlying cardiopulmonary disease and those at the extremes of age, the diagnosis may prove to be more difficult. Unlike both acute bronchitis and some cases of exacerbations of chronic bronchitis, which often are self-limited diseases, pneumonia is associated with significant morbidity and mortality.[1] Thus, the physician must be comfortable with the likely etiologies and therapeutic strategies to be utilized. Etiologic diagnosis usually rests on demonstrating the causative pathogen in respiratory secretions, blood, or pleural fluid. This process is complicated by the potential for contamination of expectorated sputum by organisms colonizing the upper respiratory tract and the fact that the majority of patients may be unable to provide a satisfactory expectorated specimen devoid of upper respiratory contaminants. Thus, many patients will have to be treated empirically based on information provided from history and physical examination.

OFFICE EVALUATION FOR SUSPECTED PNEUMONIA

The patient suspected of having pneumonia requires a comprehensive history and physical examination. The history should investigate epidemiologic issues such as recent travel, exposure to animals and birds, presence in a high-risk group for acquired immune deficiency syndrome (AIDS), recent antibiotic administration, drug allergies, and history of similar illness in family members or colleagues. Physical examination must assess the extent of pulmonary involvement, presence of disease outside the lungs, stability of vital signs, presence of known underlying disease, and the general "severity of illness" of the patient.

The presence of cough often points to infection within the chest. It represents the fifth most common reason for outpatient visits but will be associated with radiographic evidence of pneumonia in fewer than 3% of cases.[2] The clinical presence of significant sputum production, "severely ill" appearance, respiratory rate over 25/min, and temperature over 99°F are statistically associated with the presence of pneumonia by roentgenography, whereas rhinorrhea and sore throat mitigate against this diagnosis in the patient with cough as a presenting complaint.[2]

Which additional laboratory tests to order remains controversial. The physician must continually balance the risks and costs of procedures with those of empirical therapy in the absence of a specific etiologic diagnosis. Some authorities feel that "making a specific etiologic diagnosis in cases of community-acquired pneumonia is not necessary in the majority of cases."[3] Chest P–A and lateral x rays should be routinely obtained to demonstrate the presence of pneumonia, evaluate the configuration, and rule out the presence of abscess, large pleural effusion, pericarditis, etc.

Sputum evaluation should be carried out in all patients. However, the validity and reliability of the specimen may be directly related to the care used to obtain it.[3] In many clinical situations, specimen collection is not supervised, and sputa are collected from patients without overt respiratory infections.[4] Expectorated specimens will prove reliable if associated with the presence of large numbers of polymorphonuclear leukocytes, small numbers of epithelial cells, and mucous strands. Specific criteria exist for quantitative assessment of specimens.[5] Gram-stained preparations of such samples allow for the documentation of inflammatory cells and the morphology of causative pathogens and are extremely cost effective. Utilization of routine sputum culture and sensitivity is controversial. A recent publication stated "I recommend that we do away with routine sputum cultures in the initial assessment of patients with community-acquired pneumonia."[3] It is this author's opinion that the presence of organisms morphologically consistent with *S. pneumoniae* from a "quality" sputum is sufficiently diagnostic for implementation of treatment. Results of culture may only prove misleading. The presence of other organisms or the lack of an obvious causative pathogen should result in culture and sensitivity being obtained so long as the sputum specimen is considered microscopically meaningful.

In most instances, blood cultures and complete blood count will not provide useful information for patients with pneumonia being managed in the outpatient setting. The office assessment of pneumonia for pediatric patients is made even more difficult by the routine inability to document infection through sputum evaluation. It has been noted that specific etiologic diagnosis in children is made in fewer than 10% of cases.[6] Nonetheless, in older children attempts to obtain a good specimen should be made, and the results of Gram stain utilized when available. If evidence of lobar pneumonia is demonstrated, many pediatric infectious disease specialists recommend at least one blood culture, although the yield is low.[6]

Other laboratory tests should be employed as clinically indicated. Tests for cold agglutinins are positive in up to 50% of patients with pneumonia caused by *Mycoplasma pneumoniae*, are inexpensive to perform, and provide rapid and reliable data when positive in this clinical context.[7] In occasional cases, where unusual pathogens such as *Mycoplasma pneumoniae* in the patient with "negative" cold agglutinins are considered, acute and convalescent sera can be analyzed for serological evidence of infection. However, results are usually delayed to the extent that they provide little information for initial management.

DECISION TO HOSPITALIZE

A major consideration in the management of the patient with pneumonia is the need for hospitalization. Charges for the in-hospital care of a patient with pneumonia will be almost 20 times greater than care rendered at home.[8,9] Placement of a patient in an acute care institution allows for timely assessment, provides the opportunity for the easy administration of parenteral antibiotics and other fluids, allows for necessary laboratory evaluation, and generally insures compliance. However, unnecessary hospitalization is associated with large expenditures of health care dollars, the risk of nosocomial infection, and the potential for unneeded time lost from work or school. Thus, the decision to hospitalize must be undertaken judiciously; the clinician must weigh the pros of careful patient care against the cons of cost and risks for nosocomial complications. Clearly, not all patients with the diagnosis of pneumonia require hospitalization. Only about 50% of persons diagnosed with "pneumonia" will be hospitalized after assessment in an emergency room. Selected otherwise "fit" patients with pneumococcal pneumonia may be treated out of hospital.[10] However, scientifically valid criteria that evaluate the need for hospitalization are difficult to demonstrate from the literature.

The decision to hospitalize is based primarily on the severity of illness of the patient. Other issues that contribute to this decision are compliance, likely etiologic diagnosis, patient age, the presence of underlying illness, diagnostic certainty, and the availability of appropriate oral antibiotics. The latter issue has become decreasingly important with the advent of home intravenous therapy for the administration of parenteral antibiotics outside of the hospital.[11] Table 7.1 provides comparative data for individuals with community-acquired pneumonia treated on an ambulatory basis and compares them with a matched group that

Table 7.1
Clinical Characteristics of Inpatients and Outpatients with Pneumonia[a]

Characteristic	Inpatients (n = 25)	Outpatients (n = 94)
Age (years)	55.4	35.1[b]
Underlying disease (%)	100	14
Heart rate (bpm)	111	96
One lobe involvement (%)	56	20
Respiratory rate/min	29	20
Leukocyte count/mm^3	14	12
Po_2	62	72

[a]Adopted from Siegel.[11]
[b]Differences all significant at $P < 0.02$.

required hospitalization. In general, although not based on sound scientific data, the following criteria may be utilized for the treatment of patients at home: (1) compliant patient capable of taking antibiotics without nausea or vomiting, (2) available agent for use at home, (3) patient not "sick" enough to require hospitalization, (4) no likelihood of enteric gram-negative of *S. aureus* pneumonia, (5) patient not at extremes of age, (6) no evidence of cavitation, large pleural effusion, or multilobar consolidation, and (7) no evidence of extrapulmonary spread such as meningitis, septic arthritis, or endocarditis. It should be noted that these recommendations are not "independent" variables. For instance, it is highly unlikely that patients with *S. aureus* pneumonia and/or cavitary pneumonia will not be clinically sick enough to require hospitalization.

CAUSES OF PNEUMONIA IN THE OUTPATIENT SETTING

Most scientific discussions that have explored the etiology of community-acquired pneumonia in adults have analyzed only those patients who have been hospitalized. This has automatically skewed the data toward sicker patients, where more invasive diagnostic technology may be employed. Therefore, the causes of pneumonia in persons not requiring hospitalization remain uncertain. In the pediatric age group, treatable pneumonias that can be managed as outpatients will most commonly be caused by either *S. pneumoniae, H. influenzae,* or *Mycoplasma pneumoniae.*[12] However, most authorities recognize "viral" pneumonias as the most common cause of pneumonia in this age group; they may represent 70–90% of all cases.[12] Viruses most commonly implicated include respiratory syncytial virus (RSV) and parainfluenza virus in children under 2 years of age and either influenza virus or adenovirus in older children.[12] Likely nonviral etiologies vary with the age of the pediatric patient. In the child under 6 years of age, *S. pneumoniae* and *H. influenzae* (usually type b) are implicated, whereas in the older child either *S. pneumoniae* or *M. pneumoniae* is typically noted.[6,12] The role for *Mycobacterium tuberculosis* and endemic environmental fungi such has *Histoplasma capsulatum* or *Coccidioides immitis* must be explored initially through careful epidemiologic history of travel or exposure.

In adults, disease caused by *S. pneumoniae* and *Mycoplasma pneumoniae* and those that are "viral" are the most likely to meet criteria for outpatient management.[3,13] There are few data concerning the management of other pathogens in this setting: however, *H. influenzae* has occasionally been noted and successfully treated.[11] *Mycoplasma pneumoniae* is statistically more likely to be noted in the young adult, whereas infection caused by *S. pneumoniae* can occur in individuals of any age but is more common in the elderly.[14]

Disease caused by *S. pneumoniae* (pneumococcal pneumonia) can often be differentiated clinically from that caused by *Mycoplasma pneumoniae*.[15] Table 7.2 summarizes major points that allow differentiation between these two most common treatable pathogens in adults. Historically, pneumococcal pneumonia was associated with the abrupt onset of a single chill and fever in an older patient with underlying cardiopulmonary disease, splenic dysfunction, or disorder of immunoglobulin or complement production. Pleurisy was often seen, and cough was productive and "rusty" in color. More recent data, provided through evaluation of older patients often with underlying cardiopulmonary disease, now demonstrate that the disease may present in a more subtle fashion.[16] Complaints may be quite nonspecific and may mimic nonpulmonary conditions. Mental status changes may predominate. Fever may be absent or low grade, and overt respiratory distress may be easily overlooked. However, physical examination and chest x ray often corrobrate location of disease. Alternatively, disease caused

Table 7.2
Pneumococcal versus Mycoplasmal Pneumonia

	Type of pneumonia	
Feature	Pneumococcal	Mycoplasmal
Age	Older	Younger
Presentation	Acute	Subacute
Cough	Productive	Nonproductive
X ray	Local	Diffuse/local
Effusion	May be prominent[a]	Small
Abscess	Rare[a]	Rare[a]
Fever	High	Modest
Gram stain		
Cellular content	PMNs	PMNs/lymphocytes
Organisms	Gram-positive diplococci	Rare

[a]Presence is indication for hospitalization.

by *M. pneumoniae* is usually subacute in onset, associated with nonproductive cough, and is usually seen in otherwise healthy young individuals.[15] There may be a variance between findings on physical examination and chest roentgenography. However, it must be stressed that presentation of these two infections may be identical in any single patient, and clinical differentiation may by impossible.

Evaluation of quality sputum in patients with pneumococcal pneumonia will often demonstrate large numbers of PMNs and monotonous fields of lancet-shaped gram-positive diplococci. Alternatively, if sputum is available from patients with mycoplasma pneumonia, a disease caused by organisms not stained by Gram stain, it will often demonstrate PMNs in the absence of descernible pathogens.

Radiographic differentiation may prove difficult, and a great deal of overlap can be noted. Classical pneumococcal pneumonia was often associated with lobar consolidation.[17] Up to 57% of patients had associated parapneumonic effusions, but frank empyema, abscess, or other evidence of tissue necrosis was infrequent.[18] More recent studies demonstrate that most patients with this disease now have radiographic evidence of bronchopneumonia, probably related to underlying chronic obstructive pulmonary disease that prevents anatomic consolidation.[16,19] Abscess continues to be extremely uncommon and should promote a search for alternative diagnoses or additional pathogens. Radiographic presentation of disease caused by *Mycoplasma pneumoniae* often is associated with diffuse infiltrates involving most lung fields, although bronchopneumonia and even lobar consolidation have been seen.[20] Pleural effusions are seen in up to 25% of patients but are usually unpretentious.[20,21] Evidence of tissue necrosis is rare.

Subacute or chronic pneumonia in adults must prompt an evaluation for additional pathogens that include *Mycobacterium tuberculosis*, endemic environmental fungi, and oral anaerobes. In this clinical circumstance, staining and culturing for acid-fast bacilli should be performed and, if positive, may allow for outpatient management.[22] Hospitalization for tuberculosis should no longer be considered routine but should rather be limited to persons in whom the diagnosis is uncertain, if the patient is "severely ill," for failure of compliance, or if extremely young children are in the home environment.

Pneumocystis carinii pneumonia is the most common infectious etiology of AIDS[23] and should be considered as a possible etiologic agent for pneumonia in the outpatient in an appropriate high-risk group who presents with pneumonia. Typically this disease is manifested by nonproductive cough, diffuse alveolointerstitial infiltrates, and dyspnea.[24,25] Increasing numbers of such patients have been seen outside of geographic areas where AIDS has been classically noted, and it is anticipated that more patients will fall under the purview of the primary care physician. If clinically suspected, the diagnosis can be made from induced expectorated secretions over 50% of the time when they are appropriately stained.[26] The causative pathogen will not be demonstrated on routine Gram stain. Diagnosis and treatment can be rendered in the outpatient setting so long as the patient is compliant, the diagnosis is secure, and the patient's respiratory status is satisfactory. A variety of new treatment modalities for this disease are evolving that include aerosolized pentamidine isethionate and the combination of diaminodiphenylsulfone (dapsone) plus trimethoprim. Details are presented in Chapter 4 dealing with the acquired immunodeficiency syndrome.

PNEUMONIA TREATMENT IN THE OUTPATIENT SETTING

Antibiotic therapy is virtually always indicated when treatable pneumonia is suspected. Table 7.3 depicts usual outpatient treatment regimens for common pneumonias seen out of hospital. A number of antibiotic strategies can be employed when pneumococcal pneumonia is anticipated. In the absence of allergy, penicillin remains the drug of choice at this time despite the fact that strains resistant to this agent have been demonstrated in selected areas of the world.[27] For uncomplicated disease in adults, doses of no more than 2.4 million units per day should be employed.[28] Many physicians prefer to administer an initial dose of procaine penicillin G, 600,000 units intramuscularly, and then to continue treatment with penicillin VK, 250 mg p.o. four times each day.[28] Therapy should be continued for 7–10 days. Alternative agents useful especially for patients allergic to penicillin include either erythromycin or cephalexin.[28] Both

Table 7.3
Therapy of Pneumonia in Outpatients

Organism	Antibiotic	Dose	Duration
S. pneumoniae	Procaine penicillin G, then penicillin VK	600,00 U stat, followed by 250–500 mg p.o. q.i.d.	10 days
	Penicillin V	250–500 mg p.o. q.i.d.	10 days
	Erythromycin	250–500 mg p.o. q.i.d.	10 days
	Cephalexin	250–500 mg p.o. q.i.d.	10 days
M. pneumoniae	Erythromycin	500 mg p.o. q.i.d.	21 days
	Doxycycline	200 mg p.o. stat, then 100 mg p.o. b.i.d.	21 days
H. influenzae	Amoxicillin[a]	500 mg p.o. t.i.d.	10 days
	Cefaclor	500 mg p.o. t.i.d.	10 days
	Trimethoprim–sulfamethoxazole	160–800 mg b.i.d. or t.i.d.	10 days
	Amoxicillin–clavulanic acid	500 mg p.o. t.i.d.	10 days
Unknown	Erythromycin	500 mg p.o. q.i.d.	14 days

[a]Agent of choice if likelihood of ampicillin/amoxicillin resistance low.

are administered orally in doses of 250–500 mg four times each day. Tetracycline should usually be avoided because up to 10% of strains in the United States are now noted to be resistant to this class of agent.[29] Other oral preparations that may have very occasional usage include clindamycin and trimethoprim–sulfamethoxazole, although there is limited experience with both of these for this disease. The latter agent should be used with caution in patients taking other drugs because of potential interactions between many classes of agents (e.g., coumadin, phenytoins, methotrexate) and the sulfa moiety of this antibiotic combination.[30,31]

Either erythromycin or tetracycline is the drug of choice for *Mycoplasma pneumoniae* pneumonia.[32] Both may be administered orally for periods of up to 21 days. Tetracyclines should not be utilized in children because of the potential of bone and tooth derangement. Erythromycin may be associated with significant amounts of gastric upset, so compliance should be monitored closely. Doxycycline is the author's tetracycline of choice because it may be administered only twice daily and can be given with food.

Patients with *H. influenzae* pneumonia may be occasionally treated solely as outpatients[11] or more frequently have therapy initiated in hospital and completed in the ambulatory setting. In clinical situations where pneumonia with this organism is anticipated, the likelihood of antibiotic resistance must be considered in defining a drug strategy. In the United States, approximately 16% of nontypable strains and 31% of type b strains are now resistant to ampicillin/amoxicillin.[33] At least 50–64% of strains are resistant to erythromycin.[33,34] Likelihood of resistance varies considerably among geographic regions and may also vary among different hospitals within a city.[34,35] Therefore, the physician must have access to resistance rates in his area of practice in order to employ antibiotics rationally for this disease. If the likelihood of resistance is low, ampicillin or amoxicillin in doses of 250–500 mg orally three or four times each day for 10 days is sensible. However, if resistance is anticipated (and this should be the case in most instances), then alternative therapy with agents such as cefaclor, amoxicillin–clavulanic acid, or trimethoprim–sulfamethoxazole should be employed. Decisions among these agents must take into account allergies, concomitant use of other medications, acceptible side effects, cost, and likelihood of compliance.

In many circumstances the physician will have to treat pneumonia empirically, as bacteriologic confirmation will never be available. For adults, oral erythromycin, 500 mg four times daily for 14 days, is a reasonable therapeutic compromise. The use of this relatively safe agent will provide satisfactory treatment for the two most common pathogens likely to cause outpatient treatable pneumonia in adults—*S. pneumoniae* and *M. pneumoniae*. In children, empirical therapy for outpatients is the rule, and the choice of agents must be predicated on the age of the patient. In children under the age of 6, where *H. influenzae* and *S. pneumoniae* are the most likely pathogens, most authorities recommend the use of amoxicillin or ampicillin for 10 days.[6,12] In children older than 8 years of age, either erythromycin alone or in combination with sulfisoxazole has been advocated, since the most likely pathogens are similar to those seen in adults.

Ancillary treatment in addition to antibiotics should, in most instances, be limited to management of proven underlying disorders. Salicylates or other antipyretics should not be employed routinely unless temperatures in excess of 105°F are noted or unless the metabolic stress of an elevated temperature would prove deleterious. When utilized, they are best employed on a regular basis, such as every 4 hr, rather than being administered only when temperatures exceed a given limit. Patients with underlying cardiopulmonary disease will often require judicious use of "supportive" medications such as diuretics, bronchodilators, or digitalis preparations. Persons with severe obstructive lung disease being chronically managed with corticosteroids will frequently need "stress" doses of these agents. However, it should again be cautioned that most persons with major underlying diseases will be best managed initially in the hospital.

Adequate hydration should be encouraged in order to aid mobilization of secretions. There is no role for the routine use of decongestants, antihistamines, or expectorants in the management of outpatients with pneumonia. Some of these may actually prove deleterious by excessively drying secretions.

FOLLOW-UP OF OUTPATIENTS WITH PNEUMONIA

Patients treated for pneumonia in the ambulatory setting must be carefully followed to insure compliance and clinical improvement. At least telephone contact with the patient should be made by 48–72 hr to assess these issues. Failure to improve by this time should provoke an assessment for alternative diagnoses, failure of compliance, pulmonary complications, or drug-related reactions. Hospitalization will often be indicated. For persons responding satisfactorally to treatment, therapy should be continued for an appropriate length of time, and a follow-up visit scheduled thereafter to document clinical cure. Follow-up chest roentgenography is always indicated to demonstrate return to base line. In otherwise healthy individuals, repeat x rays should not be obtained until approximately 6 weeks after pneumonia was first diagnosed.[3,36] Prior to this time, residual evidence of disease may be seen that has no bearing on clinical response and therefore may only confuse the physician. In persons with underlying obstructive lung disease, time to complete radiographic resolution may be up to 16 weeks.[36] Failure of the chest x ray to return to prepneumonia status should stimulate an assessment for endobronchial lesions, tuberculosis, or other secondary processes.

In most clinical situations, follow-up sputum analyses are not indicated and may actually provide conflicting data. It is anticipated that antibiotic therapy will result in bacteriological colonization of the upper respiratory tract. Gram stains and cultures may therefore demonstrate bacteria not clinically implicated in disease. Treatment of such organisms is contraindicated. The physician should reserve follow-up Gram stains and cultures for patients who fail to respond to treatment with clinical documentation of an ongoing lower respiratory process. Similarly, it is usually unnecessary to follow complete blood counts and other blood chemistry tests regularly unless clinical evidence of untoward drug effects or failure to respond is demonstrated. The need for other laboratory studies such as serum theophylline levels and other drug levels is predicated on the utilization of such agents for underlying diseases in patients at risk.

Patients should be kept at home for an amount of time necessary for them to reacquire a sense of well-being. In most instances less than 1 week of time away from work or school will suffice. The infections that cause the vast majority of pneumonias that can be treated in outpatients will not require any form of isolation, so relative normalcy of the home situation can be maintained.

PREVENTION OF PNEUMONIAS

Otherwise healthy young individuals are unlikely to contract pneumonias except on an extremely sporadic basis. Therefore, there are no indications for antibiotic prophylaxis, immunization, or immunoglobulin administration. Elderly individuals, those with underlying cardiopulmonary disease, and others with selected hematological dysfunction are candidates to receive annual influenza vaccination and possibly a single immunization against pneumococcal pneumonia.[37,38] The use of the latter vaccine in "high-risk" individuals suffering from old age, liver or renal failure, or chronic obstructive lung disease has recently been challenged by several studies that demonstrate no significant advantage over placebo in preventing either pneumococcal bronchitis or pneumonia in these populations.[39,40] One study assessing pneumococcal bacteremia failed to demonstrate efficacy of previous pneumococcal vaccine administration.[40] Reasons for apparent failure of this vaccine are not completely known but may involve failure of hosts with multiple underlying diseases to mount an adequate antibody response to pneumococcal vaccine.[41]

There is no role for the currently available *H. influenzae* type b vaccine for adults at risk for pneumonia with this organism. The vast majority of disease related to this pathogen is caused by nontypable strains, for which vaccine usage is without benefit. The role of this vaccine in pediatric lower respiratory tract infections has not been adequately explored but probably has little value.

INDICATIONS FOR REFERRAL OR HOSPITALIZATION

Indications for hospitalization have been given earlier in this chapter. Referral to an infectious disease specialist should be strongly considered for patients who fail to respond to therapy as outlined but who are not sick enough to require hospitalization. It is usually wise to refer after a single course of ineffective antibiotic therapy rather than to attempt management by switching antimicrobials in the hope that unusual pathogens are implicated. Pulmonary input may be indicated for help with management of the adult with severe underlying obstructive pulmonary disease and in the unusual clinical situation where chest x ray fails to return to baseline following treatment and an appropriate waiting period.

REFERENCES

1. Centers for Disease Control: Years of potential life lost by principal diagnosis, United States. *Morbid Mortal Week Rep* 1984; 33:407.
2. Diehr P, Wood RW, Bushyhead J, *et al:* Prediction of pneumonia in outpatients with acute cough—a statistical approach. *J Chron Dis* 1984; 37:215–225.
3. LaForce FM: Community-acquired lower respiratory tract infections: Prevention and cost-control strategies. *Am J Med* 1985; 78(suppl 6B):52–57.
4. Jacobson JT, Burke JP, Jacobson JA: Ordering patterns, collection, transport, and screening of sputum cultures in a community hospital: Evaluation of methods to improve results. *Infect Control* 1981; 2:307–311.
5. Geckler RW, Grellion DH, McAllister CK, *et al:* Microscopic and bacteriologic comparison of paired sputa and transtracheal aspirates. *J Clin Microbiol* 1977; 6:396–399.
6. Grossman M, Klein JO, McCarthy PL, *et al:* Concensus: Management of presumed bacterial pneumonia in ambulatory children. *Pediatr Infect Dis* 1984; 3:497–500.
7. Levine DP, Lerner AM: The clinical spectrum of *Mycoplasma pneumoniae* infections. *Med Clin North Am* 1978; 62:961–978.
8. Jacobson JA, Jacobson JT: Pneumococcal vaccination of hospitalized patients. *Clin Res* 1978; 26:397.
9. Willems JS, Sanders ER, Riddiough MA, *et al:* Cost-effectiveness of vaccination against pneumococcal pneumonia. *N Engl J Med* 1980; 303:553–559.
10. Blaser MJ, Klaus BD, Jacobson JA, *et al:* Comparison of cefadroxil and cephalexin in the treatment of community-acquired pneumonia. *Antimicrob Agents Chemother* 1984; 24:163–167.
11. Siegel D: Management of community-acquired pneumonia in outpatients. *West J Med* 1985; 142:45–48.
12. Wald ER: Management of pneumonia in outpatients. *Pediatr Infect* Dis 1984; 3(suppl):S21–S23.
13. Brown RB, Landis JN: Update on non hospital-acquired pneumonias. *Prim Care* 1979; 6:463–481.
14. McHenry MC: The infectious pneumonias. *Hosp Pract* 1980; 15:41/52.
15. Donowitz GR, Mandell GL: Acute pneumonia. In: Mandell GL, Douglas RG Jr, Bennett JE, eds. *Principles and Practice of Infectious Disease,* ed 2. New York, John Wiley & Sons, 1985:394–407.
16. Ort S. Ryan JL, Barden G, *et al:* Pneumococcal pneumonia in hospitalized patients. Clinical and radiological presentations. *JAMA* 1983; 249:214–218.
17. Tilghman RC, Finland M: Clinical significance of bacteremia in pneumococcic pneumonia. *Arch Intern Med* 1957; 59:602–619.
18. Taryle DA, Potts DE, Sahn SA: The incidence and clinical correlates of parapneumonia effusions in pneumococcal pneumonia. *Chest* 1978; 74:170–173.
19. Ziskind MM, Schwartz MI, George RB, *et al:* Incomplete consolidation in pneumococcal lobar pneumonia complicating pulmonary emphysema. *Ann Intern Med* 1970; 72:835–839.
20. Murray HW, Masur H, Senterfit LB, *et al:* The protean manifestations of *Mycoplasma pneumoniae* infection in adults. *Am J Med* 1975; 58:229–242.

21. Fine NL, Smith LR, Sheedy PF: Frequency of pleural effusions in mycoplasma and viral pneumonias. *N Engl J Med* 1970; 283:790–793.
22. Glassroth J, Robins AG, Snider DE: Tuberculosis in the 1980s. *N Engl J Med* 1980; 302:1441–1450.
23. Centers for Disease Control: Update: Acquired immunodeficiency syndrome—United States. *Morbid Mortal Week Rep* 1985; 34:245–248.
24. Walzer PD, Perl DP, Krogstad DJ, *et al: Pneumocystis carinii* pneumonia in the United States. Epidemiologic, diagnostic, and clinical features. *Ann Intern Med* 1974; 80:83–93.
25. Kovacs JA, Hiemenz JW, Macher AM, *et al: Pneumocystis carinii* pneumonia: A comparison between patients with the acquired immunodeficiency syndrome and patients with other immunodeficiencies. *Ann Intern Med* 1984; 100:663–671.
26. Bigby TD, Margolskee D, Curtis JL, *et al:* The usefulness of induced sputum in the diagnosis of *Pneumocystis carinii* pneumonia in patients with the acquired immunodeficiency syndrome. *Am Rev Respir Dis* 1986; 133:515–518.
27. Jacobs MR, Path FF, Path MRC, *et al:* Emergence of multiply resistant pneumococci. *N Engl J Med* 1978; 299:735–740.
28. Roberts RB: *Streptococcus pneumoniae.* In: Mandell GL, Douglas RG Jr, Bennett JE, eds. *Principles and Practice of Infectious Disease,* ed 2. New York, John Wiley & Sons, 1985:1142–1152.
29. Cooksey RC, Facklam RR, Thornsberry C: Antimicrobial susceptibility patterns of *Streptococcus pneumoniae. Antimicrob Agents Chemother* 1978; 13:645–648.
30. O'Reilly RA, Motley CH: Racemic warfarin and trimethoprim–sulfamethoxazole interactions in humans. *Ann Intern Med* 1979; 91:34–36.
31. Cockerill FR III, Edson RS: Trimethoprim–sulfamethoxazole. *Mayo Clin Proc* 1983; 58:147–153.
32. Denny FW, Clyde WA Jr, Glezen WP: *Mycoplasma pneumoniae* disease: Clinical spectrum, pathophysiology, epidemiology, and control. *J Infect Dis* 1971; 123:74–92.
33. Doern GV, Jorgensen JH, Thornsberry C, *et al:* Antimicrobial resistance among clinical isolates of *Haemophilus influenzae:* Results of a 1986 national surveillance study. In: *27th Interscience Conference on Antimicrobial Agents and Chemotherapy,* 1987,
34. Doern GV, Jorgensen JH, Thornsberry C, *et al:* Prevalence of antimicrobial resistance among clinical isolates of *Haemophilus influenzae:* A collaborative study. *Diag Microbiol Infect Dis* 1986: 4:95–107.
35. Doern GV, Chapin KC: Susceptibility of *Haemophilus influenzae* to amoxicillin/clavulanic acid, erythromycin, cefaclor, and trimethoprim/sulfamethoxazole. *Diag Microbiol Infect Dis* 1986; 4:37–41.
36. Jay SJ, Johanson WG, Pierce AK: The radiographic resolution of *Streptococcus pneumoniae* pneumonia. *N Engl J Med* 1975; 293:798–801.
37. Centers for Disease Control: Recommendations for prevention and control of influenza. *Ann Intern Med* 1986; 105:399–404.
38. Bolan G, Broome CV, Facklam RR, *et al:* Pneumococcal vaccine efficacy in selected populations in the United States. *Ann Intern Med* 1986; 104:1–6.
39. Simberkoff MS, Cross AP, Al-Ibrahim M, *et al:* Efficacy of pneumococcal vaccine in high-risk patients. *N Engl J Med* 1986; 315:1318–1327.
40. Forrester HL, Jahnigen DW, LaForce FM: Inefficacy of pneumococcal vaccine in a high-risk population. *Am J Med* 1987; 83:425–430.
41. Simberkoff MS, Cross AP, Schiffman G, *et al:* Further analysis of antibody responses to pneumococcal vaccine among patients enrolled in a trial of efficacy. In: *27th Interscience Conference on Antimicrobial Agents and Chemotherapy,* 1987.

8

Urethral Discharge

Nelson M. Gantz

INTRODUCTION

The complaint of urethral discharge is responsible for over 1 million office visits to U.S. physicians yearly.[1] Urethral discharge refers to secretions passed through the urethral meatus at times other than voiding. The secretions may be described as clear, purulent, or bloody. The complaint of urethral discharge is generally found only in males and is rarely noted in females. The discharge arises from the urethral glands and less often represents prostatic secretions; it is usually associated with dysuria and/or meatal pruritus. Fever and flank or suprapubic pain rarely occur with urethritis and should suggest other diseases elsewhere in the genitourinary tract.

ETIOLOGIES

The causes of urethral discharge include both noninfectious and infectious etiologies. The discharge that occurs immediately after ejaculation is normal and consists of semen or seminal components. Other noninfectious causes or urethral discharge include mechanical or chemical irritation, urethral stricture, nonbacterial prostatitis, urethral diverticula, urethral caruncle, and phimosis.

In the majority of patients, the urethral discharge has an infectious etiology. Infectious causes of urethral discharge may be classified as gonococcal urethritis if caused by *N. gonorrhoeae* of nongonococcal urethritis (NGU), formerly called nonspecific urethritis, if not caused by *N. gonorrhoeae*.[2,3] It should be noted that the two forms of urethritis are not mutually exclusive, as mixed infections may be present in the same patient. Although NGU is not a reportable disease in the United States, it is estimated to be at least twice as common as gonococcal urethritis. Multiple studies in the past 20 years have defined the etiologies of NGU, which include *Chlamydia trachomatis* (30–50%), *Ureaplasma urealyticum,* formerly T-strain mycoplasma (20–40%), *herpes simplex virus* (1%), and *Trichomonas vaginalis* (1%).[2,3] In approximately 20 to 30% of cases of NGU that appear to be sexually acquired, no cause can be determined despite extensive cultures. In studies evaluating various new potential etiologies of NGU, it is critical that valid controls be included to establish the role for other potential pathogens.

Postgonococcal urethritis (PGU) refers to urethritis that occurs following therapy for gonococcal urethritis with agents such as ampicillin that are not effective for pathogens causing NGU. *Chlamydia trachomatis* is responsible for up to 80% of cases of PGU.[4] Mixed gonococcal and *Chlamydia* infections occur in 20 to 30% of heterosexual men presenting with urethritis, which explains why therapy should be directed against gonococci and *Chlamydia* to prevent PGU.[1]

CLINICAL MANIFESTATIONS

Discharge and dysuria occur in patients infected with *Neisseria gonorrhoeae* or *Chlamydia trachomatis* (see Table 8.1). The discharge in patients with gonorrhea tends to be purulent, whereas in patients with *Chlamydia* infection it is usually mucoid, thin, sticky, and watery. Dysuria is reported more often in patients with gonococcal infections. Asymptomatic infections also occur in patients with gonococcal as well as chlamydial infections, particularly among persons named as sexual contacts of culture-positive index cases. Thus, as many as 50% of male contacts of infected females with gonorrhea and 20% of male contacts of infected females with *Chlamydia* have asymptomatic infections or have minimal symptoms. The clinical manifestations of gonococcal (GC) and nongonococcal urethritis usually overlap to such an extent that a diagnosis requires laboratory tests, since the two entities cannot be distinguished on clinical grounds.[5]

Table 8.1
Clinical Distinction between Gonococcal Urethritis and NGU

Manifestation	Gonococcal	NGU
Incubation period	2–7 days	7–21 days
Onset	Abrupt	Gradual
Discharge	Yellow, profuse	Thin, clear, watery
Dysuria	Moderate	Mild

DIAGNOSIS

Examination of the urethra for the presence of discharge and microscopic examination of a Gram-stained smear of the discharge for polymorphonuclear leukocytes (PMNs) are essential to the diagnosis of urethritis (Fig. 8.1). If there is no spontaneous discharge, then have the patient try to "milk" the urethra from the base to attempt to obtain a specimen. If no urethral discharge can be obtained either spontaneously or by vigorous milking of the urethra, then the initial 5 to 10 ml of urine should be examined after centrifugation for the presence of PMNs.

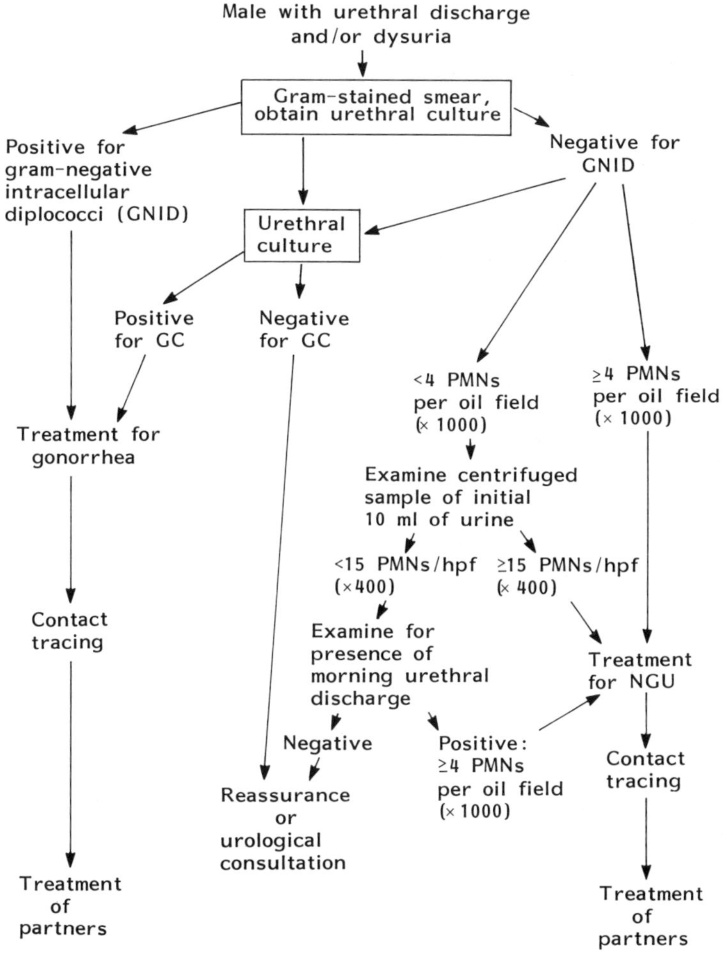

Figure 8.1. Initial presentation of a male with urethral discharge.

Uretheral leukocytocis has been defined as the presence of at least four PMNs per oil-immersion field and is diagnostic of urethritis.[6] If symptoms are present but no discharge can be obtained from the urethra and a urine specimen fails to show PMNs, then an examination of the urethra for any discharge in the morning before first micturation may be helpful.[7] Patients can be given a microscopic glass slide to try to obtain a specimen prior to voiding in the morning. A routine urinalysis is not a reliable method for detecting urethritis. Voiding within 2 to 4 hr of the examination may obscure the presence of urethral inflammation.

A presumptive diagnosis of GC urethritis can be made if the Gram stain of the material shows typical gram-negative intracellular diplococci. The sensitivity of the Gram stain of urethral discharge exceeds 95% in males with GC. The urethral culture for GC will confirm the diagnosis and detect an additional 5% of smear-negative cases. If the urethral smear reveals only extracellular or atypical gram-negative diplococci, then the diagnosis depends on the culture results. For patients in whom material cannot be obtained for examination, then a nasopharyngeal calcium alginate swab (Calgiswab®) should be inserted 2 to 3 cm into the urethra for culture. Material for GC culture should be inoculated onto selective culture medium. Plates should be incubated in an atmosphere of 3 to 5% CO_2 for 48 hr. A serological test for syphilis should also be obtained in all patients with suspected GC or NGU. Although the sensitivity of the Gram stain smear of urethral discharge is 90 to 95% in symptomatic males, it has a yield of only 50 to 70% in asymptomatic males who are named as contacts of infected females.[1] A culture for *Neisseria gonorrhoeae* is also recommended if the smear is unequivocally positive so that susceptibility testing can be performed on the isolate. In addition to examination of a Gram-stained smear of urethral discharge and culture, GC can be identified by antigen detection methods. One commercial test, known as Gonozyme®, was similar to the Gram stain in detecting urethral gonorrhea.[8] However, nonculture methods do not allow for susceptibility testing, and their role in diagnosis is unclear.

The diagnosis of NGU is usually one of exclusion. Since laboratory facilities to culture chlamydial and ureaplasmal organisms are not readily available to clinicians, the diagnosis of NGU is established by demonstrating urethral inflammation ($\geq$4 PMNs/oil-immersion field) with no evidence of *N. gonorrhoeae* by Gram-stained smear or urethral culture.

In obtaining a culture for *Chlamydia,* use a cotton-tipped swab with a metal shaft rather than a clacium alginate swab (Calgiswab®) because the latter are inhibitory to *Chlamydia*. *Chlamydia* can also be detected by noncultural methods by identifying chalamydial antigens.[9–11] To date, two tests have been marketed. One test, Micro Track®, involves direct fluorescent antibody staining of chlamydial elementary bodies in a urethral smear.[9,10] The test has a sensitivity of 70 to 90% depending on the population studied. The test has few false positives. The other test is an enzyme-linked immunoassay, which has been marketed as Chlamydiazyme®.[11] The test has a sensitivity that is comparable to the direct fluorescent antibody test and a specificity that is slightly lower. The place of these antigen tests in the diagnosis of chlamydial infection remains to be determined. Serological tests are generally not helpful in diagnosis, since testing usually cannot distinguish recent from remote infection. A negative serological test is good evidence against the presence of chlamydial infection.

THERAPY OF GONOCOCCAL URETHRITIS

Changes in the antimicrobial therapy of urethritis have occurred over the years because of stepwise increases in penicillin resistance, β-lactamase-producing *N. gonorrhoeae,* non-β-lactamase-producing penicillin-resistant *N. gonorrhoeae,* and plasmid-mediated tetracycline resistance. Today, 1% of U.S. isolates are penicillinase-producing strains of *N. gonorrhoeae* (PPNG).[12] Ceftriaxone and spectinomycin are effective against PPNG. Because of both plasmid-medited and chromosomally mediated tetracycline-resistant strains of *N. gonorrhoeae,* tetracycline can no longer be used as sole therapy for urethritis in a patient with a penicillin allergy.[13] Aqueous procaine penicillin/probenecid also has limited use today because of possible procaine reactions and resistant gonococci. For heterosexual men with urethritis, because of the high probability of mixed infections, therapy for both *Chlamydia* and GC is recommended. For homosexual men with GC, simultaneous chlamydial infection is unusual. See Table 8.2 for treatment recommendations.

THERAPY OF NGU

Optimal therapy for NGU consists of using either a tetracycline or erythromycin for a 7-day course. Therapy for 4 days is less effective than 7- to 14-day regimens, but a 21-day course offers no advantage.[1] There are no reported cases of therapy failures because of resistant chlamydial isolates. However, some

Table 8.2
Therapy of Gonococcal Urethritis[a]

1. Ampicillin,[b] 3.5 g (or amoxicillin, 3.0 g) orally, plus probenecid, 1 g orally
2. Ceftriaxone,[b,c,d] 125 mg i.m. or 250 mg i.m.
3. Spectinomycin,[c] 2 g i.m. (for penicillin-allergic patients)

[a]All treatment regimens should be followed by doxycycline, 100 mg orally b.i.d. for 7 days, or tetracycline, 500 mg orally q.i.d. for 7 days. If patients are unable to tolerate tetracycline, then use erythromycin, 500 mg orally for 7 days.
[b]Adequate therapy for incubating syphilis.
[c]Efficacy for PPNG and for concomitant anogenital infections.
[d]Efficacy for concomitant pharyngeal infections and therapy of choice for GC in homosexual men.

Table 8.3
Therapy of Chlamydial Urethritis

1. Doxycycline, 100 mg orally b.i.d. for 7 days
2. Tetracycline, 500 mg orally q.i.d. for 7 days
3. Erythromycin, 500 mg orally q.i.d. for 7 days
4. Erythromycin, 250 mg orally q.i.d. for 14 days (for patients with gastrointestinal intolerance to higher dose erythromycin)
5. Trimethoprim–sulfamethoxazole, nine regular-strength tablets orally once daily for 3 days

strains of *Ureaplasma* are resistant to tetracycline but remain susceptible to erythromycin[14] (see Table 8.3).

MANAGEMENT OF SEX PARTNERS

Sexual contacts of infected patients should be seen and treated for both *N. gonorrhoeae* and *Chlamydia.* All sexual partners within the past 30 days should be identified, examined, and treated, since asymptomatic infection occurs frequently.

FOLLOW-UP

Men with positive urethral cultures for *N. gonorrhoeae* should be seen 4 to 7 days after completing antibiotic therapy for test-of-cure cultures. Patients with NGU do not require follow-up unless symptoms persist.

PERSISTENT OR RECURRENT NGU

Patients with chlamydial urethritis will usually respond to tetracycline or erythromycin therapy. Failure to respond may result from compliance problems, tetracycline-resistant *Ureaplasma urealyticum,* which should be susceptible to erythromycin, reinfection, or other organisms such as *Trichomonas vaginalis* or herpes simplex virus. If compliance problems or reinfection do not appear to be issues, then the patient should receive a course of erythromycin. If the urethral discharge still persists, then a wet-prep examination of a urethral specimen should be examined for *Trichomonas vaginalis.* Occasionally, patients will have herpetic urethritis causing a discharge, but usually they will have obvious penile lesions. Reiter's syndrome should also be considered in a patient with a persistent urethral discharge. Patients with Reiter's syndrome note a urethral discharge, which usually begins 1 to 2 weeks after sexual intercourse. Other features of the syndrome, which often appear 1 to 5 weeks after the onset of the urethral discharge, include arthritis, mucocutaneous skin lesions called keratosis blennorrhagica and balanitis circinata sicca, as well as conjunctivitis. The findings may not be present all at once, and there is no diagnostic laboratory test. Patients with Reiter's syndrome are often positive for HLA-B27 histocompatability antigen. Patients with persistent discharge may be given a 3- to 6-week course of a tetracycline, erythromycin, or trimethoprim–sulfamethoxazole, although data supporting this recommendation are not available.

REFERENCES

1. Hooton TM, Barnes RC: Urethritis in men in sexually transmitted diseases. *Infect Dis Clin North Am* 1987; 1:165–178.
2. Holmes KK, Handsfield HH, Wang SP, *et al:* Etiology of nogonococcal urethritis. *N Eng J Med* 1975; 292:1199–1205.
3. Swartz SL, Kraus SJ, Hermann KL, *et al:* Diagnosis and etiology of nongonococcal urethritis. *J Infect Dis* 1978; 138:445–454.
4. Bowie WR, Alexander ER, Holmes KK: Etiologies of postgonococcal urethritis in homosexual and heterosexual men: Roles of *Chlamydia trachomatis* and *Ureaplasma urealyticum. Sex Transm Dis* 1978; 5:151–154.
5. Jacobs NF, Kraus SJ: Gonococcal and nongonococcal urethritis in men: Clinical and laboratory differentiation. *Ann Intern Med* 1975; 82:7–12.
6. Kraus SJ: Semiquantitation of urethral polymorphonuclear leukocytes as objective evidence of nongonococcal urethritis. *Sex Transm Dis* 1982; 9:52–55.
7. Desai K, Robson HG: Comparison of the Gram-stained urethral smear and first-voided urine sediment in the diagnosis of nongonococcal urethritis. *Sex Transm Dis* 1982; 9:21–25.
8. Danielsson D, Moi H, Forslin L: Diagnosis of urogenital gonorrhea by detecting gonococcal antigen with a solid phase enzyme immunoassay (Gonozyme). *J Clin Pathol* 1983; 36:674–677.
9. Stamm WE, Harrison HR, Alexander ER, *et al:* Diagnosis of *Chlamydia trachomatis* infections by direct immunofluorescence staining of genital secretions. *Ann Intern Med* 1984; 101:638–641.
10. Uyeda CT, Welborn P, Ellison-Birang N, *et al:* Rapid diagnosis of chlamydial infections with the MicroTrak direct test. *J Clin Microbiol* 1984; 20:948–950.
11. Howard LV, Coleman PF, England BJ, *et al:* Evaluation of Chlamydiazyme for the detection of genital infections caused by *Chlamydia trachomatis. J Clin Microbiol* 1986; 23:329–332.
12. Centers for Disease Control: Penicillinase-producing *Neisseria gonorrhoeae*—United States, Florida. *Morbid Mortal Week Rep* 1986; 35:12–13.
13. Centers for Disease Control: Tetracycline-resistant *Neisseria gonorrhoeae*—Georgia, Pennsylvanis, New Hampshire. *Morbid Mortal Week Rep* 1985; 34:563–564.
14. Evans RT, Taylor-Robinson D: The incidence of tetracycline-resistant strains of *Ureaplasma urealyticum. J Antimicrob Chemother* 1978; 4:57–63.

9

Vaginal Discharge

Nelson M. Gantz

VAGINITIS

The complaints of vaginal discharge, dysuria, vulvar pruritus, and dyspareunia account for at least 10% of all office visits to private practitioners.[1] These complaints indicate a number of possible diagnoses with overlapping symptoms, including vaginitis, cervicitis, and urinary tract infection. It is important to try to have the patient localize the site of the dysuria as being internal or external. Internal dysuria suggests that the problem relates to the urinary tract, whereas external dysuria occurs more often with vaginal disorders.

Vaginal discharge may be normal or pathological. Normal or physiological vaginal discharge is called leukorrhea and is usually nonpruritic, lacks an offensive odor, is not associated with vulvar discomfort, contains few white cells, and has a normal vaginal flora. The predominant organisms comprising normal vaginal flora are gram-positive rods, lactobacilli. Normal vaginal secretions have an acidic pH of about 4.0. An increase in physiological discharge can occur at the time of ovulation, during pregnancy, prior to menses, and with oral contraceptive use. An abnormal vaginal discharge usually has an offensive odor, often contains many polymorphonuclear leukocytes, has an abnormal vaginal microflora, and is frequently accompanied by dysuria, dyspareunia, and vulvar itching and soreness. An abnormal vaginal discharge can result from both noninfectious and infectious causes.

ETIOLOGIES

There are multiple causes for an abnormal vaginal discharge. Extravaginal disease may mimic vaginal discharge. Dermatological and psychosomatic disorders may result in vaginal complaints. Rectovaginal or vesicovaginal fistula may result in the passage of either feces or urine through the vagina. Patients with procitis may have a discharge that simulates a vaginal discharge. Noninfectious causes of vaginal discharge include chemical irritation or allergy from contraceptive foams or feminine hygiene products, a foreign body such as a forgotten vaginal tampon, contraceptive sponge, or device used for masturbation, and atrophic vaginitis. The vaginal mucosa in postmenopausal women may be deficient in estrogen, resulting in a thin, scanty discharge that may be accompanied by vulvar soreness and pruritus. The atrophic vaginal mucosa also may become secondarily infected. Vaginal discharge may be seen with gynecological neoplasms. The discharge may be scanty and blood-tinged.

The majority of patients with a vaginal discharge have an infectious etiology, and numerous organisms have been implicated. This discussion is limited to the three most common forms of infectious vaginitis, which include candidal vaginitis, trichomoniasis, and bacterial vaginosis caused by *Gardnerella vaginalis. Neisseria gonorrhoeae* rarely infects the adult vagina, and the discharge originates in the endocervix. The discharge passes through the introitus and is perceived as vaginal discharge by the patient. Similarly, chlamydial or herpetic cervicitis may have an excessive cervical discharge that is interpreted as an abnormal vaginal discharge by the patient. The diagnosis of chlamydial or herpetic cervicitis depends on the physical examination and on obtaining cultures.

Candidal Vaginitis

Candida albicans, a yeast, is the most frequent of the specific agents causing vaginitis. *Candida* yeasts are oval cells 3 to 5 μm in diameter that may form buds. The organism stains gram-positive, forms pseudohyphae, which are composed of enlongated chains of budding yeasts, and grows readily on culture media in 24 to 48 hr. Species of *Candida* other than *C. albicans* may cause vaginitis, but *C. albicans* causes 95% of vaginal yeast infections. Vaginal yeast colonization occurs commonly, yet it is unclear why some women develop symptomatic infections that respond readily to therapy and other women become symptomatic and have frequent recurrences. Factors predisposing to infection include diabetes mellitus, pregnancy, use of oral contraceptives, obseity, use of corticosteroids, and recent antibiotic use. The characteristic clinical picture such as the "cottage-cheese-like" vaginal discharge occurs in only half the patients with candidal vaginitis. Most cases are not sexually transmitted. There is no evidence to support the theory that intestinal yeasts are responsible for vaginal candidiasis.

Candida organisms can be identified on the saline wet preparation. *Candida* appear as small oval cells that may be budding or appear as filamentous forms, the so-called pseudohyphae. If the saline wet preparation is negative for trichomonads, then a drop of vaginal discharge can be placed on a slide with 10% potassium hydroxide (KOH). A cover slip is applied, and the material is gently

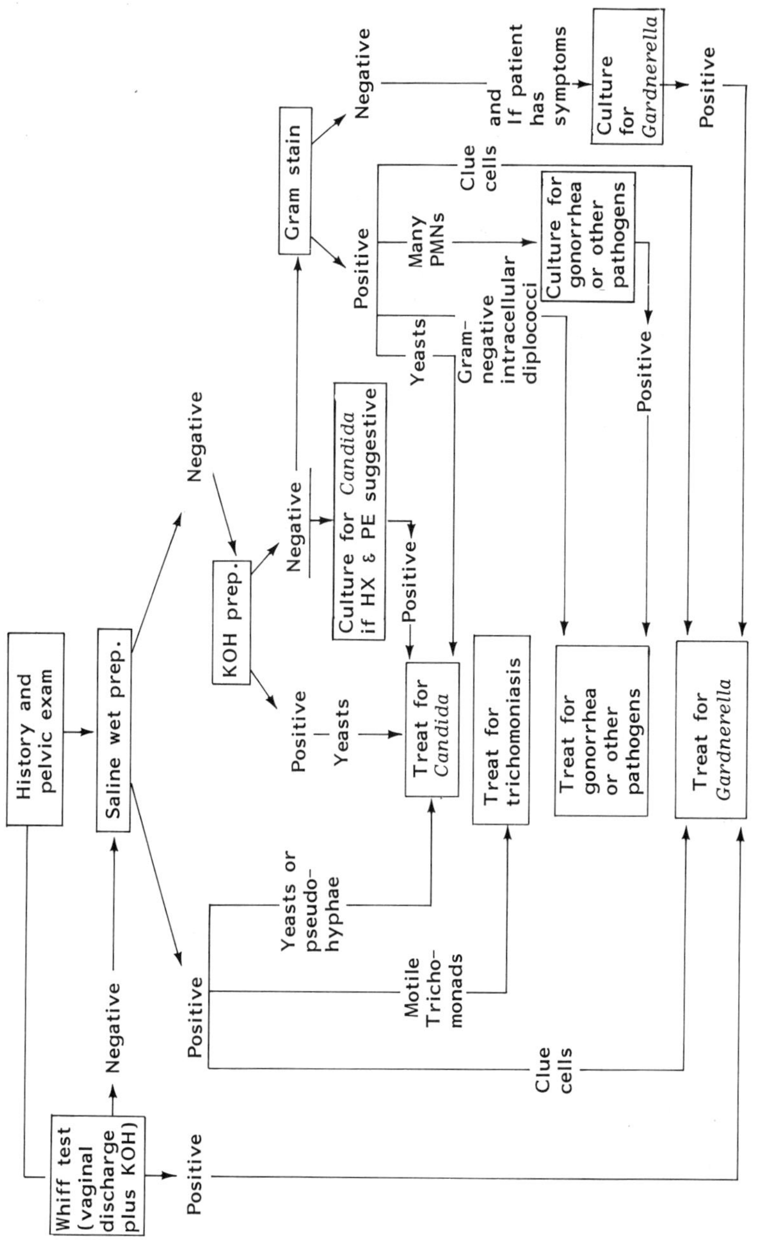

Figure 9.1. Presentation of a female with vaginal discharge.

heated. The KOH will destroy other cellular elements and debris to facilitate the diagnosis of yeast. Occasionally, symptomatic women with fungal vaginitis will have negative saline and KOH wet preparations for *Candida*. In this situation, a vaginal culture for yeast should be obtained to establish the diagnosis. Vaginal cultures for fungi should not be done on asymptomatic women, since therapy is only indicated for symptomatic patients and 25 to 30% of normal adult women will have a positive culture for *Candida* species. A smear of the vaginal discharge can also be examined for yeast by Gram stain. *Candida* appear as gram-positive oval structures that may form pseudohyphae (see Fig. 9.1).

A number of agents are effective in eradicating vaginal yeast infections including vaginal miconazole or clotrimazole. Both drugs result in cure rates of 50 to 90% when given once daily at bedtime for 1 week. Both miconazole cream and clotrimazole appear more effective than the older drug nystatin. Clotrimazole vaginally at bedtime given for three nights is highly effective, with cure rates comparable to 7 days of therapy.[2] In pregnancy, vaginal candidiasis is difficult to cure, and there is more experience with nystatin. However, micronazole and clotrimazole vaginal suppositories are probably safe in pregnancy, and no adverse effects have been reported.

The dilemma occurs in the patient with recurrent vaginal candidiasis. There is a group of women who have persistent vulvovaginal candidiasis, which recurs promptly after a course of antifungal therapy. The pathogenesis of these episodes is unclear. Most of these women lack any predisposing factors to explain the multiple recurrences. Oral nystatin aimed at reducing the intestinal reservoir of yeasts has not been effective. In evaluating a woman with possible intractable vaginal candidiasis, it is first important to establish the diagnosis by smear using a Gram stain or KOH preparation or by culture. One approach described by Sobel recommends a 2-week course of ketoconazole (400 mg) daily followed by a maintenance course of ketoconazole of 100 mg (half tablet) daily for 6 months.[3] Patients who fail on the maintenance dose of 100 mg may be given 200 mg daily of ketoconazole. Oral ketaconazole is effective in preventing recurrences, but relapse is common after the drug is discontinued. Nausea occurs in about 10% of patients receiving ketaconoazole. There is a risk of hepatitis in patients receiving ketoconazole, particularly in patients over age 50. The risk of hepatitis in patients receiving ketoconazole is one in 15,000, and hepatic function should be monitored.

Trichomonal Vaginitis

Trichomonas vaginalis is a pear-shaped flagellated protozoan with dimensions of 7 × 10 μm. This organism is responsible for approximately 25% of cases of vaginitis. *Trichomonas* is often associated with other sexually acquired pathogens such as *N. gonorrhoeae* or *Chlamydia*. The organism is usually sexually transmitted. The discharge is usually malodorous and has a pH greater than

4.5. The onset of the disease is often at the time of menses. The classic description of a profuse, often frothy yellow discharge and "strawberry cervix" as a result of punctate cervical hemorrhages is found in less than 50% of cases. Approximately 25% of patients with *Trichomonas* are asymptomatic, 25% note vulvar pruritus, and half complain of pruritus and vaginal discharge.

Specimens for examination for *Trichomonas* should be taken from the posterior vaginal fornix. The cotton-tipped swab is then placed in a tube with 1 to 2 ml of saline. After the pelvic examination is completed, the swab is placed on a slide, and a cover slip is applied. This preparation is examined as soon as possible without the use of special stains for motile trichomonads. The motile trichomonads with their flagellae can be seen best with the 40× objective (see Fig. 9.1).

About two-thirds of women who are infected with *Trichomonas* will have a positive saline wet preparation. Thus, the diagnosis of trichomoniasis cannot be ruled out without performing a culture. This involves inoculating vaginal discharge into special culture medium that will support the growth of the organism. This medium is incubated and then examined daily for motile trichomonads. Unfortunately, most laboratories do not perform cultures for *Trichomonas*. The organism can also be seen on routine Papanicolaou smears, which in some studies have a sensitivity similar to the wet preparation, but false positives occur more frequently.[4]

The diagnosis should be facilitated in the future by the development of monoclonal antibodies to *T. vaginalis* and by detecting the organisms by immunofluorescence.

The drug of choice for *T. vaginalis* vaginitis is oral metronidazole given as a single 2-g dose.[5] Asymptomatic as well as symptomatic patients should be treated. To prevent recurrences, the patient's sexual partner(s) should also be treated. Metronidazole should be avoided during pregnancy because of its potential carcinogenicity, and vaginal clotrimazole may be tried to treat trichomoniasis. Relatively resistant strains of *T. vaginalis* to metronidazole have been identified, and women infected with these strains may respond to an oral or intravenous course of metronidazole given in a dose of 2 g/day for 5 to 7 days.[1]

Gardnerella Vaginosis

Gardnerella vaginalis is a small pleomorphic gram-negative rod that causes bacterial vaginosis, formerly called nonspecific vaginitis. Previously this bacterium was named *Haemophilus vaginalis* and later *Corynebacterium vaginale*. Although *Gardnerella* is used as a marker to establish the diagnosis of bacterial vaginosis, the disease is a polymicrobic process involving in addition *Bacteroides* species, anaerobic streptococci, and *Mobiluncus,* an anaerobic curved commashaped gram-negative rod. Evidence suggests that the disease is a polymicrobial infection with the high concentration of anaerobes playing a major pathogenic role in the infection.[6] Although the infection is related to sexual activity, no corresponding illness in male partners has been described. Although *Gardnerella* can be isolated from 90% of patients with bacterial vaginosis, it is also found in 30 to 40% of normal asymptomatic women. Criteria to diagnose bacterial vaginosis include the presence of a gray homogeneous vaginal discharge, a fishy vaginal odor, pH of vaginal fluid >4.6, positive whiff test, and clue cells on microscopic examination of vaginal secretions.[7,8]

In the whiff test, a drop of vaginal discharge is mixed with 10% KOH. A distinct fishy odor is identified in 70% of patients with bacterial vaginosis. A positive test can also occur in trichomoniasis. Vaginal epithelial cells studded with tiny coccobacilli giving them a granular appearance, the clue cell, can be seen on a saline wet preparation, and this suggests a diagnosis of bacterial vaginosis. Clue cells can also be identified on Gram stain as vaginal epithelial cells studded with tiny gram-negative rods. In a typical clue cell, the borders of the vaginal epithelial cells are obscured with numerous bacteria. Vaginal epithelial cells with distinct borders and few bacteria adherent to the surface are not clue cells.

A Gram stain should also be examined for the number of PMNs. Normally a few PMNs may be present. An increase in PMNs occurs with trichomoniasis, gonococcal endocervical infection, and other infectious causes of cervicitis. In contrast, an increase in PMNs does not occur with candidiasis and *Gardnerella* infections. Finally, *Gardnerella* can be readily isolated on vaginal cultures, but, as with *Candida,* only symptomatic women should receive treatment.[9] In summary, a Gram stain of vaginal fluid showing clue cells without PMNs is the most reliable way to diagnose bacterial vaginosis. Vaginal cultures for anaerobes are inappropriate and not indicated (see Fig. 9.1).

Metronidazole is the drug of choice for bacterial vaginosis, with cure rates of approximately 90% when it is given orally for 7 days in a dose of 500 mg twice a day.[10] Single-dose metronidazole is less efficacious, and patients should be treated for 1 week. Amoxicillin given in a dose of 500 mg t.i.d. for 1 week has lower cure rates than metronidazole, but it can be an alternative drug, especially for *Gardnerella* infections in pregnancy. Vaginal creams containing sulfonamides and oral tetracycline have no place in the therapy of this disease. Treatment of male sexual partners of patients with bacterial vaginosis is not indicated, since studies fail to show a reduction in recurrence rates when the sexual partner is treated.[1] Partners should be examined, since they may have other sexually transmitted diseases.

Gonorrhea

Neisseria gonorrhoeae is a fastidious gram-negative diplococcus that frequently infects the endocervix, resulting in a discharge that is perceived as vaginal discharge by the patient. This organism does not infect the vaginal mucosa of adults. Gonorrhea should be diagnosed by obtaining an endocervical swab of material for culture for *Neisseria gonorrhoeae*. A swab for culture for this organism should be obtained from the endocervical canal and not from the posterior vaginal fornix. The sensitivity of a single endocervical culture for gonorrhea is between 80% and 90%. A rectal culture will detect an additional 5% of positive cases. A Gram stain for gonorrhea of endocervical secretions will be positive in about 50% of patients with *N. gonorrhoeae* infections. A positive smear should have gram-negative intracellular diplococci and not just extracellular diplococci.

Treatment of endocervical gonorrhea consists of using amoxicillin, 3 gm orally, plus 1 g of probenecid orally. Alternative therapy with ceftriaxone, 125 to 250 mg intramuscularly, is efficacious for endocervical gonorrhea as well as for infection at other sites such as the pharynx and rectum. Spectinomycin, 2 gm intramuscularly, is recommended for patients with a penicillin allergy. All patients treated for gonorrhea should be given therapy for chlamydial coinfection with a tetracycline, preferably doxycycline, 100 mg b.i.d. for 1 week. Erythromycin may be substituted for tetracycline in pregnancy. Neither tetracycline nor erythromycin should be given as sole therapy for gonorrhea because of tetracycline-resistant strains. The regimen using procaine penicillin is no longer recommended to treat endocervical gonorrhea. Follow-up cultures should be obtained from all infected sites including the rectum 4 to 7 days after completing treatment.

Other Causes

Two other organisms, *C. trachomatis* and herpes simplex virus, may infect the cervix, resulting in mucopurulent cervicitis. Patients may be asymptomatic or have an endocervical discharge that is perceived by the patient as vaginal discharge. Herpes simplex virus (HSV) may produce ulcerative lesions of the cervix. The presence of mucopurulent cervicitis may be seen by noting yellow or green pus on the tip of the cotton swab inserted in the endocervical canal. The diagnosis of mucopurulent cervicitis may be established by demonstrating on a Gram-stained smear of endocervical discharge ten or more PMNs per oil-immersion field.[11] To confirm the diagnosis of *Chlamydia,* obtain a culture or use an antigen detection assay such as a direct fluorescent antibody test (MicroTrak®) or an enzyme-linked immunoassay (Chlamydiazyme®). Obtain a culture for HSV if there are ulcerative lesions of the cervix or external genital lesions of the vulva suggestive of HSV infection. Therapy for mucopurulent cervicitis caused by *Chlamydia* should be treated the same as for NGU in males. Studies to demonstrate cure are not indicated for *Chlamydia* if patients are asymptomatic. The sexual partners of women with mucopurulent cervicitis should be treated empirically for chlamydial infection. Treatment of chlamydial mucopurulent cervicitis is critical to prevent the development of pelvic inflammatory disease.

REFERENCES

1. Paavonen J, Stamm WE: Lower genital tract infections in women. *Infect Dis Clin North Am* 1987; 1:179–198.
2. Masterson G, Napier IR, Henderson JN, *et al:* Three-day clotrimazole treatment in candidal vulvovaginitis. *Br J Vener Dis* 1977; 53:126–128.
3. Sobel J: Recurrent vulvovaginal candidiasis: A prospective study of the efficacy of maintenance ketoconazole therapy. *N Engl J Med* 1986; 315:1455–1458.
4. Fouts AC, Krams SJ: *Trichomonas vaginalis:* Re-evaluation of its clinical presentation and laboratory diagnosis. *J Infect Dis* 1980; 141:137–143.
5. Dykers JR: Single dose metronidazole for trichomonal vaginitis. *N Engl J Med* 1975; 293:23–24.
6. Spiegel CA, Amsel R, Eschenbach DA, *et al:* Anaerobic bacteria in nonspecific vaginitis. *N Engl J Med* 1980; 303:601–607.
7. Gardner HL, Dukes CD: *Hemophilus vaginalis* vaginitis: A newly defined specific infection previously classified ''nonspecific'' vaginitis. *Am J Obstet Gynecol* 1955; 69:962–976.
8. Taylor E, Blackwell AL, Barlow D, *et al: Gardnerella vaginalis,* anaerobes, and vaginal discharge. *Lancet* 1982; 1:1376–1379.
9. Spiegel CA, Amsel R, Holmes KK: Diagnosis of bacterial vaginosis by direct Gram stain of vaginal fluid. *J Clin Microbiol* 1983; 18:170–177.
10. Pheifer TA, Forsyth PS, Durfee MA: Nonspecific vaginitis: Role of *Haemophilus vaginalis* and treatment with metronidazole. *N Engl J Med* 1978; 298:1429–1434.
11. Paavonen J, Critchlow CW, DeRouen T, *et al:* Etiology of cervical inflammation. *Am J Obstet Gynecol* 1986; 154:556–564.

10

Outpatient Urinary Tract Infections in Young Women

Richard A. Gleckman

INTRODUCTION

It has been estimated that there are millions of office visits annually by young women who experience uncomfortable voiding symptoms. Some women experience discomfort when their urine passes over inflamed labia. These women have what has been termed "external dysuria," a condition caused by infectious vaginitis.[1] Other women manifest deep or "internal dysuria" associated with frequency and urgency. These latter women have infectious urethritis, cystitis, or pyelonephritis.

URETHRITIS

The acute infectious urethral syndrome can be defined as the presence of dysuria and urinary frequency of less than 2 weeks duration caused by a "nonsignificant" ($<10^5$ bacteria/ml of urine) number of a conventional urinary pathogen, *Neisseria gonorrhoeae* or *Chlamydia trachomatis*.[2] No evidence exists that the urethral syndrome is caused by *Ureaplasma urealyticum, Mycoplasma hominis,* or cytomegalovirus. Features that suggest a bacterial cause of the urethral syndrome include suprapubic pain and/or hematuria (microscopic or gross). When a patient with multiple or new sex partners develops dysuria, irritative voiding symptoms, and pyuria and demonstrates no bacteriuria attributed to traditional uropathogens, the diagnosis of chlamydial or gonococcal urethral syndrome should be considered. It needs to be underscored, however, that young married women engaged in a monogamous sexual relationship do not develop the urethral syndrome caused by *Chlamydia trachomatis* or *Neisseria gonorrhoeae*.[3]

For women with the urethral syndrome caused by "low-count" conventional bacterial uropathogens, single-dose or 3- to 5-day therapy is effective treatment. When the urethral syndrome is caused by *Chlamydia* sp., a 10-day course of doxycycline is indicated.[4] The drug is prescribed as 100 mg p.o. b.i.d. The optimum therapy for gonococcal urethritis has not been established. I would suggest 125 mg ceftriaxone administered once i.m.

There are some women with the urethral syndrome who have no organism identified as the cause of their irritative voiding symptoms. These women do not demonstrate pyuria, and they do not benefit from receiving an antibiotic.[4] In order to relieve their discomfort (burning, urgency), pyridium (200 mg t.i.d. p.o.) should be prescribed. They should be warned, however, that their urine will appear "bloody."

More recently a new form of urethritis has been identified.[5] These women have irritative voiding symptoms, pyuria on first-void urine specimen, bacteriuria, and recovery of *E. coli* on a urethral swab. Of note is the fact that the bladder urine is sterile, confirming a urethral infection. These women should probably receive a 10-day course of antimicrobial therapy.[5]

ACUTE BACTERIAL CYSTITIS

Traditionally a woman has been considered to have bacterial cystitis when she experiences frequency, urgency, dysuria, and suprapubic pain accompanied by pyuria and bacteriuria. The presence of fever and flank pain have conventionally been ascribed to pyelonephritis. Although statistically there appears to be evidence for these clinical impressions, it is important to appreciate that accurate techniques to identify precisely the anatomic site of urinary tract infections indicate that there is an imprecise correlation between the "classical" syndromes and the organ source of infection.[6] Frequency, dysuria, and suprapubic pain can be experienced by patients with pyelonephritis, and the presence of fever or flank pain does not exclude the diagnosis of bacterial cystitis. Twelve years ago the antibody-coated-bacteria (ACB) immunofluorescence test was heralded as a breakthrough in the effort to develop a noninvasive, accurate procedure to determine the site of a urinary tract infection. Subsequently it was appreciated, however, that there are no standards for the performance or interpretation of the test and that the ACB determination often fails to correlate with information obtained from ureteral catheterization, the most accurate method of localizing a urinary tract infection.[7]

It has been accepted practice for years for physicians to make a diagnosis of cystitis when the patient experienced voiding symptoms and had "significant" (defined as $>10^5$ bacteria/ml of urine) numbers of bacteria in the urine. This practice has been challenged, as some experts have suggested that $>10^4$ organisms/ml or even, perhaps, $>10^2$ organisms/ml represents the best diagnostic criterion for cystitis for the dysuric young woman with a coliform infection.[8,9] In either event, we know that a number of factors influence bacterial quantitation in the urine (hydration, frequency of urination, antimicrobial therapy) and that failure to recover 100,000 or more organisms does **not** rule out the diagnosis of bacterial cystitis in the woman with irritative voiding symptoms.

Most urinary tract infections in young women occur in August.[10] *Escherichia coli* is the most common cause of bacterial cystitis in women. Clinicians are often unaware of the fact that *Staphylococcus saprophyticus,* a coagulase-negative staphylococcus, is the second most common cause of acute symptomatic bacterial cystitis. Infection caused by this organism is often associated with microscopic hematuria.

Bacterial cystitis is a disease that is not life-threatening but one that can result in incapacitating symptoms. Often the disease will spontaneously resolve, in terms of both symptoms and bacteriuria.[11] The goals of treatment are to achieve a higher cure rate than the natural course of the disease and to prevent recurrent infections. When appropriate treatment is prescribed, bacteriuria is eradicated within a day, and for 80% of patients frequency, urgency, burning, and pyuria resolve within 4 days.

Prior to 1967, a 7- to 14-day regimen of an oral antimicrobial agent was standard treatment for acute bacterial cystitis. During the last 20 years the need to administer therapy for this long a period has been reassessed, and the suggestion has been offered that shorter courses of treatment are preferable. The rationale for considering a reduced treatment duration for acute symptomatic cystitis stems from the concept that the high urinary concentrations achieved by oral antimicrobial agents could be expected to eradicate a superficial mucosal infection such as cystitis. An additional impetus for exploring abbreviated treatments was the observation that when symptoms abated patients often discontinued therapy prematurely, without adverse sequelae.

Single-dose therapy has been the most intensively evaluated short-course treatment.[12] There are numerous advantages to this treatment program: enhanced compliance, reduced cost and side effects, and less selective pressure on the rectal and periurethral zone. Another potential value of single-dose treatment is that failure to achieve an immediate bacteriological response, as determined by persistent bacteriuria 2 to 3 days after therapy, could serve as an indicator that tissue invasion is present and that the woman requires more intensive drug therapy, 10 to 14 days.

Single-dose treatment is not indicated for pregnant women, women with symptoms that exceed 5 days, or women with structural abnormalities of the urinary tract. Single-dose therapy is also not indicated for women who have immunocompromising diseases (i.e., diabetes mellitus, neoplastic disorders, etc.) or infections caused by organisms resistant to the oral agent prescribed. In addition, only young women with susceptible strains of *E. coli* should be considered candidates for single-dose therapy.

A number of antimicrobial agents have been determined to be both safe and effective when prescribed in single doses: amoxicillin, 3 g; sulfisoxazole, 1 g; trimethoprim, 400 mg; trimethoprim–sulfamethoxazole, two double-strength tablets; tetracycline, 2.5 g; nitrofurantoin, 200 mg; and cephalexin, 3 g. No study has identified the optimum drug treatment of acute bacterial cystitis.

Four issues remain to be resolved concerning single-dose therapy. Is it as effective as the traditional 7- to 14-day course of treatment? The published data are not in agreement.[12] Is single-dose therapy associated with an increased number of recurrent infections? Limited data suggest that single-dose therapy exerts less suppression of enteric bacilli on the rectum, urethra, and vagina, thereby permitting perineal colonization and increased numbers of recurrent infections.[13] Does failure with single-dose therapy result in serious sequelae when relapse occurs? There are no reports of bacteremia or need for hospitalization, but, very rarely, relapsing infection has appeared as acute symptomatic pyelonephritis.[14] Does inadequately treated pyelonephritis, which clinically presented as cystitis and was managed with single-dose drug therapy, become recalcitrant to subsequent conventional treatment? Limited data suggest that this can occur.[15]

Single-dose therapy achieves a cure rate in 80–90% of patients. Diminished therapeutic response occurs in women with residual urine and patients with organisms resistant to the drug prescribed.[16] In order to reduce medical expenses, the suggestion has been made that pretreatment urine colony count, culture, and susceptibility testing not be performed, as the most common pathogens, as well as their drug susceptibility profiles, are usually predictable. However, a recent concern is the *in vitro* resistance to sulfonamide and ampicillin for 25–30% of *E. coli* strains.

The suggestion has also been made that posttreatment urine cultures need not be performed routinely, as most treatment failures will be associated with the return of symptoms.[17] Alternatively, the clinician could elect to have either the patient, the nurse, or a physician's assistant use the dip-slide test, which is inexpensive, reliable, and allows self-testing.

The dip-slide technique consists of a glass slide or plastic template coated with an agar medium on each side (Uricult®, Oxoid®). The dip-slide method correlates well with standard streak (bacteriological calibrated loop), and the results are easily quantitated by comparison with photographs or drawings of standardized bacterial cultures. In addition, colonies can be readily subcultured for identification and susceptibility testing.

The pregnant woman with bacterial cystitis should receive amoxicillin, 250 mg t.i.d. for 7 days. If the patient is allergic to penicillin, either a short-acting sulfonamide or nitrofurantoin can be prescribed. The sulfonamide should not be offered during the third trimester. There is no role for a quinolone for the pregnant woman.

ACUTE SYMPTOMATIC PYELONEPHRITIS

Young women with acute symptomatic pyelonephritis who do not require hospitalization can be adequately treated with oral antimicrobial agents.[18] Outpatient therapy, however, is restricted to women who are free of nausea and vomiting, have a secure diagnosis, will comply with the treatment program, and have no structural abnormalities of the urinary tract. Most of these infections are caused by *E. coli,* less commonly *Klebsiella* sp., *Enterobacter* sp., *Proteus* sp., *Streptococcus* sp., and *Staphylococcus saprophyticus*. It appears appropriate to treat these patients for 10–14 days.[18,19] While awaiting the identification of the uropathogen and its susceptibility profile, a clinician might obtain a urine Gram stain and consider initiating treatment with trimethoprim–sulfamethoxazole (one double-strength tablet b.i.d.) or norfloxacin (400 mg b.i.d.) if gram-negative rods appear to be the responsible pathogens.[20]

When symptomatic bacterial pyelonephritis occurs in young women who require hospitalization, initial therapy for gram-negative infection could consist of an aminoglycoside, parenteral trimethoprim–sulfamethoxazole, a parenteral third-generation cephalosporin, or aztreonam. Oral antimicrobial therapy can commence 72 hr after admission, when susceptibility data are available and it is apparent that the patient's clinical condition has improved. Drug therapy should be offered for 10 days.[21] The entire treatment program does not have to be performed in the hospital.

When a young woman with pyelonephritis complies with the treatment program, eradication of bacteriuria should be demonstrated within 1–2 days of the onset of drug administration. Failure of rapid achievement of a sterile urine often indicates inappropriate drug selection, obstructive uropathy, or renal insufficiency. The clinician should also anticipate resolution of fever within 72 hr of initiating therapy for pyelonephritis. Persistent fever in this population of young women usually suggests obstruction, diabetes mellitus, or drug reaction; less likely is intrarenal or perinephric abscess.

Patients who have been treated for acute symptomatic pyelonephritis and are noted to have recurrent disease, known as relapse or "bacterial persistence" (as determined by the detection of the original uropathogen within 2 weeks after the discontinuation of drug treatment, after it had previously been established that sterility of the urine had been achieved), are candidates for additional drug therapy, traditionally for 2–6 weeks, as well as radiographic studies of the urinary tract. The x rays are performed in order to detect potentially correctable urological abnormalities such as renal calculi, ectopic ureters, papillary necrosis in a single calyx, unilateral atrophic infected kidney, and unilateral medullary sponge kidney. Renal scarring per se is never a cause for bacterial relapse. In my experience, however, radiographic studies often fail to identify structural abnormalities in patients who relapse following treatment for acute symptomatic pyelonephritis.

RECURRENT CYSTITIS

Most recurrent infections in young women are reinfections, that is, the introduction of a new organism from the fecal–perineal flora. This phenomenon usually occurs more than 2 weeks after discontinuation of treatment for the prior infection. In premenopausal women, use of the diaphragm and sexual intercourse have been associated with recurrent urinary tract infections. A recent study indicates that oral contraception, tampon use, the frequency of washing the genital area, and the direction one wipes after defecation have no effect on the development of urinary tract infections.[23]

For 90% of women with recurrent cystitis, the concern is exclusively symptomatic morbidity and inconvenience. Therefore, these women should not be offered prolonged or potentially toxic antimicrobial programs. When a well-motivated young woman experiences a symptomatic exacerbation of acute cystitis as infrequently as once or twice a year, she can be instructed to take single-dose antimicrobial therapy to eradicate her infection.[24] For women who experience few episodes and develop these infections in relationship to sexual intercourse, postcoital voiding combined with antibiotic prophylaxis can be recommended.[25]

Chronic prophylaxis is indicated for and limited to those women who experience three or more symptomatic infections per year. Chronic prophylaxis is designed to prevent patient discomfort from recurrent cystitis and is prescribed for 6 months. A number of treatment programs are effective. These include the following: cephalexin, 125 mg h.s.; trimethoprim, 100 mg h.s.; sulfamethoxazole, 500 mg h.s.; trimethoprim–sulfamethoxazole, half tablet h.s. three times a week; nitrofurantoin, 50 mg h.s.; and methenamine hippurate, 1 g b.i.d. Chronic adminsitration of nitrofurantoin has been associated with frequent and serious adverse events (gastorintestinal disturbances, skin eruptions, peripheral neuropathy, chronic hepatitis, hematological toxicity, as well as subacute and chronic pulmonary reactions), and I feel that it should **not** be prescribed as chronic prophylaxis for otherwise healthy young women. It is important to appreciate, however, that chronic prophylaxis does not correct the basic defect that predisposes some women to recurrent symptomatic bacterial cystitis and that, unfortunately for some patients, disabling symptomatic infections return following the discontinuation of chronic prophylaxis.

Traditionally, primary care physicians and internists have referred women with recurrent symptomatic bacterial urinary tract infections to urologists for further evaluation. Assessment has usually included cystoscopy, voiding cystourethrography, and excretory urography. The literature indicates, however, that these invasive diagnostic procedures rarely identify surgically remediable disease in women who experience recurrent cystitis.[26,27] In addition, no impressive data indicate that either urethral dilatation or urethrotomy effectively prevents recurrent infections.

REFERENCES

1. Komaroff AL, Pass TM, McCue JD, *et al:* Management strageties for urinary and vaginal infections. *Arch Intern Med* 1978; 138:1069–1073.
2. Stamm WE, Wagner KF, Ansel R, *et al:* Causes of the acute urethral syndrome in women. *N Engl J Med* 1980; 303:409–415.
3. Berg AO, Heidrich FE, Fihn SD, *et al:* Establishing the cause of genitourinary symptoms in women in a family practice. *JAMA* 1984; 251:620–625.
4. Stamm WE, Running K, McKevitt M: Treatment of the acute urethral syndrome. *N Engl J Med* 1981; 304:956–958.
5. Fihn SD, Johnson C, Stamm WE: *Escherichia coli* urethritis in women with symptoms of acute urinary tract infection. *J Infect Dis* 1988; 157:196–198.
6. Busch R, Huland H: Correlation of symptoms and results of direct bacterial localization in patients with urinary tract infections. *J Urol* 1984; 132:282–285.
7. Gleckman R: A critical review of the antibody-coated bacteria test. *J Urol* 1979; 122:770–771.
8. Smith GW, Brumfitt W, Hamilton-Miller J: Diagnosis of coliform infection in acutely dysuric women. *N Engl J Med* 1983; 309:1393.
9. Stamm WE, Counts GW, Running KR, *et al:* Diagnosis of coliform infection in acutely dysuric women. *N Engl J Med* 1982; 307:463–468.
10. Anderson JE: Seasonality of symptomatic bacterial urinary infections in women. *J Epidemiol Commun Health* 1983; 37:286–290.
11. Mabeck EE: Treatment of uncomplicated urinary tract infection in nonpregnant women. *Postgrad Med J* 1972; 48:69–75.
12. Gleckman RA: Treatment duration for urinary tract infections in adults. *Antimicrob Agents Chemother* 1987; 31:1–5.
13. Counts GW, Stamm WE, McKevitt M, *et al:* Treatment of cystitis in women with a single dose of trimethoprim–sulfamethoxazole. *Rev Infect Dis* 1982; 4:484–490.
14. Hooton RM, Running K, Stamm WE: Single-dose therapy for cystis in women. *JAMA* 1985: 253:387–390.
15. Rubin RH, Fang LST, Jones SR, *et al:* Single dose amoxicillin therapy for urinary tract infection. *JAMA* 1980; 244:561–564.
16. Shand DG, O'Grady F, Nimmon CC, *et al:* Relation between residual urine volume and response to treatment of urinary infection *Lancet* 1970; 1:1305–1306.
17. Schultz HF, McCaffrey LA, Keys TF, *et al:* Acute cystitis: A prospective study of laboratory tests and duration of therapy. *Mayo Clin Proc* 1984; 59:391–397.
18. Abraham E, Baraff LJ: Oral versus parenteral therapy of pyelonephritis. *Curr Ther Res* 1982; 31:536–542.
19. Stamm WE, McKevitt M, Counts GW: Acute renal infection in women: Treatment with trimethoprim–sulfamethoxazole or ampicillin for two or six weeks. *Ann Intern Med* 1987; 106:341–345.

20. The Urinary Tract Infection Study Group: Coordinated multicenter study of norfloxacin versus trimethoprim–sulfamethoxazole treatment of symptomatic urinary tract infections. *J Infect Dis* 1987: 155:170–177.
21. Gleckman R, Bradley P, Roth R, *et al:* Therapy of symptomatic pyelonephritis in women. *J Urol* 1985; 133:176–178.
22. Shortliffe LMD, McNeal JE, Wehner N, *et al:* Persistent urinary infections in a young woman with bilateral renal stones. *J Urol* 1984; 131:1147–1151.
23. Strom BL, Collins M, West S, *et al:* Sexual activity, contraceptive use, and other risk factors for symptomatic and asymptomatic bacteriuria. *Ann Intern Med* 1987; 108:816–823.
24. Wong ES, McKevitt M, Running K, *et al:* Management of recurrent urinary tract infection with patient-administered single-dose therapy. *Ann Intern Med* 1985; 102:302–307.
25. Pfau A, Sacks T, Englestein D: Recurrent urinary tract infections in premenopausal women: Prophylaxis based on an understanding of the pathogenesis. *J Urol* 1983: 129:1153–1157.
26. Engel G, Schaeffer AJ, Grayhock JT, *et al:* The role of excretory urography and cystoscopy in the evaluation and management of women with recurrent urinary tract infection. *J Urol* 1980; 123:190–191.
27. Fowler JE Jr, Pulaski ET: Excretory urography, cystography, and cystoscopy in the evaluation of women with urinary tract infection. *N Engl J Med* 1981; 304:462–465.

11

Mononucleosis and Mononucleosislike Syndromes

Richard A. Gleckman and John S. Czachor

INTRODUCTION

The syndrome of mononucleosis evokes a stereotypic response among physicians: they are apt to think of a 19-year-old college coed with a sore throat, too fatigued to get out of bed, and worried that her boyfriend may get the same symptoms because he had kissed her. This, however, is only in part true. Acute infectious mononucleosis (AIM) has a varied presentation, and although it remains most prevalent in the second decade of life, it occurs in all age groups. In this chapter, we review the pathogenesis, clinical features, complications, and treatment of acute mononucleosis. We also review the numerous conditions that resemble this disease.

ACUTE INFECTIOUS MONONUCLEOSIS

Epidemiology and Pathology

The Epstein–Barr virus (EBV) is a double-stranded DNA-containing virus that is a member of the herpes virus family and is responsible for the infection that causes mononucleosis. In the United States, approximately 50% of individuals develop EBV seroconversion before the age 5, and another group seroconvert by the middle of the second decade.[1] The peak incidence of acute infectious mononucleosis is in the 15- to 24-year-old age group.[2,3]

The carrier state is established by one of two methods. Carriage of EBV has been detected in 15–20% of healthy individuals that have no recent history of acute clinical infection. In this instance, an asymptomatic infection is responsible for the resultant carrier state.[4] A carrier state can also develop when EBV shedding persists after the clinical expression of the infection has resolved.[4] Approximately 6% of individuals with recent EBV infection can recall contact with a patient with clinically apparent infectious mononucleosis.[3]

The transmission of EBV most commonly occurs from the exposure of a susceptible host to a carrier. Intimate contact is necessary because of the low levels of titer in oropharyngeal secretions and the intermittent nature of EBV shedding into these secretions.[4] Transmission via infected blood products has been incriminated in cases of posttransfusion, postperfusion, and hemodialysis-associated infections.[5] Mononucleosis is reported throughout the year without seasonal variation. Approximately 50% of patients undergoing immnuosuppressive therapy have positive throat washings for EBV, thereby suggesting that the virus can be reactivated.[6]

The Epstein–Barr virus is unique in that is possesses a limited host range, infecting and replicating only in B lymphocytes of man and some nonhuman primates. It has been suggested that EBV is also infective within human oropharyngeal cells.[7] The cells that have been attacked either are lysed or become infected with the virus.[8] Once infected, the cells are said to be transformed or immortalized, and this occurs in 10% of affected cells.[9] However, these transformed cells usually do not produce extracellular virions, and the EBV remains in a latent form.[10] During AIM, **one** B cell per 10^4 circulating lymphocytes is infected with EBV, whereas during the latent period, a single B cell per 10^6 circulating cells remains infected.[11]

A chain of events is produced once the lymphocytes become infected with EBV. Epstein–Barr nuclear antigens (EBNA) are found in the nuclei of these cells before viral protein synthesis begins.[12] Coincident with the infection, a polyclonal proliferation of both B and T cells occurs.[11] Because of this proliferation, specific reactions are encountered. The transformed lymphocytes produce immunoglobulin of the lgM type but can also synthesize IgG or IgA.[13] These immunoglobulins are part of the host's response to EBV infection and comprise not only the nonspecific heterophile antibodies (transient antibodies directed against unrelated antigens found on sheep, horse, and beef red cells) but also virus-specific antibodies (Table 11.1). The heterophile antibodies do not cross react with the virus-specific antibodies.[14] Heterophile antibodies are produced in 80–90% of all cases of AIM, and there appears to be no correlation between the heterophile titers and the severity of the illness.[1,11,15] In fact, the role of heterophile antibodies in pathogenesis or recovery of the illness is uncertain.

Other immunologic phenomena that occur with EBV infection include depression of cell-mediated immunity, cutaneous anergy, and decreased response to mitogens and antigens.[16,17] An increase in circulating mononuclear cells during the early stages of infection is present.[5] Numerous atypical lymphocytes are found in the bloodstream, usually bearing a suppressor (T_8) T-cell phenotype, which tend to invert the T-helper/T-suppressor ratio.[11] Cytotoxic T-cell

Table 11.1
Serological Response to Epstein–Barr Virus Infection

Antibody	Initial appearance	Duration	Percentage of cases
Viral capsid antigen (VCA)			
IgM VCA	Onset	1–2 months	100%
IgG VCA	Onset	Lifetime	100%
Early antigen (EA)			
Anti-D	4 weeks	3–6 months	70–80%
Anti-R	Variable	Variable	Uncertain but low
EB nuclear antigen (EBNA)	4 weeks	Lifetime	100%

activity is also increased.[5,11] These mechanisms are considered host defenses that limit the proliferation of the infected B cells, and with recovery from the illness, they revert to normal.

Clinical Manifestations

Once a person is exposed to and infected with EBV, there is a 30- to 50-day incubation period. The infection can take one of several courses in relation to severity, and this seems to be age related. When apparent, the infection is usually self-limiting, and it runs its course over a 2- to 3-week duration. Serious complications can develop, rarely resulting in death.[18]

The classic clinical manifestations of infectious mononucleosis consist most frequently of fever, sore throat, and lymphadenopathy. A prodrome of chills, anorexia, and malaise can occur 3–5 days prior to the onset of the traditional manifestations.

Fever lasts from 10 to 14 days but can persist for several weeks. The sore throat is often described as the worst ever experienced and is present in 80–90% of patients with mononucleosis. Pharyngitis persists for 7–10 days, and it **cannot** be distinguished clinically from other causes of pharyngitis.[5] Lymphadenopathy is usually generalized and symmetrical and preferentially involves the posterior cervical, anterior cervical, submandibular, axillary, and inguinal chains.[1,5,11,18] The affected lymph nodes can be slightly tender to palpation.

Other findings noted in EBV infection include malaise, myalgias, anorexia, headache, and rash. The rash, which develops in approximately 5% of patients with AIM, can assume many forms, including maculopapular, petechial, scarlatiniform, urticarial, or erythema-multiforme-like in nature. A maculopapular rash appears in 90–100% of patients with mononucleosis who receive ampicillin.[19] Palatal petechiae are frequently seen but are not pathognomonic.

Abdominal discomfort is sometimes experienced by patients with acute

Table 11.2
Laboratory Diagnoses in Acute Infectious Mononucleosis[a]

Finding	Percentage of cases
Lymphocytosis	70%
Leukocytosis	50–70%
Neutropenia: Mild	60–90%
Severe	<1%
Thrombocytopenia: Mild	50%
Severe	<1%
Elevated liver enzymes	60–100%
Cold agglutinins (IgM)	70–80%
Coombs-positive hemolytic anemia	½–3%
Cryoglobulins	90–95%
Heterophile antibodies	80–90%
CSF abnormalities (lymphocyte pleocytosis, protein elevation)	25%

[a]Adapted from references 1, 5, 11, and 18.

mononucleosis and, on occasion, is related to the enlarging spleen. Splenomegaly is found in approximately 50% of individuals with AIM, is maximal in size at approximately 14 days into the illness, and will usually regress the following week. Hepatomegaly is identified in 10–15% of individuals with EBV infection. Jaundice is manifest in 5–10% of patients, and this abnormality is not exclusively associated with hepatomegaly.[20] Jaundice appears to be more common in patients over the age of 30[11,20] (Table 11.2).

Mononucleosis in the postadolescent patient can present with atypical manifestations. Protracted fever, jaundice, anemia, and abdominal pain resemble cholecystitis.[20,21] Guillain–Barré syndrome can also be a prominent feature.[21] In elderly patients, fever (not associated with pharyngitis, lymphadenopathy, or splenomegaly) can present as the exclusive abnormality, thereby suggesting an FUO.

Complications

Acute mononucleosis is an infection in which the vast majority of patients undergo spontaneous and complete resolution in 2–3 weeks. Occasionally, complications do occur. However, they usually resolve without residual effects. Rarely have fatalities been documented. The existence of a chronic mononucleosis syndrome has been postulated, and this topic is addressed in a separate chapter in this book (see Chapter 12).

The most dramatic complication of AIM is splenic rupture, occurring in

0.2% of individuals between the second and third weeks of illness.[1,11,18] Trauma is associated with splenic rupture in 50% of the cases, and thus, activity restrictions are prudent in the first several weeks of the illness.[1,11,22] This complication has been known to be fatal in certain instances.

Hematological alterations of a minor degree are common (see Table 11.2), but severe cases of thrombocytopenia or granulocytopenia are found in fewer than 1% of all cases of acute EBV infection. These abnormalities can lead to bleeding dyscrasias, superinfection, or even death.[23] Autoimmune hemolytic anemia is mild in character, mediated by anti-i antibodies, and occurs in fewer than 3% of patients with mononucleosis.

Postanginal sepsis, a syndrome that typically occurs in adolescents or young adults following an oropharyngeal infection, is usually caused by anaerobes such as *Fusobacteria* sp., *Bacteroides* sp., and *Peptostreptococcus* sp. It has recently been associated with infectious mononucleosis, presumably because the EBV alters the local anatomy and allows oral commensals to become pathogens.[25] Septic thrombophlebitis occurs commonly in the wake of postanginal sepsis of the neck and is responsible for embolization to the lungs, heart, and joints.

Although neurological complications such as encephalitis, meningitis, Gullian–Barré syndrome, transverse myelitis, and seizures occur in fewer than 1% of all patients with AIM, and 85% of these patients recover completely, one report suggests that neurological complications are responsible for nearly 45% of all fatalities attributed to acute EBV infection.[26] Neurological signs, such as weakness, paralysis and paresis, or mental status changes, can dominate the clinical picture and in heterophile-negative mononucleosis can be confused with primary neurological disorders.

Hepatic abnormalities are usually limited to a modest elevation of liver enzymes. Extraordinary degrees of jaundice sometimes occur. Infrequently, reports of fatal hepatic failure have been described.[27]

Cardiological and respiratory complications are very uncommon. Pericarditis, myocarditis, and pneumonia have been reported.[11,18] Respiratory airway obstruction, particularly involving the upper tract, has resulted in fatality in patients with acute mononucleosis.

Diagnosis

In about 80–90% of the patients, the diagnosis of acute infectious mononucleosis is established by the appearance of heterophile antibodies coupled with the clinical presentation.[15] The mononucleosis spot tests (tests for the presence of heterophile antibodies) have a false-positive rate of less than 1.5%.[5,11,28] Heterophile-negative mononucleosislike syndromes fall into two categories: (1) true mononucleosis and (2) mononucleosislike syndromes. The former is diagnosed through the use of specific EBV serology. For proof of acute mononucleosis when repeated heterophile antibody tests are negative, serological evidence of IgM VCA is required. This antibody is not demonstrable in the general population, is sensitive and specific for acute EBV infection, and is virtually diagnostic of the illness. The IgM VCA is present from the onset of the illness until 2 months after the clinical syndrome has subsided. However, other antibodies are also present and can help to establish the diagnosis of AIM.

The IgG VCA antibody persists for life after the inception of EBV infection. Its value for **acute** diagnostic ability is limited because of its persistent nature. A fourfold rise in titer demonstrated in acute and convalescent sera can serve to confirm the diagnosis.[15,29]

Additional antibodies, in conjunction with IgG VCA, can suggest the existence of acute mononucleosis. Antibodies to early antigen (EA) anti-D are present in 70% of individuals and peak 3–4 weeks after the onset of the illness. Coupled with a positive IgG VCA, the detection of EA anti-D suggests recent EBV infection.

Antibody to Epstein–Barr nuclear antigen (EBNA) is found at the onset of the illness, is present for life, and can assist in the diagnosis of mononucleosis. If EBNA has recently converted to measurable levels after previously being documented as negative and IgG VCA is present, then this combination of findings suggests a recent EBV infection (Fig. 11.1). The use of the various specific EBV antibody tests, including the IgM VCA antibody, results in a 93% sensitivity for diagnosis of AIM in a heterophile-negative individual.[30]

Therapy

Supportive care is offered patients with acute mononucleosis. Analgesics/antipyretics are often successful in suppressing the fever, headache, myalgias, arthralgias, and sore throat that accompany this infection. The role of corticosteroids in uncomplicated acute infectious mononucleosis is uncertain. It has been shown that corticosteroids reduce lymphadenopathy and dissipate fever more rapidly than occurs in untreated patients and also that after 8 weeks of infection, they lowered the number of circulating lymphocytes (B cell and T cell).[31] Indications for their use include impending airway obstruction, severe thrombocytopenia, and hemolytic anemia. Some physicians choose to use these agents when cardiac or neurological findings occur, but no scientific evidence has confirmed their value for these indications. Specific antiviral therapy directed against EBV does not currently exist.

Other therapeutic considerations include the avoidance of contact sports, heavy lifting, or excessive straining when splenomegaly is present in order to reduce the likelihood of splenic rupture. Also, since EVB-infected patients continue to shed virus into the bloodstream after the clinical syndrome has resolved, these individuals should not donate blood for at least 6 months.[5]

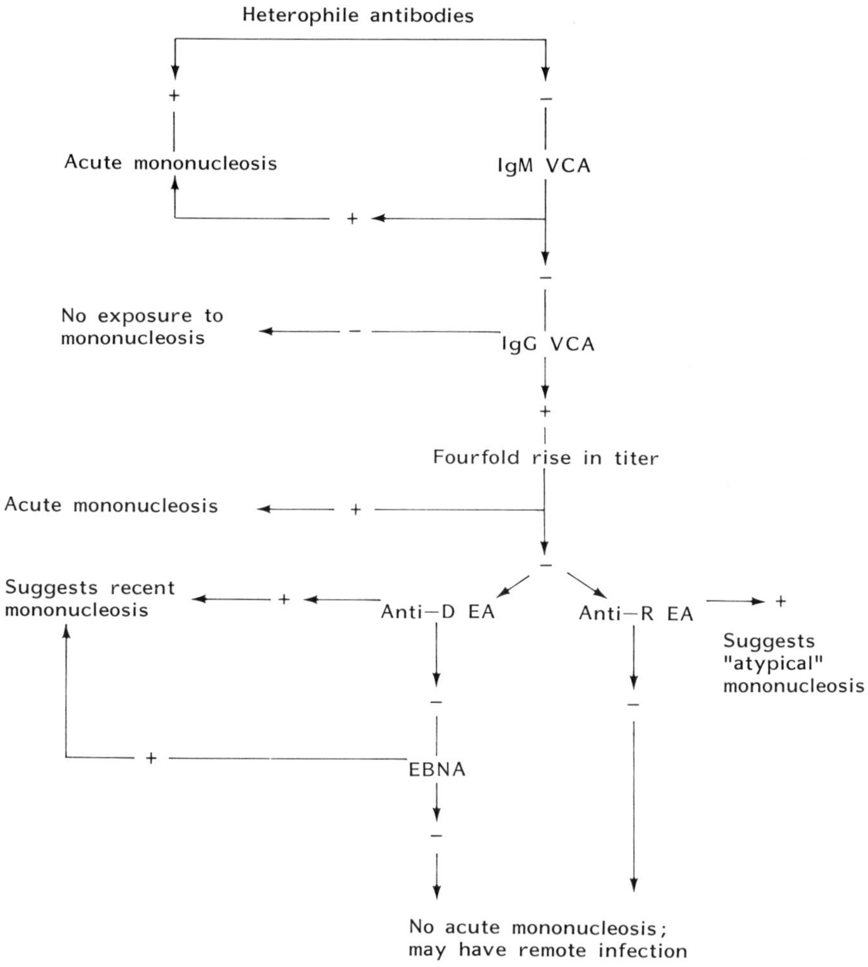

Figure 11.1. Serologic diagnosis of acute EBV infection.

MONONUCLEOSISLIKE SYNDROMES

There are a number of medical conditions that have signs and symptoms that can be confused with acute mononucleosis. When a physician encounters a patient whose clinical presentation is consistent with acute EBV infection, a rapid slide test for heterophile antibodies should be performed. If these tests are

Table 11.3
The Mononucleosislike Syndromes[a]

Entity	Fever	Pharyngitis	Lymphadenopathy	Malaise, weakness	Rash	Arthralgia, myalgia	Organomegaly
Epstein–Barr Virus	+++	++++	+++	++	+	++	+++ S
Hepatitis	++	0	0	++	++	+++	+++ H
Cytomegalovirus	+++	0	++	++	++	++	++ H,S
Human immunodeficiency virus	++	++	++++	+++	++	++	+ H,S
Trichinosis	++	0	0	+++	+	++	0
Malaria	++++	0	0	++	0	++	+++ S
Toxoplasmosis	+++	+	++++	++	0	+	+ H,S
Lymphogranuloma venereum	+	0	++	++	++	0	0
Secondary syphilis	++	+	+++	++	+++	+	+ H
Lyme disease	+++	+	++	+++	++++	++++	+ H,S
Cat scratch disease	++	+	++++	++	+	+	+ S
Subacute bacterial endocarditis	+++	0	0	++	+	++	++ S
Chronic meningococcemia	+++	0	0	++	++	+++	+ S
Acute menigococcemia	+++	+	0	++	0	++	0
Yersinia pestis (bubonic)	+++	+	+++	++	0	0	0
Yersinia enterocolitica	+++	+	+++	++	+	++	0
Brucellosis	++++	0	+	+++	0	++	+ H,S
Tularemia	++++	+	+++	++	+	++	+ H,S
Salmonella bacteremia	++++	+	0	++	+	++	++ H,S
Miliary tuberculosis	+++	0	++	++	0	0	+ H,S
Leptospirosis	+++	+	+	+++	++	+++	++ H,S
Systemic lupus erythematosus	+++	0	++	+	++	+++	+ H,S
Drug-induced mononucleosislike syndrome	+++	0	++	+	+	++	+ H,S
Juvenile rheumatoid arthritis	+++	0	+++	+	+++	++++	+++ H,S
Lymphoma	++	0	+++	++	0	+	++ H,S

[a]H, hepatomegaly; S, splenomegaly; +, rare; ++, sometimes; +++, common; ++++, very frequent.

repeatedly negative, then serological analysis for EBV antibodies is indicated. It is estimated that 10–15% of all EBV infections are not associated with heterophile antiboides and require specific serological tests for confirmation.[11] However, if these specific antibody tests are nondiagnostic or negative for acute EBV infection, then a plethora of conditions that can mimic AIM should be considered by the clinician. Syndromes caused by viruses, bacteria, parasites, and noninfectious entities are included in the differential diagnosis of the mononucleosislike syndromes (see Table 11.3).

VIRAL SYNDROMES

Hepatitis

Hepatitis infection with A, B, D, and non-A, non-B (NANB) can simulate infection with EBV.[1,32,33] A prodrome consisting of fever, malaise, arthralgias, myalgias, and rash can be demonstrated in many patients.[34] An atypical lymphocytosis can also be present. The appearance of jaundice and marked elevation of liver enzymes usually, but not always, differentiates hepatitis from mononucleosis, as these abnormalities are more commonly consistent with viral hepatitis. Pharyngitis and lymphadenopathy are not observed in hepatitis, and splenomegaly is an unusual finding. Once jaundice appears in hepatitis, the prodrome disappears.[34]

Serological tests for hepatitis A, B, and D are readily available and precise. The diagnosis of hepatitis NANB is established by the combination of clinical correlation with exclusion of other identifiable precipitating conditions. Serological markers are present prior to the onset of clinical jaundice and are used to confirm the diagnosis. Liver biopsy is seldom necessary to establish the diagnosis of viral hepatitis.

Cytomegalovirus

Cytomegalovirus (CMV) is the most commonly identified agent of heterophile-negative mononucleosislike syndromes and accounts for up to 7–10% of these cases.[11,35] Often, CMV and AIM are confused because of the similarity of the laboratory and clinical findings. Complications of the CMV mononucleosislike syndrome include pneumonia, myopericarditis, CNS diseases, thrombocytopenic purpura, hemolytic anemia, and retinitis. An atypical lymphocytosis can be present. Many of these complications are also noted with EBV infection, although exudative tonsillitis or pharyngitis is not usually seen with CMV infection.

The specific diagnosis is made either by isolation of the virus from infected tissues, such as blood (not urine, however), or by serological methods. An IgM specific antibody is diagnostic of recent/acute CMV infection. There have, however, been reports of cross reaction between the IgM antibody of CMV and IgM antibody of EBV, again underscoring the difficulty of differentiating these two entities.[33] A fourfold or greater increase of IgG specific antibody titers also confirms the diagnosis.

Human Immunodeficiency Virus

Patients with primary human immunodeficiency virus (HIV) infection can manifest a constellation of signs and symptoms that simulate the acute infectious mononucleosis syndrome.[36,37] The HIV-related acute viral syndrome develops weeks after the acquisition of infected body fluids. Needlestick accidents with blood from HIV-infected individuals, transfusion of contaminated blood products, and sexual intercourse with partners with the virus have all served to transmit the infection.

The full clinical syndrome consists of fever, sore throat, sweats, anorexia, malaise, headache, weight loss, arthralgias, myalgias, pharyngitis, diffuse lymphadenopathy, and splenomegaly. A unique component of primary HIV infection is the presence of an erythematous maculopapular rash that is usually, but not exclusively, truncal in distribution. The HIV-related infectious mononucleosis syndrome resolves spontaneously and completely within 3 weeks. The diagnosis of primary HIV syndrome requires isolation of the virus from the blood (currently a research technique) or the demonstration of seroconversion, that is, the detection of antibody development when a acute-phase serum that is obtained 8–12 weeks following the onset of the illness. At the time of the acute HIV-related viral illness, when tests for HIV antibody are negative, some patients will have detectable HIV antigen.[36] Unfortunately, antigen testing is only available at a limited number of research laboratories.

PARASITIC DISEASES

Trichinosis

This disease remains transmissible through the ingestion of improperly cooked meat containing the encysted larvae of *Trichinella spiralis*.[39] The initial phase of the disease begins 24 hr after larval ingestion and varies from asymptomatic to mild/moderate gastrointestinal manifestations, including nausea, vomiting, diarrhea, and abdominal pain. However, it is the stage of muscle invasion that can present as a mononucleosislike syndrome. At this time, prominent features include fever, myositis with myalgias, and periorbital edema; the latter finding is also seen in acute mononucleosis in nearly one-third of the cases.[1,18] Differential features that separate trichinosis from EBV infection include eosinophilia, low erythrocyte sedimentation rate, elevated serum creatinine kinase levels, and absence of lymphadenopathy, hepatosplenomegaly, and pharyngitis. Occasionally, splinter hemorrhages in subungual or conjunctival areas can be found in infection with *T. spiralis.*

The diagnosis of trichinosis is made by the use of the bentonite flocculation antibody test, which becomes positive after the third week of the infection. Sometimes a muscle biopsy is needed to secure the diagnosis; a swollen tender muscle is chosen for the biopsy site to enhance the detection of the organism.

Malaria

The **history** is the most important signal to alert the physician to consider the diagnosis of malaria, specifically the patient's travel in an endemic malarial region, the receipt of blood transfusions, or the use of intravenous drugs.[40–42] Malaria can present with fever, chills, headache, fatigue, anemia, splenomegaly, jaundice, and thrombocytopenia. Occasionally, arthralgias and myalgias are present. Often, however, physical findings of acute malarial infection are absent except for paroxysms of fever.[42]

Features that help to distinguish malaria from AIM include the presence of shaking chills, profuse diaphoresis, and the absence of pharyngitis and lymphadenopathy. With the historical information of exposure, the diagnosis is confirmed by the identification of *Plasmodium* species on thick- and thin-smear blood films.

Toxoplasmosis

The association of a mononucleosislike syndrome with acute toxoplasmosis infection has been well documented.[39,43–45] *Toxoplasma* infections account for fewer than 1% of heterophile-negative mononucleosislike syndromes.[11] Serological studies suggest that 30–40% of the adult population are infected with toxoplasmosis, and the majority are asymptomatic and never seek medical attention.[39,43] Approximately 15% of individuals, however, are symptomatic.[38] The most common manifestation is asymptomatic lymphadenopathy of the head and neck. Associated manifestations are fever, generalized lymphadenopathy, hepatomegaly, splenomegaly, myalgias, malaise, and atypical lymphocytosis; many of these findings are also present in AIM, thereby explaining the confusion that exists between the two diseases. Ocular findings, specifically chorioretinitis, can help to suggest toxoplasmosis.[33,46] Epidemiologic factors that would enhance the suspicion for toxoplasmosis include contact with cats and their feces, ingestion of undercooked meats, transfusion-acquired disease, transplant-acquired disease, or reactivation of toxoplasmosis through immunosuppression (such as AIDS or posttransplant immunosuppressant therapy).

Diagnosis of toxoplasmosis is made through the use of serological methods, which include IgM antibody to *Toxoplasma,* either by immunofluorescence or immunosorbent assay. The immunofluorescent test remains positive for only 3–4 months after the infection and may be of value to help date the onset of infection. High levels of IgG specific antibody directed against toxoplasmosis can block the reaction of this antibody test, thus necessitating the use of the immunosorbent IgM, which persists for longer periods of time than the immunofluorescent IgM and is not blocked by IgG. Serological diagnosis of acute or recent toxoplasmosis rests on the demonstration of IgM antibody, IgG antibody, and the proper clinical correlation.[47] With the high incidence of lymphadenopathy in this disease, lymph node biopsy had been advocated for diagnostic purposes, but the results can be nonspecific or confused with other diseases such as cat scratch disease.

CHLAMYDIA INFECTIONS: LYMPHOGRANULOMA VENEREUM

Lymphogranuloma venereum (LGV), caused by the organism *Chlamydia trachomatis,* is a sexually transmitted disease that has an incubation period of weeks to months. The primary lesion is a transient, painless herpetiform vesicle or nonindurated ulcer at the point of contact in the anogenital area. This lesion commonly heals quickly, seldom makes the individual seek medical attention, and can even go unnoticed. Only 5–25% of patients possess a primary lesion. The presence of this lesion can help to separate LGV from acute EBV infection.[48]

The invasive stage or secondary stage produces systemic symptoms such as fevers, chills, malaise, headache, fatigue, myalgias, anorexia, and lymphadenopathy, usually regional in distribution.[49] Occasionally arthritis, meningitis, and hepatitis may complicate this syndrome. However, draining sinus tracts involving inguinal lymph nodes, the "groove sign" (enlargement of inguinal lymph nodes above and below Poupart's ligament), rectal involvement, and the absence of pharyngitis are features that differentiate LGV from mononucleosis.

The diagnosis is established by isolation of the organism from draining sinus tracts of lymph nodes or, alternatively, by the demonstration of a fourfold rise or a single titer of ≥1:64 in the complement-fixation test. A microimmunofluorescent antibody titer of greater than 1:512 is also regarded as diagnostic. The latter test, however, remains a research technique that is not widely available.[48]

BACTERIAL INFECTIONS

Syphilis

Once *Treponemia pallidum* has penetrated the epithelium, a chance of primary syphilis is formed. The chancre can be overlooked if it is in an inaccessible area such as the vagina, cervix, or rectum.[50] Once dissemination via the lymphatics or the bloodstream has taken place, secondary syphilis has occurred. It is in this secondary stage that the disease can resemble infectious mononucleosis.

Common findings of secondary syphilis include maculopapular rash, malaise, fever, diffuse painless lymph node enlargement, arthralgias, headache, and sore throat.[50,51] Hepatitis with an elevated alkaline phosphatase concentration out of proportion to the other liver function tests is manifested at this stage of the disease and superficially resembles EBV-related hepatitis.

Differentiating aspects of syphilis include persistent rash, condyloma lata, and periosteal involvement of the bones. Serological testing (RPR,VDRL), in patients without HIV-related disease, is **always** positive, usually at a high dilution.[50,51] The FTA-ABS, a test that measures surface antigens of *T. pallidum,* and the hemagglutinin assay are **always** positive.[50] Thus, serology is the foundation for confirming the diagnosis of secondary syphilis and effectively separates this entity from AIM.

Leptospirosis

Humans acquire leptospirosis through contact with urine, blood, or tissues of infected animals (dogs, cats, rodents, livestock, wild mammals) or through contact with environments contaminated by *Leptospira.*[45] Person-to-person transmission is rare. There are two forms of the disease, an anicteric form and severe disease with jaundice, also known as Weil's disease. It is the anicteric form that resembles acute EBV infection.

An incubation period of 10–14 days precedes the spread of the leptospires. Fever, headache, myalgias, abdominal pain, nausea, and vomiting last for 4–7 days in the primary phase; after antibody to the leptospires is formed, the immune stage begins. Again, prominent clinical features mimic AIM and include fever, lymphadenopathy, hepatosplenomegaly, myalgias, rash, headache, and, rarely, meningitis. Discriminating features of leptospirosis include the intense headache, uveitis, conjunctival suffusion, and raised pretibial erythematous lesions (if present). Atypical lymphocytosis is **not** present, though there may be a leukocytosis.

Diagnosis is made by the combination of clinical correlation and serological tests. The microscopic agglutination test is very specific, can quantitate antibody titers, and gives preliminary organism serotypes. A fourfold rise over 2 weeks or a titer of 1 : 100 or greater is confirmatory of leptospirosis. Macroscopic agglutination tests have become useful screening agents, but other more specific tests (indirect hemagglutination and enzyme-linked immunosorbent assay for IgM of *Leptospira*) are also available.[31,43] Dark-field evaluation is difficult and not particularly helpful. Special culture techniques are available to grow the organism but can take several weeks.[45]

Lyme Disease

Lyme disease is a recently described syndrome caused by the spirochete, *Borrelia burgdorferi,* which is transmitted by a tick bite. The characteristic skin lesion, erythema chronicum migrans (ECM), is found in about 75% of all patients.[52] In the remaining 25% of individuals, or in people in which ECM went unnoticed, the potential for confusion with acute EBV infection exists because the early manifestations of Lyme disease simulate acute mononucleosis. Malaise, headache, fever, chills, and arthralgias are common in the early stage; less frequently noted findings are lymphadenopathy (sometimes generalized), anorexia, and pharyngitis.[52,53] A distinct mononucleosislike syndrome has been described, and the malaise of Lyme disease has indeed been likened to that of mononucleosis.[52,53] A mild leukocytosis without an atypical lymphocytosis is usually present. Separation of Lyme disease and acute EBV infection is accomplished by assessment of the clinical, epidemiologic, and serological findings.

Diagnosis of Lyme disease in the absence of ECM is based on clinical correlation and the presence of the IgM antispirochete antibody.[33] Titers of IgM rise within the first 2 weeks of the illness and remain elevated for an indefinite period afterward. An IgG response occurs at the end of the first month of infection with Lyme disease.[54]

Cat Scratch Disease

Special stains have detected small pleomorphic bacilli in the tissues of people with cat scratch disease. This illness is self-limited, and currently no specific treatment exists. Contact with a cat and the presence of a scratch or primary dermal or eye lesion is invaluable information to explain a patient's manifestations. However, infections that are not apparent may be more frequent than originally thought, as 4–6% of the general population have positive skin tests to cat scratch antigen.[45] If the association of a cat scratch with the patient's disease is not appreciated, or the primary lesion goes unnoticed, the potential for confusion between cat scratch disease and acute mononucleosis exists. Symptoms associated with typical cat scratch disease include fever, malaise, fatigue, myalgias, arthralgias, headache, splenomegaly, pharyngitis, and skin eruptions.[55]

The diagnosis of cat scratch disease is suggested by a history of exposure to cats, a positive skin test, a negative evaluation for other causes of lymphadenopathy, and characteristic histopathological findings in lymph node biopsy.

Subacute Bacterial Endocarditis

Subacute bacterial endocarditis occurs most frequently in people with preexisting heart disease. Its onset is insidious, and, on occasion, the infection can be ushered in as a ''flulike'' syndrome. Remittent fever, malaise, weakness, myalgias, arthralgia, petechiae, and splenomegaly are common manifestations in SBE, but these findings can also suggest acute mononucleosis. Leukocytosis is usually present but is not associated with atypical lymphocytes. Pharyngitis and lymphadenopathy, typical features of AIM, are not part of the SBE complex. Roth spots, Osler's nodes, Janeway lesions, splinter hemorrhages, and diastolic heart murmurs, classic signs of endocarditis in some patients, do not occur in acute mononucleosis.

The diagnosis of SBE is made via the constellation of history and physical and laboratory findings. Blood cultures are usually positive in this disease. However, they may fail to isolate fastidious or unusual microorganisms and often will not recover pathogens when previous antimicrobial therapy has been administered. Echocardiographic studies for vegetations on heart valves can be of value in the diagnostic evaluation; unfortunately, some lesions may be below the limit of resolution of currently available technology and remain undetected.[33]

Meningococcemia

Bacteremia with *Neisseria meningitidis* can produce a syndrome that consists primarily of nonspecific systemic symptoms.[56] This entity can take several forms: a mild acute form, a fulminant course (the Waterhouse–Friderichsen syndrome), and a chronic meningococcemia. The mild acute and chronic variations of meningococcemia demonstrate some features that merit differentiation from acute mononucleosis.

Acute meningococcemia most commonly follows an upper respiratory illness and generally remains mild. Headache, pharyngitis, spiking fever, chills, malaise, arthralgias, and myalgias are hallmark findings that can simulate AIM. Chronic meningococcemia can be present for an extended time period (weeks to months) and bears a closer resemblance to acute EBV infection than acute meningococcemia. In addition to fever, chills, arthralgias, and malaise, a maculopapular rash and, on occasion, splenomegaly are present.[57]

The absence of lymphadenopathy helps to differentiate meningococcemia from acute infectious mononucleosis. The diagnosis of meningococcemia depends on the isolation of *N. meningitidis* from blood or skin lesions.[33,56,57]

Yersinia

Yersinia-species-related infections can mimic acute mononucleosis. *Yersinia pestis* is the etiologic agent that causes plague; both the bubonic and speticemic forms present with fever, chills, malaise, weakness, nausea, and vomiting.[58] Travel to an endemic area with exposure to the vectors or the animals harboring the bacterium initiates the infection. Bubonic plague has accompanying painful regional lymphadenopathy, but this can also at times present in a generalized fashion. The absence of rash and organomegaly help to eliminate plague from the differential diagnosis of the mononucleosislike syndromes.

Yersinia enterocolitica sporadically is responsible for an infectious enterocolitis in human beings, manifested by abdominal pain, fever, nausea, vomiting, diarrhea, and headache. Recently, however, this organism has been associated with acute pharyngitis and fever unaccompanied by diarrhea.[57] This form of *Y. enterocolitica*-associated infection could cause confusion with acute EBV infection. Distinguishing features of *Y. enterocolitica* infection include abdominal pain (which may mimic appendicitis), moderate to severe diarrhea, and, rarely, intestinal perforation.[60]

The diagnosis of *Yersinia* sp. infection is made from historical and epidemiologic information, aspiration and direct fluorescent antibody staining of involved lymph nodes (*Y. pestis*), and culture of the organism from stool (*Y. enterocolitica*). Blood cultures are invaluable in septicemic patients with either *Y. pestis* or *Y. enterocolitica*. Serological methods are also available for diagnostic confirmation.[33]

Brucellosis

The *Brucella* sp.—*melitensis, suis, abortus,* and *canis*—all cause human disease.[45] Brucellosis demonstrates protean manifestations, and it can exist as an acute, subacute, relapsing, or chronic disease. Both acute and subacute forms of brucellosis can simulate infectious mononucleosis. Brucellosis is acquired through contact with infected animals or their secretions.[45] Transmission occurs via occupational exposures (abattoir workers, veterinarians) or through ingestion of contaminated dairy products.

Acute brucellosis, when it presents as a mild illness of brief duration over a few days, and subacute brucellosis, with its gradual onset, may have signs and symptoms that mimic acute EBV infection. Fever, chills, malaise, fatigue, weakness, myalgias, anorexia, and diaphoresis are common. Less frequent but similar mononucleosislike features include splenomegaly, lymphadenopathy, and relative lymphocytosis. Discriminating symptoms that help to distinguish brucellosis as the diagnosis include testicular pain, ocular pain, visual blurring, and dysuria, though these features occur infrequently.[32]

The diagnosis is established by isolation of *Brucella* sp. from the blood or bone marrow of the affected individual. The organisms are notorious for slow, fastidious growth, and they can be difficult to isolate. Serological testing is positive when a fourfold or greater rise in antibody titer is present. Presumptive diagnosis of brucellosis, as determined by serological methods, requires an agglutination titer of 1 : 160 or greater (either in single or serial specimens) accompanied by the appropriate clinical features.[33]

Tularemia

Francisella tularensis is the organism that causes tularemia, and transmission occurs through direct contact with infected animals or their secretions or through a vector.[61,62] Numerous distinct clinical forms of tularemia are recognized. Asymptomatic infection can develop. The most common symptoms consist of fever, chills, malaise, fatigue, and cough, features that occur in all clinical subgroups. Four of the tularemia subgroups—ulceroglandular, glandular, typhoidal, oropharyngeal—have mononucleosislike syndromes.

Ulceroglandular and glandular forms of tularemia share identical clinical characteristics except for the presence of ulcerated skin lesions in the former entity. Pharyngitis can develop in ulceroglandular tularemia.[62] Both syndromes can be accompanied by regional or generalized lymphadenopathy.

Typhoidal or septicemic forms of tularemia can mimic EBV infection, as they can manifest fever, chills, headache, abdominal pain, and vomiting. There often is no exposure history in this type of tularemia. The absence of lymphadenopathy, splenomegaly, rash, and pharyngitis may be useful in differentiating these forms of tularemia from AIM.

Oropharyngeal tularemia can occur after ingestion of infected meat.[61,62] An erythematous exudative or membranous pharyngotonsillitis with cervical adenopathy is usually present.

Francisella tularensis infections are usually diagnosed through serological methods, and high rates of infectivity exist in laboratory personnel that handle this organism. In addition, it has very fastidious growth requirements and is difficult for inexperienced laboratories to culture. Serological tests include the agglutination determination, which becomes positive shortly after infection and peaks at 1 month. A single titer of 1 : 160 or greater is consistent with acute or past infection; a fourfold or larger rise in titer is consistent with recent tularemia. Serological cross reactivity may be present with *Brucella, Mycoplasma, Legionella,* and *Proteus* X-19.[61]

Salmonella Bacteremia

Bacteremia caused by *Salmonella* species is responsible for typhoid and paratyphoid fevers. By definition, blood cultures are positive unless there has been previous antimicrobial therapy. Diarrhea is not necessarily part of this syndrome, and the stool cultures may not reveal the infecting strain of *Salmonella*.[33] Enteric fever can present as a nonspecific febrile illness of varying levels of severity (though paratyphoid fever classically produces a milder illness than typhoid fever) and in the early stages can simulate acute mononucleosis. Remittent fever, chills, nausea, vomiting, headache, myalgias, malaise, and anorexia are common to both disorders.[61,62] Typhodial hepatitis usually results in serum liver enzyme elevations without serum bilirubin elevation, a pattern similar to that found in acute EBV infection. Pharyngitis and rash are infrequent manifestations. Lymphadenopathy seldom if ever occurs and is restricted to the cervical region when present. Classically, a neutropenia is found, but in the early stages of enteric fever, a leukocytosis without atypical lymphocytosis can exist. If present, a pulse/temperature disparity can be a finding consistent with *Salmonella* bacteremia. Though not pathognomonic for enteric fever, rose spots can be found in the upper abdomen in a minority of patients.[33,63]

The diagnosis is made by the recovery of the *Salmonella* species in the blood. Stool cultures will only be positive in one-third to two-thirds of patients later in the illness. Serological studies are not reliable, as approximately 50–60% will **not** show a fourfold rise in titers during treatment for enteric fever.[65]

Tuberculosis

Miliary tuberculosis can be associated with nonspecific signs and symptoms that can resemble acute EBV infection: fever, chills, malaise, weakness, splenomegaly, and hepatomegaly. Lymphadenopathy is generalized but may be regionally limited to the cervical and axillary regions. The diagnosis of miliary tuberculosis is hampered by the fact that 20% of patients will have negative tuberculin skin tests, half the patients will **not** have a miliary pattern on chest radiographs, few patients recall an antecedent TB infection, and many patients will have negative sputum smears for acid-fast bacilli.[66] Rash and pharyngitis are not characteristic features of miliary tuberculosis. The presence of meningitis, peritonitis, and pleuritis, however, suggests the diagnosis of miliary disease.[33] Coexistent conditions such as a history of intravenous drug abuse, malignancy, and alcoholism are often found in patients with miliary tuberculosis.

The diagnosis of miliary tuberculosis is strongly suggested by demonstration of the acid-fast bacillus in biopsy. Definitive diagnosis requires culture. Though many have negative sputum smears, almost two-thirds will have positive sputum cultures. Bone marrow biopsy using the trephine needle is a sensitive method to detect miliary TB. However, liver biopsy remains the most sensitive diagnostic procedure to establish the diagnosis.[31,64]

NONINFECTIOUS MONONUCLEOSISLIKE SYNDROMES

Systemic Lupus Erythematosus

Lupus remains an illness with protean manifestations, a serum abundant with immunologically derived proteins, and an uncertain etiologic agent. Many of the symptoms of SLE are nonspecific and may resemble those of acute mononucleosis. Fever, arthralgias, myalgias, malaise, and lymphadenopathy are common in this disorder as well as in acute EBV infection. Hepatomegaly and splenomegaly are found in 25% and 10% of lupus patients, respectively. Cutaneous manifestations are uncommon but tend to be somewhat specific for SLE. Malar rash, dermal infarctions (vasculitis) of the digits, and telangiectasias are the usual skin findings. Alopecia, renal abnormalities, leukopenia, thrombocytopenia, and cardiopulmonary disorders suggest the diagnosis of lupus.

The diagnosis of lupus is established through a combination of rather distinctive clinical and laboratory findings. Positive tests for antinuclear antibody (ANA) are found in almost every individual with active lupus. However, there have been ANA-negative patients described; tests for antibodies to double-stranded DNA, Smith antigen, Ro antigen, and La antigen can establish the diagnosis in these individuals. Biological false-positive VDRL can occur in this syndrome as well as in infectious mononucleosis.[1,5,11,33] Urinalysis, evaluation of the urinary sediment, and renal function tests are of value when assessing a patient with presumed SLE.

Medications and the Mononucleosislike Syndromes

Adverse drug reactions can produce nonspecific signs and symptoms that can be confused with acute EBV infection. Features commonly reported include fever, arthralgias, myalgias, lymphadenopathy, anorexia, skin rashes, and, on occasion, splenomegaly. Drugs that have been implicated with this clinical complex include procainamide, isoniazid, and phenytoin.

Juvenile Rheumatoid Arthritis

This disorder can present with abnormalities that mimic acute EBV infection. Intermittent fever, chills, generalized lymphadenopathy, myalgias, and hepatosplenomegaly precede the appearance of profound arthritis.[67] Once the arthritis has manifested itself, the systemic symptoms usually fade to some degree. An evanescent, pale erythematous macular rash found on the trunk and proximal extremities can appear during febrile periods but can be present at other times as well. Mild hepatic dysfunction can simulate the liver function derangements that occur in patients with acute mononucleosis. Differentiation from AIM includes the presence of pleuritis, pericarditis, severe arthritis, and iridocylitis and the recurrent nature of juvenile rheumatoid arthritis.

The diagnosis depends on the protean clinical findings combined with the exclusion of other diseases. A successful trial of salicylate therapy strongly supports the diagnosis.[67]

Lymphoma and Leukemia

Hodgkin's disease, non-Hodgkin's lymphoma, and chronic leukemia can present with signs and symptoms that resemble acute EBV infection. Insidious onset of generalized lymphadenopathy, fever, night sweats, malaise, weakness, and hepatosplenomegaly mimic acute mononucleosis. The absence of joint complaints, pharyngitis, and rash may help separate these hematological neoplasms from acute EBV infection. The diagnosis of lymphoma or leukemia is confirmed by biopsy of enlarged lymph nodes or bone marrow aspiration and biopsy. Supporting evidence is provided by associated laboratory and radiologic studies.

REFERENCES

1. Schooley RT, Dolin R: Epstein–Barr virus (infectious mononucleosis). In: Mandell GL, Douglas RG, Bennett JE, eds. *Principles and Practice of Infectious Disease,* ed 2. New York, John Wiley & Sons, 1985:971–978.
2. Sumaya CV, Ench Y: Epstein–Barr virus infectious mononucleosis in children: I. Clinical and general laboratory findings. *Pediatrics* 1985; 75:1003–1010.
3. Heath CW, Brodsky AL, Potolsky AI: Infectious mononucleosis in a general population. *Am J Epidemiol* 1972; 95:46–52.
4. Niederman JC, Miller G, Pearson HA, *et al:* Infectious mononucleosis: Epstein–Barr virus shedding in saliva and the oropharynx. *N Engl J Med* 1976; 294:1355–1359.
5. Sabetta JR: Diagnosis: Infectious mononucleosis. *Hosp Med* 1984; March:109–143.
6. Straunch B, Andrews LL, Siegal N, *et al:* Oropharyngeal excretion of Epstein–Barr virus by renal transplant recipients and other patients treated with immunosuppressive drugs. *Lancet* 1974; 1:234–237.
7. Purtillo DT, Tatsumi E, Manolov G, *et al:* Epstein–Barr virus as an etiologic agent in the pathogenesis of lymphoproliferative and proliferative diseases in immune deficient patients. *Int Rev Exp Pathol* 1985; 27:113–183.
8. Aaberg TM, O'Brien WJ: Expanding opthalmologic recognition of Epstein–Barr virus infections [Editorial]. Am J Opthalmol 1987; 104:420–423.
9. Henderson E, Miller G, Robinson J, *et al:* Efficiency of transformation of lymphocytes by EB virus. *Virology* 1977: 76:152–163.
10. Miller G, Lipmann M: Release of infectious EBV by transformed marmoset leukocytes. *Proc Natl Acad Sci USA* 1973; 70:190–194.
11. Purtillo DT: Epstein–Barr virus: The spectrum of its manifestations in human beings. *South Med J* 1987; 80:943–947.
12. Robinson J, Smith D: Infection of human B lymphocytes with high multiplicities of Epstein–Barr virus: Kinetics of EBNA expression, cellular DNA synthesis, and mitosis. *Virology* 1981; 109:336–343.
13. Brown NA, Miller G: Immunoglobulin expression by human B lymphocytes clonally transformed by Epstein–Barr virus. *J Immunol* 1982: 28:24–29.
14. Henle W, Henle G. Hewetson J, *et al:* Failure to detect heterophile antigens in Epstein–Barr

virus infected cells and to demonstrate interaction of heterophile antibodies with Epstein–Barr virus. *Clin Exp Immunol* 1974; 17:281–286.

15. Nikoskelainen J, Leikola J, Klemola E: IgM antibodies specific for Epstein–Barr virus in infectious mononucleosis without heterophile antibodies. *Br Med J* 1974; 4:72–75.
16. Haider S, Coutinho M de L, Emond RTD, *et al:* Tuberculin anergy and infectious mononucleosis. *Lancet* 1973; 2:74.
17. Mangi RJ, Neiderman JC, Kelleher JE, *et al:* Depression of cell mediated immunity during acute infectious mononucleosis. *N Engl J Med* 1974: 291:1149–1153.
18. Gates RN, McCall CE: Infectious mononucleosis. In: Cluff LE, Johnson JE III, eds. *Clinical Concepts of Infectious Diseases,* ed 3. Baltimore, Williams & Wilkins, 1982:166–172.
19. Pullen H, Wright N, Murdoch J: Hypersensitivity reactions to antibacterial drugs in infectious mononucleosis. *Lancet* 1967; 2:1176–1178.
20. Furhman SA, Gill R, Horwitz CA, *et al:* Marked hyperbilirubinemia in infectious mononucleosis: Analysis of laboratory data in seven patients. *Arch Intern Med* 1987; 147:850–853.
21. Horwitz CA, Henle W, Henle G, *et al:* Infectious mononucleosis in patients aged 40 to 72 years: Report of 27 cases, including 3 without heterophil-antibody responses. *Medicine (Baltimore)* 1983; 62:256–262.
22. Smith EB. The anatomic pathology of infectious mononucleosis and its complications. In: *Proceedings of the International Infectious Mononucleosis Symposium.* Washington, American College Health Association. 1967:109.
23. Katner HP, Pankey GA: Fatal mononucleosis. In: Pankey GA, ed. *Ochsner Clinic Reports on Serious Hospital Infections,* Vol 3. Newtown, PA, Associates in Medical Marketing. 1987:1–7.
24. Wilkinson CS, Petz LD, Garraty G: Reappraisal of the role of anti-i in hemolytic anemia in infectious mononucleosis. *Br Med J Haematol* 1973; 25:715–722.
25. Dagan R, Powell KR: Postanginal sepsis following infectious mononucleosis. *Arch Intern Med* 1987; 147:1581–1583.
26. Penman HG: Fatal infectious mononucleosis: A critical review. *J Clin Pathol* 1971; 23:765–771.
27. Allen VR, Bass BH: Fatal hepatic necrosis in glandular fever. *J Clin Pathol* 1963; 16:337–341.
28. Seitanidis B: A comparison of the monospot with the Paul–Bunnell test in infectious mononucleosis and other diseases. *J Clin Pathol* 1969; 22:323–328.
29. Sumaya CV, Ench Y: Epstein–Barr virus infectious mononucleosis in children: II. Heterophile antibody and viral specific responses. *Pediatrics* 1985; 75:1011–1019.
30. Fleisher GR, Collins M, Fager S: Limitations of available tests for diagnosis of infectious mononucleosis. *J Clin Microbiol* 1983: 17:619–624.
31. Brandfonbrener A, Epstein A, Wu S, *et al:* Corticosteroid therapy in Epstein–Barr virus infection: Effect on lymphocyte class, subset, and response to early antigen. *Arch Intern Med* 1986; 146:337–339.
32. Schleupner CJ, Overall JC Jr: Infectious mononucleosis and Epstein–Barr virus: 1. Epidemiology, pathogenesis, immune response. 2. Clinical picture, diagnosis, management. *Postgrad Med* 1979; 65:83–89,95–105.
33. Bergman MM, Gleckman RA: Heterophile negative infectious mononucleosislike syndrome. *Postgrad Med* 1987; 81:313–322.
34. Gall EP. Clues that suggest viral arthritis. *Diagnosis* 1987; 9:31–37.
35. Horowitz CA, Henle W, Henle G: Diagnostic aspects of the cytomegalovirus mononucleosis syndrome in previously healthy persons. *Postgrad Med* 1979; 66:153–158.
36. Kessler HA, Blaauw B, Spear J, *et al:* Diagnosis of human immunodeficiency virus infection in seronegative homosexuals presenting with an acute viral syndrome. *JAMA* 1987; 258:1196–1199.
37. Cooper DA, Gold S, Maclean P, *et al:* Acute AIDS retrovirus infection: Definition of a clinical illness associated with seroconversion. *Lancet* 1985; 1:537–540.
38. Lange Wantzin GR, Orskov Lindhardt B, Weismann K, *et al:* Acute HTLV-III infection associated with exanthema, diagnosed by seroconversion. *Br J Dermatol* 1986; 115:601–606.

39. Tan JS: Common and uncommon parasitic infections in the United States. *Med Clin North Am* 1978; 62:1059–1081.
40. Guerrero IC, Weniger BC, Schultz MG: Transfusion malaria in the United States 1972–1981. *Ann Intern Med* 1983; 99:221–226.
41. Barrett-Conner E: Malaria: An ''imported'' disease to be reckoned with in the U.S. *Calif Med* 1971; 115:19–24.
42. Harris LF, Shasteen WJ, Lampert R: Malaria: Recent experience in a community. *South Med J* 1984; 77:1121–1123.
43. McCabe RE, Brooks RG, Dorfman RF, *et al:* Clinical spectrum of 107 cases of toxoplasmic lymphadenopathy. *Rev Infect Dis* 1987; 9:754–774.
44. Remington JS, Barnett CG, Meikel M, *et al:* Toxoplasmosis and infectious mononucleosis. *Arch Intern Med* 1962; 110:250–259.
45. Elliot DL, Tolle SW, Goldberg L, *et al:* Pet-associated illness. *N Engl J Med* 1985; 313:985–995.
46. deLuise VP: Toxoplasmosis: An update and overview. *Res Staff Physician* 1983; 29:62–68.
47. Brooks RG, McCabe RE, Remington JS: Role of serology in the diagnosis of toxoplasmic lymphadenopathy. *Rev Infect Dis* 1987: 9:1055–1062.
48. Krockta WP, Barnes WC: Genital ulceration with regional adenopathy. *Infect Dis Clin North Am* 1987; 1:217–234.
49. Levine JF, Gross PA: Infectious diseases: Sexually transmitted diseases. In: *Roche Handbook of Differential Diagnosis,* Vol 6. Nutley, NJ, Hoffman–LaRoche, 1984:3–19.
50. Musher DM: Syphilis. *Infect Dis Clin North Am* 1987; 1:83–96.
51. Drusin LM: Syphilis: Clinical manifestations, diagnosis, treatment. *Urol Clin North Am* 1984; 11:121–130.
52. Schmed ES, Williams DN: Lyme disease: The tick bite, the rash, and the sequelae. *Postgrad Med* 1985; 77:303–310.
53. Steere AC, Bartenhagen NH, Craft JE, et al: The early clinical manifestations of Lyme disease. *Ann Intern Med* 1983; 99:76–82.
54. Zemel L: Lyme disease: Ten years later. *Infect Med* 1986; 3:202–207.
55. Margileth AM, Wear DJ, English CK: Systemic cat scratch disease: A report of 23 patients with prolonged or recurrent severe bacterial infection. *J Infect Dis* 1987; 155:390–402.
56. Wolf RE, Birbara CA: Meningococcal infections at an army training center. *Am J Med* 1968; 44:243–255.
57. Frank ST, Gomez RM: Chronic meningococcemia. *Medit Med* 1968; 133:918–920.
58. Koster FT: Plague: Peripatetic pest of the American west. *Drug Ther* 1984; Sept:64–72.
59. Tacket CO, Davis BR, Carter GP, *et al: Yersinia* enterocolitis pharyngitis. *Ann Intern Med* 1983; 99:40–42.
60. Rabinowitz M, Stremple JF, Wells KE, *et al: Yersinia enterocolitica* infection complicated by intestinal perforation. *Arch Intern Med* 1987; 147:1662–1663.
61. Harrell R, Bates JH: Clinical recognition and treatment of tuleremia. *Intern Med* 1987; 8:115–123.
62. Evans ME, Gregory DW, Schaffner W, *et al:* Tularemia: A 30 year experience with 88 cases. *Medicine (Baltimore)* 1983; 64:251–269.
63. Klotz SA, Jorgensen JH, Buckwold FJ, *et al:* Typhoid fever: An epidemic with remarkably few clinical signs and symptoms. *Arch Intern Med* 1984; 144:533–537.
64. Rubin RH, Weinstein L: *Salmonellosis.* New York, Straton Intercontinental Medical Book Corp, 1977.
65. Hoffman TA, Ruiz CJ, Counts GW, *et al:* Waterborne typhoid fever in Dade County, Florida: Clinical and therapeutic evaluations of 105 bacteremic patients. *Am J Med* 1975; 59:481–487.
66. Weir MR, Thornton GF: Extrapulmonary tuberculosis: Experience of a community hospital and review of the literature. *Am J Med* 1985; 79:467–478.
67. Bujak JS, Aptekar RG, Decker JL, *et al:* Juvenile rheumatoid arthritis presenting in the adult as fever of unknown origin. *Medicine (Baltimore)* 1973; 52:431–444.

12

Chronic Fatigue Syndrome

Nelson M. Gantz

INTRODUCTION

In most textbooks, infectious mononucleosis is described as a self-limited acute illness lasting 2 to 3 weeks. In the vast majority of patients, recovery occurs uneventfully without specific therapy. Recurrent and chronic forms of the illness are not described in textbooks, although a more gradual resolution of the illness has been noted. Recently, on television, in newspapers, and in numerous popular magazines, an illness called chronic Epstein–Barr virus (CEBV), or the ''yuppie flu'' because it often attacks better-educated, hard-driving, young professionals, has been described. This has been called by some writers as ''the malaise of the 80s'' and support groups have sprung up throughout this and other countries around the world. The practicing clinician has been besieged by patients seeking relief for this illness with little guidance from the usual medical sources. This has been an extremely frustrating situation for both patients and clinicians.

In daily practice, clinicians are called on the manage ''CEBV'' despite controversy over its existence. The occurrence of persistent or recurrent symptoms, which may include fatigue, low-grade fever, myalgias, depression, headaches, sore throat, paresthesias, dizziness, impaired cognition, sleep disorders, arthralgias, and painful lymphadenopathy, can be debilitating, life wrecking, and for many patients totally disabling. Patients often note that after waking up in the morning and showering, they are so exhausted that they are forced back to bed to rest for the remainder of the day. This chapter focuses on a number of questions regarding this syndrome. Is this a real illness? Is this a new syndrome? What is the cause of this syndrome? What is the relationship of EBV to chronic infectious mononucleosis? How can the syndrome be diagnosed? What laboratory studies should be obtained to establish a diagnosis? What illnesses should be included in the differential diagnosis? How should this syndrome be managed? How is the illness transmitted?

Chronic infectious mononucleosis can be classified into at least three syndromes.[1] In the first, patients develop typical acute infectious mononucleosis as a result of a primary EBV infection. However, unlike the vast majority of patients, recovery fails to occur for months to years. There is no explanation why most patients recover whereas for others the symptoms and signs are persistent. In the second syndrome, which is extremely rare, patients have a severe chronic EBV infection with interstitial pneumonia, pancytopenia, hepatitis, uveitis, and fever.[2] In the second syndrome, exceedingly high titers of EBV antibodies are noted, such as a VCA IgG of 1 : 10,240 and and EA-D of >1 : 640. Of the two patients reported with severe chronic EBV infection, neither developed an antibody response to the Epstein–Barr nuclear antigen. The third syndrome, which has been called chronic EBV, is probably best designated as the chronic fatigue syndrome (CFS).[3–6] The etiology of this last syndrome is unknown.

IS THIS A REAL DISEASE?

Although the syndrome is characterized by relatively nonspecific symptoms and normal laboratory findings, there are at least four reasons to consider the chronic fatigue syndrome to be a real organic illness. First, the main symptom complex develops over a few hours to a few days. Second, although many of the symptoms are seen with psychoneurotic disorders, several others are not, including low-grade fevers (<101°F), recurrent cervical adenopathy, and pharyngitis. Third, patients give a consistent description of how their illness began and report a list of multiple but similar complaints. Patients usually state that they were in the prime of their life, became ill, and never recovered from what seemed like a "cold" or the "flu." Fourth, there are a number of neurological features including abnormal results on psychological testing, particularly in the tests of recent memory and concentration.

IS THIS A NEW DISEASE?

Since the 1930s, a number of reports describing similar syndromes characterized by fatigue, malaise, myalgias, neurological complaints, and low-grade fever have been published. These illnesses have been described by various names such as atypical poliomyelitis, Akureyri disease, Iceland disease, benign myalgic encephalomyelitis, royal free disease, epidemic neuromyasthenia, and postviral fatigue syndrome.[7–16] Despite extensive studies, the eiology of all these illnesses has remained unknown. More recently, chronic fatigue has been referred to as "CEBV," and an outbreak in Incline Village, a resort community in Nevada, as Lake Tahoe disease.[17] Both sporadic and epidemic illnesses with fatigue as a central feature have been reported. There have been over 30 outbreaks of epidemic neuromyasthenia since 1934. A few of the outbreaks involve nearly 1000 cases. Typically, after a 2- to 3-week incubation period, young to middle-aged adults, mostly female, develop an illness of unknown etiology characterized by fatigue, fever, and malaise. In addition, persistent fatigue following an acute episode of an infectious disease such as viral hepatitis, brucellosis, or influenza has been well described. Prolonged recovery from primary EBV infection has also been reported. All these reports describing individuals with similar complaints underscore that this is not a new syndrome.

WHAT IS THE CAUSE OF THIS SYNDROME? WHAT IS THE ROLE OF EBV IN CHRONIC INFECTIOUS MONONUCLEOSIS?

The etiology of the chronic fatigue syndrome is unknown. Although recent reports have described patients with prolonged illness characterized by nonspecific constitutional symptoms attributed to EBV, the serological profiles reported do not differ statistically from those seen in normal patients with no complaints. The diagnosis of "CEBV" was based according to several reports on an elevated anti-VCA IgG and anti-EA levels and descreased or absent EBNA antibodies.[4–6] In a general medical clinic in Boston, 21% of patients were suffering from a chronic fatigue syndrome, but the EBV antibody levels were not statistically different from those from age- and sex-matched controls.[18] This study and the report from Lake Tahoe in which patients had elevated antibody levels against cytomegalovirus, herpes simplex virus, and measles virus make the case that this syndrome is unlikely to be linked to EBV. It is also recognized that EBV serology is poorly reproducible, and results between laboratories are not comparable. At this point, it is premature to claim that EBV is responsible for this syndrome. Another virus that was first described in 1986 is human B lymphotrophic virus (HBLV), or human herpesvirus VI.[19] Further studies are needed to assess the role of this virus in the chronic fatigue syndrome.

HOW CAN THIS SYNDROME BE DIAGNOSED?

This syndrome, characterized by debilitating fatigue combined with multiple other complaints, is a diagnosis of exclusion. A working case definition has been developed by Dr. Gary Holmes at the Centers for Disease Control and colleagues to provide a basis for evaluating patients who have unexplained chronic fatigue. The case definition was designed to foster clinical research and epidemiologic studies. A case of CFS must fulfill the following criteria, which have been published in the *Annals of Internal Medicine* in 1988.[20] Weight change of $>10\%$ in the absence of dieting should suggest other diagnoses. A detailed personal and family psychiatric history is important, since affective disorders may be inherited.

CASE DEFINITION FOR CHRONIC FATIGUE SYNDROME

A case of CFS must fulfill major criteria 1 and 2, at least six of the 11 symptoms criteria, and at least two of the three physical criteria or at least eight of the 11 symptom criteria.

Major Criteria

1. New onset of persistent or relapsing debilitating fatigue or easy fatigability in a person who has no previous history of similar symptoms, that does not resolve with bedrest, and that is severe enough to reduce or impair average daily activity below 50% of the patient's premorbid activity level for a period of at least 6 months.
2. Other clinical conditions that may produce similar symptoms have been excluded by thorough evaluation based on history, physical examination, and appropriate laboratory findings; these include (1) malignancy, (2) autoimmune disease, (3) localized infection (such as occult abscess), (4) chronic or subacute bacterial disease (such as endocarditis, Lyme disease, or TB), fungal disease (such as histoplasmosis, blastomycosis, or coccidioidomycosis), and parasitic disease (such as toxoplasmosis, amebiasis, giardiasis, or helminthic infestation), (5) disease related to human immunodeficiency virus (HIV) infection, (6) chronic psychiatric disease, either newly diagnosed or by history (such as endogenous depression, hysterical personality disorder, anxiety neurosis, schizophrenia, or chronic use of major tranquilizers, lithium, or antidepressive medications), (7) chronic inflammatory disease (such as sarcoidosis, Wegener's granulomatosis or chronic hepatitis), (8) neuromuscular disease (such as multiple sclerosis or myasthenia gravis), (9) endocrine disease (such as hypothyroidism, Addison's disease, Cushing's syndrome, or diabetes mellitus), (10) drug dependency or abuse (such as alcohol, controlled prescription drugs, or illicit drugs), (11) side effects of a chronic medication or other toxic agent (such as a chemical solvent, pesticide, or heavy metal), or (12) other known or defined chronic pulmonary, cardiac, gastrointestinal, hepatic, renal, or hematological disease.

If any of the results from these tests are abnormal, the physician should search for other conditions that may cause such a result. If no such conditions are detected by a reasonable evaluation, this criterion is satisfied.

Minor Criteria

Symptom Criteria

To fulfill a symptom criterion, a symptom must have begun at or after the time of onset of increased fatigability and must have persisted or recurred over a period of at least 6 months (the individual symptoms may or may not have occurred simultaneously).

1. Mild fever: oral temperature between 99.4°F and 101°F, if measured by patient, and/or chills. (Note: oral temperature of >101°F is less compatible with CFS and should prompt studies for other causes of illness.)
2. Sore throat.
3. Painful lymph nodes in the anterior or posterior cervical or axillary distribution.
4. Unexplained generalized muscle weakness.
5. Muscle discomfort/myalgias.
6. Prolonged (>24 hr) generalized fatigue following levels of exercise that would have been easily tolerated in the patient's premorbid state.
7. Generalized headaches of a type, severity, or pattern that is different from headaches the patient may have had in the premorbid state.
8. Migratory arthralgias without joint swelling or redness.
9. Neuropsychological complaints (one or more of the following: photophobia, transient visual scotomata, forgetfulness, excessive irritability, confusion, difficulty thinking, inability to concentrate, depression).
10. Sleep disturbance (hypersomnia or insomnia).
11. Description of the main symptom complex as initially developing over a few hours to a few days (this is not a true symptom but may be considered as equivalent to the above symptoms in meeting the requirements of the case definition).

Physical Criteria

Documented by a physician on at least two occasions at least 1 month apart:

1. Low-grade fever: oral temperature between 99.5°F and 101°F, or rectal temperature between 100°F and 101.5°F. (See note under symptom criterion 1.)
2. Nonexudative pharyngitis.
3. Palpable and/or tender anterior or posterior cervical or axillary lymph nodes (Note: lymph nodes >2 cm in diameter suggest other etiologies. Further evaluation is warranted).

Table 12.1
Evaluation of a Patient with Unexplained Fatigue

CBC and differential
Electrolytes
Glucose
Creatinine
Liver function tests
Calcium, phosphorus
Aldolase or creatine phosphokinase (CK)
Urinalysis
Chest x ray
Erythrocyte sedimentation rate
Antinuclear antibody
Thyroid-stimulating hormone (TSH)
HIV antibody

WHAT LABORATORY STUDIES SHOULD BE OBTAINED TO ESTABLISH A DIAGNOSIS OF CFS?

Table 12.1 lists studies that are recommended in evaluating a patient with unexplained fatigue. Presently, there are no laboratory tests to establish the diagnosis of CFS. Interestingly, the erythrocyte sedimentation rate is generally low normal, usually 1 to 5 mm at 1 hr. If practical, it may be helpful to save a red-top tube of serum for future studies when a diagnostic test is devised. Skin testing for tuberculosis with appropriate controls is also indicated. In the meanwhile, it is important to exclude any other occult illness that may be responsible for the fatigue. Psychological testing can also provide documentation of a number of the complaints such as the memory problems and concentration defects that are extremely troublesome for the patient.

WHAT ILLNESSES SHOULD BE INCLUDED IN THE DIFFERENTIAL DIAGNOSIS OF CFS?

These entities are listed under the second major criteria of the case definition. Appropriate laboratory studies should be obtained if the history or physical examination suggests any of these disorders. Another disorder, fibromyalgia or fibrositis, shares many features with the chronic fatigue syndrome.[21] Finally, depression and somatization should also be considered in the differential diagnosis of patients with CFS.

HOW SHOULD THIS SYNDROME BE MANAGED?

In evaluating a patient with unexplained fatigue, it is important to establish a diagnosis using criteria in the case definition. Patients should be reassured that the symptoms are real and that they are not "crazy." Patients often see skeptical physicians and leave their offices frustrated after being told that they have a psychosomatic disorder. Activity should be recommended as tolerated, avoiding excesses. Symptomatic therapy is indicated for the sleep disorder (e.g., triazolam), for the myalgias (e.g., amitriptyline in a dose of 10 to 20 mg administered 1 hr before bedtime), for headaches, and for depression (e.g., desipramine or phenelzine given in the usual doses). Psychiatric consultation can also be invaluable. It is essential that patients have an appointment made for a regular follow-up evaluation so that the illness can be monitored and support provided. Since the etiology is unknown, no specific therapy is available. Acyclovir administered in high doses for 1 month in an unpublished study by Dr. Stephen Strauss was no more effective than placebo in a controlled study. Intravenous γ-globulin has also been used to treat this disorder with anecdotal responses, but controlled studies are lacking. Similarly, some individuals advocate diet modification as well as high-dose vitamins, but again support for this approach from controlled trials is nonexistent. Referral of patients to established support groups can be extremely beneficial in helping patients cope with their life-wrecking illness.

The natural history of this disorder has not been well characterized. Approximately one-third of patients spontaneously get better. In another two-thirds of individuals, the illness appears to persist with waxing and waning periods.

HOW IS THIS DISORDER TRANSMITTED?

Since the etiology is unknown, it is unclear how this syndrome is transmitted. There appears to be no intrafamilial spread of this disorder, since more than one case in a family is extremely unusual.

SUMMARY

The chronic fatigue syndrome is real. The etiology is unknown, but an illness with multiple causes would not be surprising. It is probably not caused by EBV. The diagnosis is one of exclusion. It is important to use symptomatic therapy and to provide reassurance and support as well as regular follow-up for the patients.

REFERENCES

1. Komaroff AL: The "chronic mononucleosis" syndromes. *Hosp Pract* 1987; May:71–75.
2. Schooley RT, Carey RW, Miller G, *et al:* Chronic Epstein-Barr virus infection with interstitial pneumonitis. *Ann Intern Med* 1986; 104:636–643.
3. Tobi M, Morag A, Ravid Z, *et al:* Prolonged atypical illness associated with serologic evidence of persistent Epstein–Barr virus infection. *Lancet* 1982; 1:61–64.
4. DuBois RE, Seeley JK, Brus I, *et al:* Chronic mononucleosis syndrome. *South Med J* 1984; 77:1376–1382.
5. Jones JF, Ray CG, Minnich LL, *et al:* Evidence for active Epstein–Barr virus infection in patients with persistent unexplained illnesses: Elevated anti-early antigen antibodies. *Ann Intern Med* 1985; 102:1–7.
6. Strauss SE, Tosato G, Armstrong G, *et al:* Persisting illness and fatigue in adults with evidence of Epstein–Barr virus infection. *Ann Intern Med* 1985; 102:7–16.
7. Sigurdsson B, Sigurjonsson J, Sigurdsson JH, *et al:* A disease epidemic in Iceland simulating poliomyelitis. *Am J Hyg* 1950; 52:222–238.
8. Sigurdsson B, Gudmundsson KR: Clinical findings six years after outbreak of Akureyri disease. *Lancet* 1956; 1:766–767.
9. White DN, Burtch RB: Iceland disease: New infection simulating acute anterior poliomyelitis. *Neurology (Minneap)* 1954; 4:506–516.
10. Gilliam AG: *Epidemiologic Study of Epidemic Diagnosed as Poliomyelitis, Occurring among Personnel of Los Angeles County General Hospital during the Summer of 1934*. Bulletin 240. Washington, US Public Health Service, Division of Infectious Diseases, Institute of Health, 1938.
11. Galpine JF, Brady C: Benign myalgic encephalomyelitis. *Lancet* 1957; 1:757–758.
12. Shelokov A, Habel K, Verder E, *et al:* Epidemic neuromyasthenia: An outbreak of poliomyelitis-like illness in student nurses. *N Engl J Med* 1957; 257:345–355.
13. Poskanzer DC, Henderson DA, Kunkle EC, *et al:* Epidemic neuromyasthenia: An outbreak in Punta Gorda, Florida. *N Engl J Med* 1957; 257:356–364.
14. Dillon MJ, Marshall WC, Dudgeon JA, *et al:* Epidemic neuromyasthenia: Outbreak among nurses at a children's hospital. *Br Med J* 1974; 1:301–305.
15. The Medical Staff of the Royal Free Hospital: An outbreak of encephalomyelitis in the Royal Free Hospital Group, London, in 1955. *Br Med J* 1957; 2:895–904.
16. Behan PO, Behan WMH, Bell EJ: The postviral fatigue syndrome—an analysis of the findings in 50 cases. *J Infect* 1985; 10:211–222.
17. Holmes GP, Kaplan JE, Stewart JA, *et al:* A cluster of patients with a chronic mononucleosis-like syndrome: Is Epstein–Barr virus the cause? *JAMA* 1987; 257:2297–2302.
18. Buchwald D, Sullivan JL, Komaroff AL: Frequency of "chronic active Epstein–Barr infection" in a general medical practice. *JAMA* 1987; 257:2303–2307.
19. Salahuddin SZ, Ablash DV, Markham PD, *et al:* Isolation of a new virus, HBLV, in patients with lymphoproliferative disorders. *Science* 1986; 234:596–601.
20. Holmes GP, Kaplan JE, Gantz NM, *et al:* Chronic fatigue syndrome: A working case definition. *Ann Intern Med* 1988; 108: 387–389.
21. Buchwald D, Goldenberg DL, Sullivan JL, *et al:* The "chronic, active Epstein–Barr virus infection" syndrome and primary fibromyalgia. *Arthritis Rheuma* 1987; 30(10):1132–1136.

ADDITIONAL READING

Straus SE: The chronic mononucleosis syndrome. *J Infect Dis* 1988; 157:405–412.

13

Management of Infectious Diarrhea

Richard B. Brown

INTRODUCTION

Diarrhea is an extremely common disorder that represents one of the most important reasons for which patients seek medical attention. Although most publications fail to define this entity adequately, the following discussion employs a working definition as follows: a change in bowel habits resulting in an increase in the frequency and liquidity of fecal discharges.[1] It accounts for approximately 4% of acute illness, ranks second only to the common cold with regard to time lost from work, and accounts for approximately 2% of all ambulatory visits.[2] Diarrhea appears as a principal diagnosis on 1–2% of hospital discharges.

Most instances of diarrhea are self-limited and presumed to be infectious in etiology. The practicing clinician must be able to distinguish among those cases that require antimicrobial agents, those that can be handled supportively, and those for which full evaluation, possibly including invasive procedures, is indicated.

FACTORS CONTRIBUTING TO DIARRHEA

Relationships between the host and the pathogen are extremely important in defining the likelihood of diarrhea. Table 13.1 depicts several of the most important host and microbial factors that are involved.[3] Persons at the extremes of life appear at risk for selected forms of gastrointestinal disease. Young children appear predisposed to infections with rotavirus and enteropathogenic *E. coli*[4] The elderly may become infected more easily with species of *Salmonella*. Rea-

Table 13.1
Factors Contributing to Diarrhea[a]

Microbial factors	Host factors
Toxin production	Patient age
Organism attachment	Personal hygiene
Other virulence factors	Gastric acidity
Intestinal immunity	Normal enteric flora
Intestinal motility	

[a]Adopted from Guerrant.[3]

sons for these age-associated relationships are not completely known but are probably related the presenced or absence of gastric acid, local gastrointestinal production of IgA, and perhaps subtle adherance interactions at the level of the gastrointestinal mucosa.[3]

Gastric acidity plays a major role in host susceptibility to infectious diarrhea. Normal gastric pH provides significant protection to the gastrointestinal tract. Values of less than 4.0 result in the killing of over 99% of ingested *E. coli* in less than 30 min. Similarly, patients with achlorhydria or pharmacological manipulations that raise gastric pH appear far more susceptible to disease caused by a variety of pathogens that include *Salmonella* and *Vibrio cholerae.*

The "normal flora" of the gastrointestinal tract is of extreme importance in providing protection against exogenous pathogens. Under most circumstances anaerobes such as *B. fragilis* peptostreptococci and peptococci are present in concentrations of up to 10^{11}/g of feces while facultative anaerobes such as *E. coli* and *S. faecalis* are found in concentrations of up to 10^{7}/g of stool.[5] Older studies have demonstrated that small doses of antimicrobial agents are capable of disrupting this protective flora, allowing colonization with more resistant enterobacteraciae that include *P. aeruginosa* and *Klebsiella* species, and may allow infection with far fewer organisms than seen under normal circumstances. Reasons for this protection are multiple and probably involve production of by-products that are toxic for selected pathogens and utilization of binding sites so that they are unavailable for attachment.

The role of intestinal motility is evident from studies that have shown that infections caused by *Salmonella* and *Shigella* species behave more aggressively when treated with antimotility compounds and that intestinal overgrowth occurs in clinical situations of hypomotility.[3] Intestinal immunity consists of usual systemic factors and special features inate to the gastrointestinal tract. Active intestinal humoral immunity is provided through secretory IgA, formed in the lamina propria, which can be directed against selected antigens in the cell walls of bacterial pathogens. The lamina propria also provides less specific immunity through availability of large numbers of polymorphonuclear leukocytes, which appear to help prevent transgressions by potential pathogens.[3]

Factors present in potential pathogens include toxins, adhesiveness factors, and invasiveness factors.[3] Toxins include neurotoxins, cytotoxins, and enterotoxins and may either be ingested preformed or elucidated after ingestion of the organism. Toxins can function by directly affecting intestinal secretion/ absorption, altering peristalsis, effecting mucosal destruction, or acting centrally on vomiting centers. Selected bacterial species must be able to adhere to cell walls in order to provoke diarrhea. This has been best demonstrated for certain strains of enterotoxigenic *E. coli.* Toxigenicity may not be able to occur in the absence of prior adhesion. Invasiveness is noted in species of bacteria that include most strains of *Shigella* and *Salmonella* and is probably related to cell wall antigens.[3] It must be acknowledged, however, that for many organisms the mechanisms for disease production are unknown.

APPROACH TO THE PATIENT WITH DIARRHEA

Several basic questions must be addressed prior to initiating optimal management for the patient with diarrhea. Initial decisions to be made include need for hospitalization and need for any strategies other than supportive management. No scientifically valid data exist that aid the physician in assessing the need for hospitalization. In general, major reasons include the "toxicity" of the patient and presence of significant dehydration, both of which can be noted on initial physical examination. These problems occur more commonly in patients at the extremes of life. Other reasons to consider hospitalization include the possibility of early life-threatening disease and the lack of patient compliance. Additional issues that must ultimately be considered include need for either antibiotics or invasive procedures. Decisions will be based on the results of a careful appraisal of the patient that should include history and physical examination and simple gross and microscopic evaluation of the stool. In some instances, failure to respond to a trial of supportive therapy may indicate need for further assessment.

Patients with the chief complaint of diarrhea should have a careful epidemiologic history that takes into account (1) recent travel, (2) similar illnesses in the family, (3) exposure to improperly prepared or nonpasteurized foods or beverages, (4) recent intake of medications, especially antibiotics, and (5) homosexuality. Attention must be paid to the patient's description of the frequency and character of the bowel movements. Individuals with greater than 15 movements per day and a duration of diarrhea of less than 1 week are more likely to have a bacterial etiology.[6] A history of frequent stools containing blood, mucus, or pus should be noted, as well as complaints of abdominal discomfort, rectal urgency, and nausea or vomiting. A history of fever and rigors may also point toward an identifiable bacterial pathogen.

Physical examination should assess the hydration status of the patient with careful attention paid to skin turgor and blood pressure. Because several types of diarrheal illness may be accompanied by extraintestinal manifestations (e.g., rash or arthritis), a comprehensive evaluation is indicated for all patients. Especial attention should be paid to the abdomen and rectum, and an actual specimen of stool should be sought for gross and microscopic evaluation as well as for testing for occult blood. The presence of abdominal guarding or rebound tenderness could indicate an early surgical process.

Laboratory evaluation should be based on clinical presentation, history, and physical examination. Routine studies such as complete blood count and serum electrolytes are not routinely indicated. However, such testing should be considered in patients who are hospitalized with diarrhea, and tests that include serum electrolytes should be employed in patients with clinical dehydration. Blood cultures should be reserved for patients who are constitutionally ill and possibly bacteremic and probably should be obtained on all febrile hospitalized patients. However, the absence of fever (especially in those at the extremes of life) should not mitigate against obtaining blood cultures.[7]

Appropriate assessment of stool can provide much meaningful and cost-effective information. Gram stains to define organism morphology are rarely useful since stool is loaded with various bacteria. However, occasionally, useful information can be gathered if overwhelming numbers of organisms with uniform morphology (i.e., *Staphylococcus, Candida,* or *Campylobacter*) are noted.[6] Microscopic evaluation for fecal leukocytes provides rapid and inexpensive information concerning the possibility of invasive diarrhea.[8] However, correlation with an identifiable cultural pathogen has given conflicting results, and some data now demonstrate that the presence of fecal leukocytes fails to correlate with culture positivity.[9] This study documented that only 70% of patients with shigellosis and about 35% of those with salmonellosis had fecal leukocytes demonstrated. Alternatively, however, absence of fecal leukocytes strongly mitigates against an invasive pathogen. Clearly, use of fecal leukocytes as an indicator of need for culture has shortcomings. It is the opinion of the author that stool cultures should be obtained under the following circumstances: (1) patients hospitalized for diarrhea, (2) patients with fever and diarrhea lasting more than 1–2 days, (3) diarrhea unresponsive to a reasonable course (i.e., 2–3 days) of supportive therapy, (4) patients with diarrhea who are returning from foreign travel, (5) food handlers with diarrhea, and (6) homosexuals with diarrhea.

Clinical laboratories must test for pathogens other than *Salmonella* and *Shigella. Campylobacter, Aeromonas,* and *Yersinia* species, recently recognized pathogens in diarrhea, require special media and environmental conditions that should be available in all microbiology laboratories (*vide infra*).

Other tests should be obtained as necessary but may not be routinely ordered unless epidemiologically indicated. Stools for "ova and parasites" are frequently ordered by physicians as a knee-jerk reflex but will not routinely be positive and are extremely labor intensive to perform. This study should be reserved for patients with diarrhea who have recently returned from travel to an endemic area or who have other unusual epidemiologic exposures, those with unresponsive diarrhea, especially with negative cultures for bacteria, and homosexuals who practice anal intercourse. It is generally not indicated as a study for patients who develop diarrhea during hospitalization. Stools for *C. difficile* toxin should be ordered in patients who develop diarrhea while taking antibiotics or cancer chemotherapeutics and can be considered in selected other cases of diarrhea unresponsive to therapies being employed.

Occasional patients will require invasive studies, such as proctosigmoidoscopy or colonoscopy with biopsy, or radiologic evaluations that can include barium enema or upper gastrointestinal series with small bowel follow-through. The decision to employ such procedures is based on the clinical presentation of the patient that includes chronicity, toxicity of the patient, response to specific or nonspecific therapy, and results of other noninvasive evaluations. The most common reason for such invasive or radiographic procedures is to rule out inflammatory but noninfectious conditions such as ulcerative colitis or Crohn's disease. However, they may also be useful in evaluation for pseudomembranous colitis, malignancy, and diverticulitis, which may occasionally present with diarrhea. Patients with either Crohn's disease or ulcerative colitis often present with constitutional symptoms, bloody stools, and subacute or chronic complaints. Significant overlap exists between infectious diarrheas and inflammatory bowel diseases, and reports exist that demonstrate barium enema results and proctosigmoidscopic changes consistent with ulcerative colitis in patients with *Campylobacter,* amebic, and *Salmonella* gastroenteritis.[4,10,11] Thus, it is always important to rule out infectious gastroenteritides in patients being evaluated for the possibility of inflammatory bowel disease.

GENERAL MANAGEMENT OF DIARRHEA

Supportive care for the patient with diarrhea must consider needs for fluid and electrolyte replacement, relief of abdominal pain or discomfort, and possibly amelioration of the diarrhea itself. Needs for intravenous or oral replacement of fluids must take into account the degree of dehydration of the patient, age, compliance, and severity of underlying illness. Most individuals will be noted to have only modest dehydration and can be successfully managed with oral replacement outside of the hospital. For mild diarrhea, replacement with carbonated beverages, tea, clear soups, and water taken with salted crackers will usually suffice.[12] Moderate disease should be treated with more physiological replacements available as Gatorade®, Pediolyte®, or the mixture outlined in Table 13.2. Severe diarrhea in patients who cannot be hospitalized requires

Table 13.2
Oral Rehydration Regimen[a]

Amount	First glass	Amount	Second glass
8 oz	Fruit juice	8 oz	Pure water
1/2 tsp	Honey or corn syrup	$\frac{1}{4}$ tsp	Baking soda
1 pinch	Table salt		

[a]Drink alternately from each glass; supplement with carbonated beverages, boiled water, tea, or coffee. Adopted from Kimmey.[13]

treatment with the World Health Organization formula (available in packets) consisting of NaCl (3.5 g), $NaHCO_3$ (2.5 g), KC1 (1.5 g), and 20 g glucose in water to make 1 liter. It should be given with free water or other liquids. Although not scientifically validated, most authorities recommend that dietary restrictions accompany fluid rehydration. Initially, intake should be limited to clear soups, plain toast or bread, salted crackers, and sherbet. As the rate of stooling decreases, baked potatoes, chicken soups, and rice or noodles can be added. As stools regain normal shape, baked fish and chicken, applesauce, and bananas can also be added.[12]

Need to control diarrhea must be individualized and must take into account that most cases are self-limited and mild. However, many authorities routinely utilize some form of symptomatic treatment in addition to fluid therapy for patients with moderate or severe diarrhea.[12] A variety of agents are available and are summarized in Table 13.3. Anticholinergic agents that include paregoric and codeine reduce intestinal motility and should generally be avoided because they may increase the time that bacteria and their toxins remain within the gastroin-

Table 13.3
Symptomatic Therapy for Diarrhea[a]

Class of agent	Examples
Antimotility	Loperamide Tincture of Opium ?Bismuth subsalicylate
Adsorption	Kaolin, pectin Cholestyramine ?Bismuth subsalicylate
Antiprostaglandin	Aspirin Indocin

[a]Adopted from Ericsson and Dupont.[12]

testinal tract.[12–14] Loperamide may be an exception, since it also has antisecretory activity and has been shown to be at least as effective as bismuth subsalicylate (Pepto-Bismol®) in traveler's diarrhea.[12] Use of absorbants such as kaolin and pectin compounds may provide modest relief of diarrhea in mild cases and can usually be safely utilized. However, they may not alleviate cramping. Bismuth subsalicylate has been utilized for many years and appears to result in clinical improvment in many cases. Patients should be counseled, however, that full doses of this agent provide the equivalent of six to seven adult aspirins.[12] Adults receiving usual doses of 1 oz every half hour for up to 8 oz note decrease in stooling rate and in cramping and nausea. Whether tablets of this agent are as successful as the liquid is unknown. Issues related to antibiotic therapy are addressed under the sections that follow dealing with specific infectious diarrheas.

DIARRHEAS CAUSED BY SPECIFIC INFECTIOUS AGENTS

Salmonella

Salmonella species are a classical cause of gastroenteritis and are currently thought to comprise 1–2% of all cases.[15] Acute diarrheal illness represents the most common manifestation of infections with *Salmonella*. Disease with organisms of this genus can be episodic and has been associated with a variety of foods including poultry, beef, and raw milk.[16] A variety of serotypes have been implicated including *S. typhimurium, S. enteritidis, S. heidelberg,* and *S. newport.*[17] Serotypes such as *S. typhi, S. paratyphi,* and *S. cholerasuis* rarely produce this syndrome. Gastroenteritis caused by serotypes of *Salmonella* occur 8–48 hr after ingesting contaminated foods or liquids and is associated with abdominal cramping, fever, and diarrhea in most instances.[18] Severity of the diarrhea can range from modest to fulminant, and degree of constitutional complaints is similarly quite variable. In general, stools are of moderate volume, and blood is not identified grossly. Historically, gastrointestinal syndromes caused by *Salmonella* were thought to involve primarily the small intestine. However, recent investigations now demonstrate that colonic disease is common and that pathological changes consistent with and mimicking ulcerative colitis have been noted.[17]

A variety of risk factors for disease have been identified and include extremes of age, integrity of the gastric hydrochloric acid defense mechanism, underlying reticuloendothelial disease, intactness of the gastrointestinal flora, and load of ingested organisms.[18] Volunteer studies strongly suggest that healthy individuals must ingest 10^7–10^8 organisms to develop clinical infection. Infection with serotypes of *Salmonella* represents a truly invasive diarrhea, and many cases will be accompanied by fecal leukocytosis. Transient bacteremia is noted in 5–10% of adults and a higher percentage of children but does not necessarily mandate use of antibiotics.[18] Bloodstream invasion may not be recognized until after clinical disease has improved.

Abdominal pain is common and may be localized to the right lower quadrant, suggesting appendicitis. Fever lasts less than 3 days in most circumstances, and diarrhea tends to disappear within a week. In unusual cases it can last for prolonged periods. In otherwise healthy individuals, fluid and electrolyte disturbances are unusual but can be severe in patients at the extremes of age.

Patients diagnosed with *Salmonella* gastroenteritis should be managed supportively. Antibiotics should be witheld except in unusual circumstances of sepsis or in the presence of significant host risk factors. Studies demonstrate that use of antimicrobial agents prolongs the carrier state of this disease and does not impact on clinical outcome.[19] In unusual circumstances where antibiotics are to be employed, choice should be governed by suceptibility patterns, and use should be continued for 7–10 days. Resistance has been noted to antibiotics such as ampicillin and tetracycline. However, in the United States most strains remain susceptible to chloramphenicol and trimethoprim–sulfamethoxazole.[20] A summary of treatment regiments for selected infectious diarrheal illnesses is provided in Table 13.4.

Clinicians should report cases of documented *Salmonella* gastroenteritis to local health departments for follow-up epidemiologic studies and stool analyses. If disease has occurred in selected groups such as food handlers, patients may be

Table 13.4
Treatment Regimens for Specific Diarrheal Illnesses

Organism	Antibiotic treatment
Salmonella	None
Shigella	Trimethoprim–sulfamethoxazole
	Aminoglycosides
	?Quinolones
Campylobacter	Erythromycin
	?Quinolones
Aeromonas sp.	Trimethoprim–sulfamethoxazole
	Aminoglycosides
	?Quinolones
Yersinia	Trimethoprim–sulfamethoxazole
	Tetracyclines
	Aminoglycosides
	?Quinolones
Pseudomembranous colitis	Metronidazole
	Vancomycin
	Bacitracin

required to refrain from work until stool carriage has cleared. In general, stools will become negative within several weeks. However, carriage for up to 3 months has been seen. Unlike disease with *S. typhi,* chronic carriage within the biliary tract is not noted. For patients with intestinal carriage where early eradication may decrease lost employment time, a 5- to 7-day course of a nonabsorbable antibiotic such as paromomycin can be considered. Such an agent has activity against many enteric gram-negative bacilli but leaves other organisms such as anaerobes and *S. faecalis* intact.

Shigellosis

Diarrheal syndromes caused by *Shigella* species are globally recognized and are thought to be the most communicable of the infectious diarrheas.[21] In the United States over 93,000 isolates were reported between 1974 and 1980. Highest rates were from children less than 5 years of age.[22] However, persons of all ages can be infected, intrafamilial spread is common, and clinical manifestations can be severe and life-threatening. Studies demonstrate that ingestion of only 10^1–10^2 organisms is necessary to produce clinical disease in 25% of human volunteers.[23] After ingestion, organisms initially multiply in the small intestine but can no longer be found there after several days. Thereafter, disease is caused by local invasion of the distal colon and rectum, and classical symptoms that include tenesmus, bloody diarrhea, and severe constitutional illness are caused by organism replication and invasion in this anatomic area. By the time that clinical disease is present, 10^6–10^{10} organisms/g stool will be noted.

Disease occurs more frequently in lower socioeconomic groups and in travelers returning from areas with poor sanitation but can be seen endemically and sporadically in the absence of these conditions. Clinical presentation is usually that of crampy abdominal pain and diarrhea after an incubation that is usually under 3 days.[23] Diarrhea may initially be watery but often changes to include blood and pus after several days. Rectal urgency is often noted. Fever may be high, and prostration can be seen, but bacteremia is noted rarely. Fecal leukocytosis is often demonstrated but is not diagnostic. Cultures are usually positive if stools are appropriately managed and plated on selective *Salmonella/Shigella* media. It is of the utmost importance that stool specimens be plated promptly, because delays of only several hours can decrease the yield. A variety of transport media are available if prompt plating is impossible.

Symptomatic treatment of dehydration is indicated. Antibiotics are utilized both to decrease time of fecal shedding and to shorten the clinical course of disease. Although most patients have self-limited disease and improve within 7–10 days, occasional individuals progress to complications and may continue to have diarrhea for many weeks. The antimicrobial agents employed depend on the susceptibility pattern of the organism identified and are summarized in Table 13.4. Although many strains may remain susceptible to either ampicillin/amoxicillin or tetracyclines, increasing numbers have been shown to be resistant to these agents. Alternatives include trimethoprim–sulfamethoxazole and probably quinolones such as ciprofloxacin. Dose of the former is a single DS tablet b.i.d. for 5–7 days, whereas the latter could be administered in a dose of 250–500 mg b.i.d.

Campylobacter Species

Campylobacter fetus ss. *jejuni* represents a recently appreciated cause of acute diarrheal illness in the United States. Data demonstrate that 3–4% of patients with diarrhea may harbor this pathogen compared to 1–2% for *Salmonella* and *Shigella* combined.[15,24] The organism is rarely isolated in the absence of diarrhea.[24] Microbiologically, campylobacters are motile, comma-shaped gram-negative rods. Epidemiolically, most cases occur as a result of ingestion of contaminated food, water, or milk.[24,25] *Campylobacter jejuni* was previously underreported because of its fastidious growth requirements. Special antibiotic-impregnated media must be employed, and an environment of CO_2 and temperatue of 42°C should be provided in order optimally to isolate this organism.

Clinical disease may begin with a short, nonspecific prodrome; however, frank, often bloody diarrhea is usually noted by the second day. Lower abdominal cramping, tenderness, and occasional rebound may also be seen. Occasional patients may develop severe constitutional symptomatology. Examination of the stool often reveals fecal leukocytosis, and occasionally characteristic gram-negative "gull-wing" organisms consistent with *Campylobacter* will be seen. Proctoscopy and other invasive procedures are rarely employed but have demonstrated changes consistent with ulcerative colitis in selected patients.[10] Rare cases mimicking pseudomembranous colitis and Crohn's disease have also been reported.

Therapy is controversial. Many cases appear to be mild and self-limited and probably do not require antibiotics.[26] Organisms disappear from the stool shortly after symptoms subside, and thus neither carriage not transmission is routinely noted after clinical disease has ended. More severely ill patients should be treated with erythromycin in doses of 250–500 mg q.i.d. for periods of 5–7 days as summarized in Table 13.4.[26,27] Such treatment appears to decrease the length of diarrhea and to increase rate of clearance of the organisms.

Antibiotic-Associated Diarrhea

Diarrhea associated with the use of antimicrobial agents is common and represents one of the usual complaints referable to the use of these agents. Up to 25% of hospitalized patients treated with antibiotics may develop this condition, and the incidence in outpatients is unknown.[14] Data generated within the past decade have demonstrated the important role for *C. difficile* in many cases of antibiotic-associated diarrhea.[28] However, there is no easy method to differentiate diarrhea caused by *C. difficile* from that related to ''other'' etiologies for antibiotic-associated diarrhea. Clinical manifestations for both can include mild, insignificant illness. That associated with the presence of *C. difficile* and its toxin may also be fulminant and life-threatening. Constitutional complaints may be absent or severe, with high-grade fever, chills, and severe abdominal tenderness being occasionally noted.

Clostridium difficile is an anaerobic spore-forming gram-positive rod and has been implicated as being responsible for most cases of pseudomembraneous colitis.[28] It is found as part of the normal gastrointestinal flora in fewer than 5% of healthy adults but may be more common in patients who are hospitalized.[14] Healthy newborns are colonized in over 50% of instances and actually produce large amounts of toxin but rarely develop clinical manifestations. Use of antimicrobial agents alters normal intestinal microflora and allows colonic overgrowth with this organism. Toxin may be elaborated, and clinical disease ensues. A wide variety of antibiotics have now been shown to cause this disease. Although clindamycin received initial notoriety as being associated with it, more recent data demonstrate strong associations with the use of ampicillin or various cephalosporins. Virtually all antibiotics have been noted to cause this. However, aminoglycosides, metronidazole, and vancomycin are far less commonly associated than others. Pseudomembranous colitis has been documented following either parenteral or oral therapy. Circumstances that favor the clinical expression of disease include (1) elderly or debilitated patients, (2) patients with cancer, and (3) patients in intensive care units. In patients who are hospitalized, most cases will be noted on surgical services. Nosocomial spread has been well documented, and the organism has been identified on the hands of selected hospital personnel.[29,30]

Colitis is caused by the elaboration of at least two toxins that directly impact on the colonic epithelium. Clinical symptoms are variable. Most patients develop diarrhea, but occasional individuals may develop constitutional symptoms, abdominal discomfort, and even frank colonic perforation without any diarrhea. Typical disease begins within 1–2 weeks of initiating antibiotic therapy, and cramping accompanied by profuse diarrhea will be seen. Blood in the stools may be noted, but frank pus is unusual. Some cases will not be noted until antibiotics have been discontinued, so clinicians must be aware of the need for a careful history to document prior antibiotic usage.

Clinical management of patients with antibiotic-associated diarrhea is dependent on the severity of disease. All patients in whom this problem is noted should have the offending antibiotic discontinued. In general, there is no role for antispasmodics, optiates, or anticholinergics, since they may prolong disease. Mild disease that is unassociated with significant constitutional, abdominal, or chemical symptoms or signs is usually self-limited and requires no other specific therapy.[31] Disease associated with bloody diarrhea, major constitutional symptoms, or persistence should be assessed for the presence of *C. difficile*. Evaluation of stools for the presence of fecal leukocytes is rapid and inexpensive. Absence of these cells makes the diagnosis of pseudomembranous colitis improbable. Proctosigmoidoscopy is the safest and most timely way to establish the diagnosis.[14,31] The presence of characteristic pseudomembranes is virtually pathognomonic and allows the initiation of appropriate treatment. However, some cases have disease limited to the ascending or transverse colon and may require other studies that include colonscopy or barium enema.

Demonstration of the toxin is now accomplished through assays available commercially and stocked in most hospitals and other commercial laboratories. Results are available in 1 day. Toxin neutralization by antitoxin is necessary to confirm all positive cytotoxic tests. Optimally, tests positive by this method should be confirmed by culturing the organism on selective media, but in practice this is rarely performed. Merely isolating *C. difficile* from stools of symptomatic individuals is insufficient for diagnosis because of the possibility of carriage of this organism.

Whether to sigmidoscope all patients with significant diarrhea who receive antibiotics or whether to treat empirically and await results of toxin studies remains controversial. Clinical practice when dealing with sick patients is often to discontinue the likely offending antibiotic, assess for presence of the toxin, and initiate appropriate treatment while awaiting the results. More invasive testing should be considered if there is a specific contraindication to the use of the treatment regimens or if therapy fails to result in a timely response. Occasional patients who satisfy clinical criteria for pseudomembranous colitis may be candidates for empirical therapy despite the lack of diagnosis by invasive or laboratory means.

Specific therapy should be administered to all but the least symptomatic patients. Orally administered metronidazole or vancomycin should be considered an agent of choice and generally results in clinical improvement within 72 hr and eradication of toxin during a similar time period.[31] For patients unable to receive oral medications, there is no role of parenteral vancomycin because it does not achieve therapeutic concentrations in the gut when given by this route. Therapeutic failures have been noted with this regimen. Intravenous metronidazole should be considered the agent of choice for patients who must be treated intravenously. Oral vancomycin in doses of 125–500 mg q.i.d. for 5–7 days has generally been considered to be the ''gold standard'' of treatment for this disease; however, extremely high costs associated with the oral use of this agent spawned studies to define other therapeutic modalities. Matronidazole given in doses of 500 mg t.i.d. for 5–7 days has resulted in clinical cures in 80–90% of cases. It is generally considered to be the most cost-effective means of treatment, and studies have confirmed it to be as effective as vancomycin.[32] Oral bacitracin administrered in doses of 25,000 units q.i.d. for at least 7 days has also been proven to be as efficacious as vancomycin in alleviating diarrhea and other clinical symptomatology but is probably less effective in eradicating the organism from stool.[33] There is currently no role for anion-exchange resins such as cholestyramine.

Up to 30% of patients diagnosed with pseudomembranous colitis develop recurrences following discontinuation of the treatment agent. A second 7- to 10-day course of therapy with oral vancomycin is usually recommended and is associated with an excellent rate of response.[31] Rarely, individuals have been known to develop repeated relapses. Recommendations for these unfortunate individuals are less structured, but anecdotal evidence has suggested the use of prolonged courses of oral vancomycin for periods of up to several weeks.

Occasional individuals with pseudomembranous colitis related to *C. difficile* have developed either abdominal perforation requiring surgical exploration or bacteremia with an enteric pathogen such as *S. faecalis*.[34] The possibility of these life-threatening conditions requires constant vigilance on the part of the clinician.

Selected Other Bacterial Pathogens

Species of *Aeromonas,* a gram-negative bacillus, have been implicated as an important emerging cause of diarrheal illness. Selected data claim that it may be among the most common causes of diarrhea in the United States, and the clinical symptomatology can range from acute self-limited disease to chronic diarrhea.[35] Numerous studies now indicate that this organism is isolated more commonly in patients with diarrhea than in normal controls.[36] Identification of *Aeromonas* can be accomplished either by selective media or by further assessing organisms that are oxidase positive—a trait that distinguishes this species from most other causes of enteric illness.[36] Fecal leukocytes are uncommonly noted, and diarrhea tends to be watery. Drinking well water has been commonly implicated. Most strains are resistant to β-lactam antibiotics, but trimethoprim–sulfamethoxazole appears to result in symptomatic improvement when compared to untreated individuals.

Hemorrhagic colitis caused by *E. coli* 0157:H7 has been recognized for several years and constitutes an unusual form of diarrheal illness caused by *E. coli*. Initially recognized because of several outbreaks, it is now known to be associated with episodic disease as well.[37] Outbreaks have been associated with undercooked hamburger served in nursing homes, and this condition has been demonstrated to mimic ischemic colitis.[38] Clinically, onset is usually abrupt, with bloody diarrhea, little or absent fever, and severe abdominal cramping. Older individuals may often present without blood in stools, and the diagnosis may be difficult unless noted in an epidemic situation. Original epidemiologic assessment incriminated undercooked meat at fast-food chain restaurants, and hence the name ''Big Mac attack.'' Although the disease may be self-limited, patients considered to have this illness may benefit from antibiotic therapy with either trimethoprim–sulfamethoxazole or doxycycline. Use of antimicrobials, however, remains controversial. A recently reported outbreak of hemorrhagic colitis in a nursing home noted that mortality among residents was 35% and that antibiotic therapy was associated with higher mortality.[39] However, it appears that antibiotics may have been employed in sicker patients, and that may provide the reason for higher adverse outcome.

Diarrheal illness caused by *Yersinia enterocolitica* has been demonstrated to be the third most commonly isolated stool pathogen in selected studies, representing up to 0.7% of isolates.[40] It is a gram-negative non-lactose-fermenting rod that requires special laboratory measures to be isolated. Serological studies employing agglutinating antibody titers can also be employed for diagnosis, and titers above 1 : 128 are often noted in acute disease in otherwise healthy individuals.[41] Enteric disease caused by this organism is often seen in rural areas, and transmission has been associated with contaminated water and chocolate milk.[42] Fever, abdominal pain, and bloody diarrhea are characteristically present, although up to 10% of individuals in whom *Y. enterocolitica* is isolated are asymptomatic. Adolescents and adults may have a syndrome mimicking appendicitis with severe right lower quadrant pain, tenderness, and guarding.[43] Ileocolitis has been noted radiographically and pathologically in many individuals, and this illness should be considered in the differential diagnosis of ulcerative colitis, Crohn's disease, and appendicitis. Untreated patients with diarrhea may have illness last for many weeks. Although the organism is usually sensitive to aminoglycosides, chloramphenicol, tetracyclines, and trimethoprim–sulfamethoxazole, antibiotic efficacy for diarrhea caused by this agent is unproven.

Many younger individuals sick with this pathogen will develop extraintestinal manifestations that include reactive arthritis and erythema nodosum. The presence of such complaints make the clinician more strongly consider this pathogen, although similar problems can also be noted with *Salmonella, Shigella,* and both Crohn's disease and ulcerative colitis.

Diarrhea Caused by Cryptosporidiosis

Cryptosporidia are small protozoa that were first described as a cause of human diarrhea approximately a decade ago and were historically associated with disease in immunosuppressed patients, expecially those with AIDS. More recent data demonstrate the capacity of this protozoan to cause diarrhea in otherwise healthy individuals. Recent investigations documented that cryptosporidia were found in the stools of 2.8–4.3% of samples submitted for ova and parasite studies, that it was the most common parasite recognized, and that over 80% of isolates were from immunocompetent individuals.[44,45] It is recognized primarily in children and young adults and may be more prevalent in summer and fall. An association with *Giardia lamblia* may also exist.[45]

Disease in immunocompetent individuals presents typically with watery diarrhea, abdominal discomfort, and occasionally nausea and weight loss.[44–46] Disease is self-limited but may last for 2–4 weeks. Outbreaks associated with contaminated drinking water have been reported. Diagnosis requires that the laboratory be informed about the possibility of disease with this organism, because special methods are necessary for documentation. Although biopsy of intestinal tissue can be utilized, the protozoan can now be demonstrated in stool specimens by utilizing a modified acid-fast smear and concentration techniques.

Treatment consists of supportive therapy and withholding antibiotics. Occasional patients may require hospitalization for volume replacement.

REFERENCES

1. *Dorland's Illustrated Medical Dictionary,* ed 25. Philadelphia, W B Saunders, 1974:438.
2. Dingle JH, McCorkle LP, Badger GF, *et al:* A study of illness in a group of Cleveland families: XIII. Clinical description of acute nonbacterial gastroenteritis. *Am J Hyg* 1956; 64:368–375.
3. Guerrant RL: Principles and definition of syndromes. In: Mandell GL, Douglas RG Jr, Bennett JE, eds. *Principles and Practice of Infectious Disease,* ed 2. New York, John Wiley & Sons, 1985:635–646.
4. Gurwith M, Wenman WH, Hinde D, *et al:* A prospective study of rotavirus infection in infants and children. *J Infect Dis* 1981; 144:218–224.
5. Nichols RL: Intraabdominal sepsis: Characterization and treatment. *J Infect Dis* 1977; 135(suppl):S54–S57.
6. Blaer MD, Wells JG, Feldman RA, *et al: Campylobacter* enteritis in the United States. *Ann Intern Med* 1983; 98:360–365.
7. Gleckman RG, Hibert D: Afebrile bacteremia: A phenomenon in geriatric patients. *JAMA* 1982; 248:1478–1481.
8. Harris JC, Dupont HL, Hornick RB: Fecal leukocytosis in diarrheal disease. *Ann Intern Med* 1972; 76:697–703.
9. Pickering LK, Dupont HL, Olarge J, *et al:* Fecal leukocytes in enteric infections. *Am J Clin Pathol* 1977; 68:562–577.
10. Kaplan K: Infections caused by *Campylobacter* and *Yersinia enterocolitica. Infect Dis Pract* 1982; 5(11):1–7.
11. Speelman P, Kabir I, Islam M: Distribution and spread of colonic lesions in shigellosis: A colonoscopic study. *J Infect Dis* 1984; 150:899–902.
12. Ericsson CD, Dupont HL: Travelers diarrhea: Recent developments. In: Remington JS, Swartz MN, eds. *Current Clinical Topics in Infectious Diseases,* Vol 6. New York, McGraw-Hill, 1985:66–84.
13. Kimmey M: Infectious diarrhea. *Emerg Clin North Am* 1985; 3:127–142.
14. Fekety R: Antibiotic-associated colitis. *Infect Dis Pract* 1981; 4(4):1–7.
15. Drake AA, Gilchrist MJR, Washington, JA II, *et al:* Diarrhea due to *Campylobacter fetus* subspecies *jejuni. Mayo Clin Proc* 1981; 56:414–423.
16. Taylor DN, Bied JM, Munro S, *et al: Salmonella dublin* infections in the United States, 1979–1980. *J Infect Dis* 1982; 146:322–327.
17. Guerrant RL: Inflammatory enteritides. In: Mandell GL, Douglas RG Jr, Bennett JE, eds. *Principles and Practice of Infectious Disease,* ed 2. New York, John Wiley & Sons, 1985:660–669.

18. Rubin RH: Humanh Salmonellosis: Epidemiology, pathogenesis, and clinical syndromes. *Infect Dis Pract* 1982; 6(2):1–8.
19. Rosenthal SL: Exacerbation of *Salmonella* gastroenteritis due to ampicillin. *N Engl J Med* 1969; 280:147–148.
20. Bissett ML, Abbott SL, Wood RM: Antimicrobial resistance and R factors in *Salmonella* isolated in California (1971–1972). *Antimicrob Agents Chemother* 1974; 5:161–168.
21. Butler T, Mahmoud AAF, Warren KS: Algorithms in the diagnosis and management of exotic diseases: XXVII. Shigellosis. *J Infect Dis* 1977; 136:465–468.
22. Blaser MJ, Pollard RA, Feldman: *Shigella* infections in the United States, 1974–1980. *J Infect Dis* 1983; 147:771–777.
23. Dupont HL: *Shigella* species (bacillary dysentery). In: Mandell GL, Douglas RG Jr, Bennett JE, eds. *Principles and Practices of Infectious Disease,* ed 2. New York, John Wiley & Sons, 1985:1269–1274.
24. Blaser MJ, Reller LB: *Campylobacter* enteritis. *N Engl J Med* 1981; 305:1444–1452.
25. Blaser MJ, Cravens J, Powers BW, *et al: Campylobacter* enteritis associated with unpasteurized milk. *Am J Med* 1979; 67:715–718.
26. Blaser MJ, Berkowitz ID, LaForce FM, *et al: Campylobacter* enteritis: Clinical and epidemiologic features. *Ann Intern Med* 1979; 91:179–185.
27. Pitkanen T, Ponka A, Pettersson T, *et al: Campylobacter* enteritis in 188 hospitalized patients. *Arch Intern Med* 1983; 143:215–219.
28. Bartlett JG: Antibiotic-associated pseudomembraneous colitis. *Rev Infect Dis* 1979; 1:530–539.
29. Kim K-H, Fekety R, Batts DH, *et al:* Isolation of *Clostridium difficile* from the environment and contacts of patients with antibiotic-associated colitis. *J Infect Dis* 1981; 143:42–50.
30. Savage AM, Alford RH: Nosocomial spread of *Clostridium difficile. Infect Cont* 1983; 4:31–33.
31. Fekety R: Antibiotic-associated colitis. In: Mandell GL, Douglas Jr RG, and Bennett JE, eds. *Principles and Practice of Infectious Disease,* ed 2. New York, John Wiley & Sons, 1985:655–659.
32. Teasley DG, Olson MM, Gebbhard RL, *et al:* Prospective randomised trial of metronidazole versus vancomycin for *Clostridium-difficile*-associated diarrhoea and colitis. *Lancet* 1983; 2:1043–1046.
33. Dudley MN, McLaughlin JC, Carrington G, *et al:* Oral bacitracin vs vancomycin therapy for *Clostridium difficile*-induced diarrhea. *Arch Intern Med* 1986; 146:1101–1104.
34. Franson TR, Nelson JW, Rose HD: Pseudomembranous colitis complicated by bacteremia due to *Streptococcus faecalis. J Infect Dis* 1983; 147:165.
35. George WL, Nakata MN, Thompson J, *et al: Aeromonas*-related diarrhea in adults. *Arch Intern Med* 1985; 145:2207–2211.
36. Holmberg SD, Schell WL, Fanning GR, *et al: Aeromonas* intestinal infections in the United States. *Ann Intern Med* 1986; 105:683–689.
37. Remis RS, MacDonald KL, Riley LW, *et al:* Sporadic cases of hemorrhagic colitis associated with *Escherichia coli* 0157:H7. *Ann Intern Med* 1984; 101:624–626.
38. Ryan CA, Tauxe RV, Hosek GW, *et al: Escherichia coli* 0157:H7 diarrhea in a nursing home: Clinical, epidemiological, and pathological findings. *J Infect Dis* 1986; 154:631–638.
39. Carter AO, Borczyk AA, Carlson JAK, *et al:* A severe outbreak of *Escherichia coli* 0157:H7-associated hemmorrhagic colitis in a nursing home. *N Engl J Med* 1987; 317:1496–1500.
40. Snyder JD, Christenson E, Feldman RA: Human *Yersinia enterocolitica* infections in Wisconsin. *Am J Med* 1982; 72:768–774.
41. Bottone EJ, Sheehan DJ: *Yersinia enterocolitica:* Guidelines for serologic diagnosis of human infections. *Rev Infect Dis* 1983; 5:898–906.
42. Black RE, Jackson RJ, Tsai Y, *et al:* Epidemic *Yersinia enterocolitica* infection due to contaminated chocolate milk. N Engl J Med 1978; 298:76–79.

43. Vantrappen G, Agg HO, Ponette E, *et al: Yersinia* enteritis and enterocolitis: Gastrointestinal aspects. *Gastroenterology* 1977; 72:220–227.
44. Holley HP Jr, Dover C: *Cryptosporidium:* A common cause of parasitic diarrhea in otherwise healthy individuals. *J Infect Dis* 1986; 153:365–368.
45. Wolfson JS, Richter JM, Waldron MA, *et al:* Cryptosporidiosis in immunocompetent patients. *N Engl J Med* 1985; 312:1278–1782.
46. Weller PF: Giardiasis and cryptosporidiosis. *Infect Dis Pract* 1986; 9:1–8.

14

Cutaneous Infections in the Office Setting

Nelson M. Gantz

INTRODUCTION

The practicing clinician frequently encounters skin and soft tissue infections, which vary in severity from localized infections such as folliculitis to invasive and life-threatening illnesses such as necrotizing fasciitis. Factors that determine the extent of an infection include the infecting organism, predisposing conditions, and immunologic status of the host. A cutaneous rash may indicate a systemic disease such as toxic shock syndrome or reflect a localized process such as cellulitis. Systemic manifestations such as chills and fever may or may not be present in patients with skin and subcutaneous infections. The clinician must determine if hospitalization is indicated as well as which diagnostic studies and therapy should be initiated. Infections resulting from animal bites are discussed in Chapter 15. This chapter focuses on the common skin infections seen in the office practice.

CELLULITIS

Cellulitis is an acute inflammatory process involving the skin and deeper subcutaneous tissue. In adults who are not immunocompromised hosts, infection not involving the face is most often caused by *Staphylococcus aureus* and/or group A β-hemolytic streptococci. Less often other streptococci, particularly groups C and G, have been implicated in patients with cellulitis. Uncommon pathogens that can cause cellulitis in normal hosts include *Erysipelothrix* species,[1] *Vibrio vulnificus*,[2] *Mycobacterium marinum*,[3,4] and *Aeromonas hydrophilia*.[5]

Erysipelothrix species are gram-positive bacilli that produce a cellulitis of the extremities usually following a traumatic injury from shellfish or salt-water fish. The acute lesion is often purplish. Penicillin is the drug of choice.

Vibrio vulnificus is a curved gram-negative rod that produces cellulitis associated with exposure to salt-water or shellfish. Classically, cellulitis results from an injury sustained while cleaning crabs, peeling shrimp, shucking oysters, or with wounds exposed to sea water. The organism can produce a progressive cellulitis characterized by overlying bullae, which may be hemorrhagic. The process can extend to involve the fascia and muscle with large areas of tissue necrosis. Disease tends to be more extensive in patients with underlying illness such as liver disease. The diagnosis of *Vibrio vulnificus* infection should be suspected when any clinician encounters a progressive cellulitis with bullae formation following a salt-water or shellfish-related injury. An aspirate of the bullae may reveal curved gram-negative bacilli. A culture of fluid from a bullae aspiriate as well as blood cultures, which are positive in 38% of patients, should establish the diagnosis. Treatment consists of adequate debridement and parenteral tetracycline.

Another organism that can produce cellulitis following salt- or fresh-water exposure is *Mycobacterium marinum.* This acid-fact bacillus causes disease following a wide variety of injuries such as handling or cleaning fish, puncture wounds secondary to fish hooks, abrasions while exposed to fresh or salt water, or submersion of an open wound in a fish tank. The disease is relatively common along the Gulf Coast. The key to diagnosis is the presence of a nonpyogenic lesion of an extremity with an appropriate epidemiologic exposure history. Local dissemination of the infection can result in subcutaneous nodules that mimic sporotrichosis. The diagnosis is usually made by culturing a surgical specimen of a lesion for *Mycobacteria.* Histological examination shows granulomas, but acid-fast bacilli are not usually seen on special stains. The organism grows readily on Lowenstein–Jensen agar at 32°C but not at the usual temperature (35° to 37°C) used for most cultures. Optimal treatment for this disease is unknown, but single-drug therapy with trimethoprim–sulfamethoxazole or doxycycline has been efficacious. The usual duration of therapy is 3 months.[4]

Aeromonas species are gram-negative bacilli that can cause cellulitis associated with a traumatic injury related to fresh-water exposure. *Aeromonas hydrophilia* are usually susceptible to the aminoglycosides or the third-generation cephalosporins.

In evaluating a normal host with cellulitis, it is important to search for a portal of entry for the organism such as an ulcer, fissure, or abrasion. Underlying illnesses including drug addiction, diabetes mellitus, and alcoholism predispose a patient to develop cellulitis. Local factors such as peripheral vascular disease or lymphedema secondary to surgery for breast cancer also predispose a patient to develop cellulitis. It is helpful to delineate the margins of the cellulitis with a skin marker in order to follow the response to therapy. The temperature, white blood cell count, and sedimentation rate are not invariably elevated in a patient with cellulitis. An aspirate of the area of cellulitis is rarely helpful in identifying the cause of the cellulitis in a normal host. Similarly, blood cultures are usually sterile but are indicated if hospitalization is deemed necessary.

Cellulitis in a granulocytopenic host generally should be treated in the hospital. One has to consider the usual pathogens such as *S. aureus* and streptococci as well as gram-negative aerobic bacilli, anaerobes, *Candida* species, and *Cryptococcus neoformans*. Diagnosis requires that blood cultures be obtained and that a surgical wedge biopsy of the area be cultured for aerobes, anaerobes, fungi, and mycobacteria. A portion of the biopsy should be sent for histological examination including special stains.

In a normal host with cellulitis in the hospitalized setting, administration of oxacillin or nafcillin would be appropriate. Alternative agents include cefazolin, erythromycin, or clindamycin. A cephalosporin such as cefazolin should be avoided if a patient has a history of an immediate reaction to penicillin. Suitable outpatient antibiotic agents include cloxacillin, dicloxacillin, cephalexin, cephradine, cefadroxil, erythromycin, or clindamycin. In a patient with cellulitis that fails to respond to ''appropriate'' therapy, consider the possibility of a resistant pathogen or an alternative process such as gout, phlebitis, vasculitis, or underlying osteomyelitis. In patients with a coexistent tinea pedis infection and cellulitis, it is critical to treat the superficial fungal infection to prevent recurrences. Recurrent cellulitis may also occur in hospital workers who produce the cellulitis factitiously. Recurrent streptococcal cellulitis is especially a problem in patients with imparied lymphatic drainage secondary to nodal dissection, irradiation, or an abnormal perineal lymphatic system.

ERYSIPELAS

Erysipelas is a form of cellulitis involving primarily the superficial layers of the skin. There is marked swelling with a sharp demarcation between normal skin and the involved tissue. Classically, erysipelas occurs on the face and is caused by group A streptococci. Certain patients will have frequent recurrences of erysipelas at the same site. Penicillin is the drug of choice, given intravenously in a dosage of 12 million units per day. During the convalescent stage, desquamation often occurs.

TOXIC-SHOCK-LIKE ILLNESS

A toxic-shock-like syndrome in patients with group A β-hemolytic streptococci has been described that resembles staphylococcal toxic shock syndrome except that the strawberry tongue and desquamation are lacking.[6]

FOLLICULITIS

Folliculitis is an inflammatory process localized to the hair follicles. Most infections are caused by *S. aureus,* but *Pseudomonas aeruginosa* has been associated with many outbreaks involving whirlpools, hot tubs, and swimming pools.[7] The incubation period for *P. aeruginosa* folliculitis is about 48 hr and ranges from 8 hr to 5 days. The rash typically involves the buttocks, hips, axilla, arms, and thighs and spares the palms and soles. The rash is usually pruritic. Associated features may include earache, malaise, headache, mastitis, and low-grade fever. The rash can be confused with lesions caused by insect bites, scabies, contact dermatitis, or staphylococcal folliculitis. The rash heals without scarring, and specific anti-*Pseudomonas* therapy is not required. The use of topical corticosteroids to treat the disease should be avoided. Outbreaks can be prevented by maintenance of proper pH and appropriate chlorine levels of greater than 0.5 mg per liter of the whirlpool water.[8] Topical antistaphylococcal ointments such as bacitracin ointment are often used to treat staphylococcal folliculitis, but controlled studies are lacking. Use of hexachlorophene or chlorhexidine solution may facilitate healing and prevent recurrences. However, controlled trials using hexachlorophene or chlorhexidine are not available.

FURUNCULOSIS

Furunculosis, a deeper inflammatory process than folliculitis, and cutaneous abscesses, localized collections of pus, are two problems frequently encountered by the practicing clinician. *Staphylococcus aureus* is involved most often. Predisposing factors include obesity, diabetes mellitus, corticosteroid therapy, and patients with granulocyte function defects. For most patients with furunculosis, no predisposing risk factors can be identified, particularly in those individuals with recurrent furunculosis. Many furuncles drain spontaneously or following the application of moist heat. Larger abscesses require a surgical incision for drainage. Penicillinase-resistant penicillins such as oral dicloxacillin or cloxacillin are indicated for therapy of larger lesions if there is an associated cellulitis present. Oral antibiotics are also indicated if there is fever or if the process involves the midface area or hands. Management of the patient with recurrent furunculosis is not satisfactory, and various strategies have been employed including use of intranasal antibiotic ointments, continuous antistaphylococcal suppressive therapy at low doses, hexachlorophene or chlorhexidine showers to reduce staphylococcal skin counts, and combinations of antibiotics such as antistaphylococcal penicillins plus rifampin. Clindamycin in combination with rifampin may also be tried for patients with recurrent furunculosis.[9,10]

VARICELLA–ZOSTER

Varicella–zoster, or recrudescent chickenpox, generally presents few diagnostic problems for the clinician. However, the rash may be preceded by pain and paresthesias. The initial lesions can be macules, but eventually vesicles develop. Herpes simplex virus can also produce vesicles in a dermatomal distribution. Predisposing factors for varicella–zoster include increasing age, lymphoproliferative neoplasms, irradiation, and chemotherapy. However, 40% of cases of zoster occur in persons under 40 years of age. In a patient with zoster, there is no need to undertake a work-up for an occult neoplasm. Two therapeutic problems in patients with zoster are the risk of dissemination of the virus in an immunocompromised host and the prevention of postherpetic neuralgia. In immunocompromised patients, acyclovir prevents both cutaneous and visceral dissemination of the zoster virus and results in a more rapid resolution of the pain compared with a placebo. Acyclovir has to be given within 72 hr of the onset of infection and should be administered every 8 hr in a dose of 10 mg/kg if renal function is normal.[11] Postherpetic pain occurs in 50% of persons at 1 month and 25% of individuals at 3 months among those with herpes zoster above 60 years of age. Although corticosteroids have for years been recommended to prevent postherpetic pain, in a recent randomized controlled study, prednisolone did not prevent this complication.[12] Preliminary data suggest that oral acyclovir can reduce the severity of the pain in a normal host with zoster if given in a dose of 800 mg five times each day for a week in patients with normal renal function.[13] Zoster immune globulin does not prevent dissemination, nor does it prevent the development of postherpetic pain. Agents that can reduce the postherpetic pain of zoster include antidepressants such as amitriptyline, anticonvulsants, and local and regional anesthetics.

LYME DISEASE

Annular lesions that vary from a few centimeters in diameter to as many as 68 cm (average 16 cm) following a tick bite should suggest a diagnosis of Lyme disease. The lesion expands over the next 3 to 32 days and has a ringlike border and a pale center. The lesion has a predilection for intertriginous areas such as the thighs, groin, and axillae. The lesion contains the spirochete *Borellia burgdorferi*. The tick is tiny, and only half the patients can recall a tick bite. Secondary annular lesions unrelated to a tick bite occur in half the patients. The lesions persist for about 3 weeks and may recur. A flulike illness can accompany the cutaneous manifestations. The diagnosis can be confirmed by detecting specific antibody, IgM and IgG, to *B. burgdorferi* and noting a fourfold change in titer.[14] The antibody test can be negative during the first 2 weeks of the infection.

Tetracycline is the drug of choice in nonpregnant adults and children over 8 years of age. Treatment with tetracycline will prevent the later complications of the disease—cardiac disease, neurological disease, or arthritis. Tetracycline should be given in a dosage of 250 mg orally four times a day for 10 days. Alternative agents that can be used when a tetracycline is contraindicated include penicillin or ceftriaxone.[15,16]

ERYTHEMA NODOSUM

Erythema nodosum is the most common cause of inflammatory nodules of the legs. This cutaneous reaction is associated with a number of different underlying disorders.[17–19] Although the mechanism responsible for the syndrome remains unknown, it is probably an immunologically mediated host reaction to a number of unrelated infectious, inflammatory, or hormonal disorders. The lesions consist of discrete, tender, erythematous, indurated nodules, 1 to 5 cm in diameter, with a bruised appearance, occurring predominantly in the pretibial areas and lasting 3 to 6 weeks. Variations on this theme occur occasionally, and adjacent nodules may coalesce into larger lesions. They may also evolve without the bruised appearance and last several months. Although much less common, erythema nodosum may occur on the buttocks, soles, and the extensor surface of the arm. In addition to the specific lesions, patients commonly have constitutional symptoms of chills, fever, and malaise. There may be an associated edema of the legs and arthralgias usually involving the ankles or knees. Radiologically, hilar lymphadenopathy may occur. Laboratory abnormalities frequently include an elevated sedimentation rate, leukocytosis, mild anemia, and an increase in γ-globulin. Other laboratory abnormalities may provide a clue to the specific disorder associated with erythema nodosum.

The disease occurs predominantly in women. During its peak incidence in the third and fourth decades of life, women account for 90% of cases. The sex ratio is nearly equal in other age groups. The disease is uncommon in children younger than 15 years old. The female predominance also occurs in patients with histoplasmosis and coccidioidomycosis. The epidemiology of disorders associated with erythema nodosum also has changed in recent years. Before the 1950s, tuberculosis was a common cause associated with erythema nodosum, whereas today this is an infrequent cause. In Europe, infection with *Yersinia* species is a common cause of erythema nodosum.

Usually the diagnosis of erythema nodosum is made by the clinical appearance of the lesions, but since the differential diagnosis of tender nodules on the legs includes erythema induratum, nodular vasculitis, panniculitis secondary to pancreatitis or pancreatic carcinoma, polyarthritis nodosa, leukemic infiltrates, superficial thrombophlebitis, cryptococcal cellulitis, Sweet's syndrome, and factitial disease, it is best to confirm the diagnosis by a skin biopsy. The pathological changes that occur primarily in the subcutaneous tissue consist of lymphocytic and neutrophilic cell infiltration around the small vessels of the fibrous septa as well as between the individual fat cells at the periphery of the lobule. Some areas may show histiocytes, giant cells, and extravasation of red blood cells. It should be emphasized from a technical standpoint that the findings vary within each nodule so that an ellipse biopsy containing subcutaneous fat is essential to supply a large enough specimen to make an adequate diagnosis. The smaller punch biopsy is usually inadequate.[20]

Once a diagnosis of erythema nodosum is made, a search for an underlying disorder must begin.[21,22] In approximately one third to one half of the patients, no precipitating disorder can be identified. The most common disorders that are associated with erythema nodosum with decreasing frequency are infections, sarcoidosis, inflammatory bowel disease, drug reactions, and hormonal disturbances (Table 14.1).

Streptococcal infections probably account for the majority of the cases of erythema nodosum in the United States. Typically, lesions occur about 2 weeks after streptococcal pharyngitis or less commonly after cellulitis. Especially in children, but also in adults, erythema nodosum may develop with onset of primary tuberculosis at the time of or slightly prior to the conversion of the PPD

Table 14.1
Disorders Associated with Erythema Nodosum

Infections/agent
Group A β-hemolytic streptococci
Yersinosis
Salmonellosis
Chlamydial
Campylobacter
Mycobacterial
Histoplasmosis
Coccidioidomycosis
Syphilis
Lymphogranuloma venereum
Psittacosis
Drugs
Estrogens
Oral contraceptives
Sulfonamides
Iodides
Bromides
Miscellaneous
Inflammatory bowel disease, ulcerative colitis
Sarcoidosis
Behcet's disease

skin test. Geographic considerations are important in pursuing the etiology. For example, coccidioidomycosis frequently causes erythema nodosum in the San Joaquin Valley of California. Histoplasmosis is a common cause of erythema nodosum in the Mississippi and Missouri Valleys. In Scandinavian countries, *Yersinia enterocolitica,* which may produce symptoms of gastroenteritis and mesenteric arthritis, has been associated frequently with erythema nodosum. Other infectious diseases less commonly reported with erythema nodosum include infectious mononucleosis, toxoplasmosis, *Salmonella* gastroenteritis, leptospirosis, hepatitis B, syphilis, and recently *Campylobacter* gastroenteritis. The erythema-nodosum-like lesions occurring with leprosy are unique in that the mycobacterial organisms are found in the lesions, a finding limited to this infection. Special stains for acid-fast bacilli should be obtained on a portion of the skin biopsy specimen.

After infectious disorders, the next most common cause of erythema nodosum is sarcoidosis. Erythema nodosum is an early manifestation of sarcoidosis and occurs in approximately 20% of patients. The typical patient has erythema nodosum, bilateral hilar adenopathy, arthralgias, and a low-grade fever.

Approximately 10% of patients with ulcerative colitis and less often with regional enteritis will have erythema nodosum. Early in the course of inflammatory bowel disease, the activity of erythema nodosum parallels the activity of the gastrointestinal disease; however, after approximately 2 years, this is no longer true. Erythema nodosum has also been associated with Behçet's disease and Reiter's syndrome.

With the exception of oral contraceptives, drugs very seldom cause erythema nodosum. Those drugs that infrequently have been implicated are sulfonamides, iodides, and bromides.

The pathogenesis of erythema nodosum remains an enigma.

The evaluation of erythema nodosum should include a detailed study of antecedent illnesses, a complete physical examination, complete blood count, sedimentation rate, intermediate PPD skin test, chest x ray, and possibly a skin biopsy. With the appropriate geographical history, a fungal etiology should be pursued with complement-fixation titers for histoplasmosis or coccidioidomycosis. An ASLO titer or streptozyme test may be helpful in establishing a streptococcal etiology. If gastrointestinal complaints are present, then the patient should have stool cultures for *Salmonella, Campylobacter,* and *Yersinia* species. Barium studies are indicated for possible inflammatory bowel disease. A scalene node biopsy is helpful in distinguishing patients with sarcoidosis who have bilateral hilar adenopathy from those with idiopathic erythema nodosum.

Presently, there is no established treatment for erythema nodosum. The skin lesions are usually self-limited and resolve without therapy within 3 to 6 weeks. Bruiselike lesions may persist for months, but recurrences are rare. Specific therapy, if available, should be directed at the underlying disorder. Some patients may benefit from rest and salicylates for pain. Corticosteroids are only marginally effective and may worsen the underlying illness. Corticosteroids are contraindicated if the underlying illness is unknown. The role of the nonsteroidal antiinflammatory agents, such as indomethacin or naproxen, also remains unclear.

REFERENCES

1. Grieco M, Sheldon C: *Erysipelothrix rhusiopathiae. Ann NY Acad Sci* 1970; 174:523–532.
2. Wickbolt LG, Sanders CV: *Vibrio vulnificus* infection. A case report and update since 1970. *J Acad Dermatol* 1983; 9:243–251.
3. Grange JM: Mycobacteria and the skin. *Int J Dermatol* 1982; 21:497–503.
4. Wallace RJ: Nontuberculous mycobacteria and water: A love affair with increasing clinical importance. *Infect Dis Clin North Am* 1987; 1:677–686.
5. Hanson PG, Standridge J, Jarrett F, *et al:* Freshwater wound infection due to *Aeromonas hydrophilia. JAMA* 1977; 238:1053–1054.
6. Hirsch ML, Kass EH: An annotated bibliography of toxic shock syndrome. *Rev Infect Dis* 1986; 8:51.
7. Feder HM Jr, Grant-Kels JM, Tilton RC: *Pseudomonas* whirlpool dermatitis: Report of an outbreak in two families. *Clin Pediatr* 1983; 22:638–642.
8. David BJ. Whirpool operation and the prevention of infection. *Infect Control* 1985; 6:394–397.
9. Wheat LJ, Kohler RB, White AL, *et al:* Effect of rifampin on nasal carriers of coagulase-positive staphylococci. *J Infect Dis* 1981; 144:177.
10. McAnally TP, Lewis MR, Brown DR: Effect of rifampin and bacitracin on nasal carriers of *Staphylococcus aureus. Antimicrob Agents Chemother* 1984; 25:422–426.
11. Shepp DH, Dandliker PS, Meyers JD: Treatment of varicella–zoster virus infection in severely immunocompromised patients: A randomized comparison of acyclovir and vidarabine. *N Engl J Med* 1986; 314:208–212.
12. Esmann V, Geil JP, Kroon S, *et al:* Prednisolone does not prevent post-herpetic neuralgia. *Lancet* 1987; 2:126–129.
13. Bean B, Braun C, Balfour HH Jr: Acyclovir therapy for acute herpes zoster. *Lancet* 1982; 2:118–121.
14. Shrestha M, Grodzicki RL, Steere AC: Diagnosing early Lyme disease. *Am J Med* 1985; 78:235–240.
15. Steere AC, Green J, Shoen RT, *et al:* Successful parenteral penicillin therapy of established Lyme arthritis. *N Engl J Med* 1985; 312:869–874.
16. Steere AC, Hutchinson GJ, Rahn DW, *et al:* Treatment of the early manifestations of Lyme disease. *Ann Intern Med* 1983; 99:22–26.
17. Weinstein L: Erythema nodosum. *Disease-a-Month* 1969; 1–30.
18. Weinstein AJ: Erythema nodosum. *Infect Dis Pract* 1981; 5:2–4.
19. Soderstrom RM, Krull EA: Erythema nodosum: A review. *Cutis* 1978; 21:806–810.
20. Winkelmann RK: New observations in the histopathology of erythema nodosum. *J Invest Dermatol* 1975; 65:441–446.
21. White JW Jr: Erythema nodosum. *Dermatol Clin* 1985; 3:119–127.
22. Bullock WE: The clinical significance of erythema nodosum. *Hosp Pract* 1986; 21:102E–102H, 102K–102L, 102Q–102R.

ADDITIONAL READING

Strams SE, Ostrove JM, Inchsupé G, *et al:* Varicella–zoster virus infections. Biology, natural history, treatment and prevention. *Ann Intern Med* 1988; 108:221–237.

Watson PN, Evans RJ: Postherpetic neuralgia: A review. *Arch Neurol* 1986; 43:836–840.

Ginsberg MB: Cellulitis: Analysis of 101 cases and review of the literature. *South Med J* 1981; 74:530–533.

15

Management of Bites from Dogs, Cats, and Humans

Richard B. Brown

INTRODUCTION

Bites constitute an important cause of morbidity and occasional mortality and are responsible for a significant percentage of health care costs in the United States. Best data suggest that approximately 1% of emergency room visits are for this problem and that at least one million such injuries occur each year.[1,2] This may result in direct health care costs of at least $30 million annually.[3] These numbers may be major understatements, since many persons with bite injuries may never seek medical attention.

Bites may be attributable to a diverse variety of creatures that include sharks, monkeys, camels, rats, snakes, spiders, and farm animals. However, in the United States, bites from humans, dogs, and cats comprise well over 90% of all such incidents.[4] Dog bites are most common and probably account for 80–90% of this percentage.[4,5] Although most bites are clinically unimportant, up to 10% may require the placement of sutures, and 2% of patients are hospitalized.[6] The primary care practitioner must be well trained in the assessment and management of this rather common problem, because misjudgment may result in significant infectious complications that can result in need for major surgical debridement, amputation, and occasionally death. However, a truly scientific approach is hindered by the lack of sound prospective investigational data. As a result, decisions regarding matters as important as the indications and timing of suturing, use of antimicrobial agents, and indications for hospitalization are based on anecdotal experiences and retrospective analyses that are flawed by both small numbers of patients and many uncontrolled variables.

Nevertheless, evaluation of the bite wound must recognize the potential for several important infectious complications. All must be assessed in every patient who presents with this problem:

1. Potential for bacterial and other infections.
2. Possibility of tetanus.
3. Likelihood of rabies in the biting animal.

Different bite injuries carry variable risks with regard to the three items listed above. The following discussion covers issues relevant to the management of bites, with especial regard to the wide variety of potential infectious complications. Specifics detailing management of rabies and tetanus are not presented at this time. A general discussion concerning management of bites is followed by sections dealing specifically with those from humans, dogs, and cats. Each of these has unique features that include likely bacteriology of bite wound infections, likely types of wounds, and implications for debridement and antibiotic usage.

INITIAL BITE WOUND MANAGEMENT

Persons recently bitten usually seek medical attention either through the office of a primary practice physician or through some form of urgent care center. Initial assessment must take into account a variety of factors that are summarized in Table 15.1. A careful history of the events that led to the bite, the

Table 15.1
Initial Assessment of Bite Wounds

- I. History
  - A. Cause of the bite
  - B. Type of provocation
  - C. Immune status of patient and biter
  - D. Elapsed time since bite
  - E. Management prior to medical attention
  - F. Allergic history (esp. tetanus, rabies, antibiotics)
- II. Physical examination
  - A. Presence of active infection
    - 1. Purulence
    - 2. Cellulitis, lymphangitis
  - B. Extent of wound
    - 1. Through skin
    - 2. Involvement of tendons, bone, joint space
    - 3. Presence of tissue crush injury
  - C. Clinical "toxicity" of patient

underlying conditions of the patient, and prior management of the bite are essential pieces of information. The source of the bite provides data concerning the likelihood of infection and the probable pathogens. Risk of rabies will be made available through information concerning the type of biting animal and the degree of provocation, The tetanus status of the patient and an allergic history regarding tetanus or rabies immunization and antibiotics is essential. Time elapsed since the bite provides important information concerning the likelihood of infection and the type of surgical closure that can be safely utilized (*vide infra*). In general, bite wounds can be broken down into those seen within 8 hr and those seen after 12 hr. Those seen earlier are less likely to be clinically infected, and the patient usually seeks medical attention for rabies or tetanus prophylaxis and surgical wound closure.[5] Those patients with wounds seen more than 12 hr after the bite are most often demonstrated to be infected and to require aggressive medical and surgical management.[5]

Physical examination must always evaluate the severity of illness of the patient; however, the vast majority of individuals who present with bites are not clinically toxic.[7] The presence of infection must be assessed on clinical grounds, and the examiner should especially seek to document the presence of purulent material, cellulitis, or lymphangitis. A putrid smell or the presence of crepitus makes anaerobic infection likely. The extent of the bite must be carefully ascertained. Many types of bite wounds may appear far more innocuous to casual inspection than they actually are, and complications will undoubtedly occur if initial assessment underestimates the needs for drainage and debridement. The physician must compulsively evaluate the bite wound for depth. It is critical to determine if the injury involved full skin thickness and whether deeper structures, such as joints or bones, were compromised. In all cases, except for the most trivial injuries, wound assessment should be carried out with the use of a regional block employing 1% procaine and the use of either a tourniquet or an inflated blood pressure cuff to provide a bloodless field. The area of injury should be put through range of motion maneuvers, and it will often be necessary to extend the original lesion to evaluate better underlying tissues. All areas of injury should be carefully charted; pictures provide important documentation of extent of injury and can be utilized for later comparisons if necessary.

The wounds should be carefully cleansed and irrigated with large volumes of sterile saline employing a 19-gauge needle and a large syringe. A pressure of approximately 10–20 psi is advisable and may reduce wound infections by up to 80%.[8] With regard to tear injuries, any necrotic or devitalized tissue should be debrided to prevent later infection. Debridement of puncture wounds is more controversial; however, some authorities recommend complete surgical excision of all puncture wounds.[1] Depending on the extent of the bite wound, this may be performed in the outpatient setting or may require a formal operative procedure. Any evidence of joint penetration or bone compromise is grounds for hospitalization and operation.[3,9] Wounds in proximity to bones and joints should be x-rayed to evaluate compromise to these areas and to act as baseline studies in the event of later complications such as septic arthritis or osteomyelitis. If infection is present, Gram stains and cultures for both aerobic and anaerobic organisms should be obtained. In most instances, the presence of frank infection will be an indication for hospitalization, surgical debridement, and intravenous antibiotics.

Suturing of wounds is controversial. Most physicians will suture wounds of the face if less than 8 hr old because of the potential cosmetic consequences of doing otherwise.[4] Those wounds that are obviously infected and those that are more than 12 hr old should generally be left to heal either by secondary intention or by delayed primary closure after 3–5 days.[4,5,9] Infections of the hand may prove to be an exception to this rule—most authorities recommend against primary suturing. Final steps should consist of elevation and immobilization of the area, if possible, in a functional position and the initiation of an exercise program by a physical therapist.

An antibiotic will usually be prescribed, although there have been few well-controlled studies demonstrating their utility in the absence of frank infection, and the efficacy of selected agents has been poorly studied. Those injuries that present with overt infection will always require antibiotic treatment. However, it must be stressed that antibiotics should never be considered a substitute for optimal drainage or debridement, as it is unlikely that sufficient amounts of antimicrobial agent can penetrate through pus or dead and devitalized tissue to effect cure. In all instances, the bite wound must be carefully and regularly reassessed to document healing and freedom from infection. Evaluation of the patient's immune status against tetanus and the rabies status of the biter, when appropriate, should not be omitted, and appropiate measures to deal with these issues should be initiated at the time of the first visit. Immunization is discussed in Chapter 1.

HUMAN BITES

Human bites constitute an increasingly important form of bite injury, with a rate of at least 60 bites/100,000 population reported from some areas.[10] In New York City human bites are the third most common form of bite injury (following those caused by dogs and cats) and comprise 10% of all mammalian bites.[10] Although 40–80% of human bite injuries are secondary to altercations between two persons,[11,12] other causes include self-infliction through nail or lip biting, "love nips" incurred during sexual activities, and as part of the battered-child syndrome. Wounds that are received from fights can result in either puncture wounds, tear injuries, or a specific form of trauma known as clenched-fist injuries. With regard to the latter, although any part of the body may be potentially affected, at least 60% involve the hand or upper extremity. Most frequently the terminal phalanges of the long or index fingers of the dominant hand are involved. Other sites include the head or neck (15–20%), trunk (10–20%), lower extremities (5%), and other locations (5–10%).[13] In general, wounds that result from human bites are more likely to become infected than those inflicted by other mammals.[3] Risks appear to range from 25 to 50% and to correlate with length of time until medical therapy, extent of the wound, and the causative pathogens.[14–16] Those patients who defer treatment for more than 8 hr have at least a 27% incidence of infection despite hospitalization and parenteral antibiotic therapy. This is in part because of the extremely high levels of bacteria seen in the human mouth, the poor resistance of some areas of the body (such as the joint space) to infection, and a more prolonged delay in seeking medical attention.[3,9]

Human bite infections result from the inoculation of large numbers of oropharyngeal flora into normally sterile tissue spaces. Less important is contamination resulting from skin flora. The mouth houses several hundred different varieties of aerobic and anaerobic bacteria, the largest numbers of which exist in plaque and in the gingival crevices.[9] Numbers of up to 10^{11} organisms/g of tissue have been observed and are at least 10^5 higher than the amount necessary to cause significant soft tissue infection.

Organisms most likely to be implicated in human bite wound infections are summarized in Table 15.2. Historically, *S. aureus* and the viridans streptococci ("α-hemolytic streptococci") were most commonly implicated.[17,18] More recent data demonstrate a major role for oral anaerobes, *Eikenella corrodens,* and spirochetes.[18–21] Most commonly implicated anaerobes include *Bacteroides* species (especially *B. melaninogenicus*), *Fusobacterium nucleatum,* and species of *Peptococcus* and *Veillonella.* The increased role of anaerobes has been noted in bites in children as well as adults.[21] In many instances, cultures of human bites will reveal combinations of pathogens, all representing "oral flora"; however, *Eikenella corrodens* may assume a major role in selected human infections.[19,22] This slow-growing fastidious aerobic gram-negative rod may be iso-

Table 15.2
Bacteriology of Human Bite Wounds

Aerobes and facultative organisms	Anaerobes
Common	
Viridans streptococci	*B. melaninogenicus*
S. aureus	*B. intermedius*
Eikenella corrodens	Other *Bacteroides* sp.
	Flavobacterium nucleatum
Less common	*Veillonella* spp.
S. epidermidis	*Peptococcus* spp.
β- and γ-Hemolytic streptococci	Actinomyces
Corynebacterium species	Spirochetes
Other	

lated in pure culture, although more commonly it will exist in mixtures with other aerobic and anaerobic organisms. One study of 30 patients with clenched-fist injuries demonstrated that 20% of such injuries where *E. corrodens* was implicated may demonstrate this pathogen in pure culture.[19] The consideration of this organism will prompt specific antibiotic therapy (*vide infra*). Of note, there is little evidence for a major role of enteric gram-negative rods in the pathogenesis of human infection. Thus, organisms such as *E. coli, K. pneumoniae, P. aeruginosa,* and others do not need to be routinely covered in initial antibiotic management. Rarely, cases of tuberculosis, herpetic whitlow, syphilis, and other uncommon illnesses may be transmitted by human bites. Their presence should be suspected on the basis of an appropriate history and physical examination.

Clenched-fist injuries represent a common and frequently complicated form of human bite that more often results in infection than other forms of human bites.[22] They result from the closed fist impacting on the teeth of a second person and can cause 1/4 to 1/2-inch lacerations over the metacarpophalangeal joints of the dominant hand.[6] In many instances, the person does not seek early medical attention because the injury appears trivial and the patient may be embarrassed to explain the details of the injury. It is only when symptoms of infection arise, typically 12–24 hr later, that the patient is seen in a medical facility. The lesion that appears superficial may actually represent the tip of a much more significant iceberg because of the limited amount of subcutaneous tissue that separates the skin from the web spaces, tendons, bones, and joints of the hand. The seemingly trivial superficial insult may allow large numbers of bacteria from on or around the teeth to enter these deeper structures. Actual fracture may occur but is not necessary for the pathogenesis of this infectious problem. Because of dissimilarities of hand anatomy in the clenched and open positions, the physician may fail to recognize the tissue planes that were violated and thus overlook the true extent of the injury. Additionally, the changes in anatomic relationships may prevent drainage and allow still deeper entry of bacteria into tissues.

Most patients who develop complications of clenched-fist injuries will present, after a period of at least 12 hr, with established infection.[3,5,6] The wound will typically demonstrate a malodorous gray discharge, and the patient will complain of swelling, tenderness, and diminished movement of the afflicted region of the hand. In most instances, neither severe patient "toxicity," lymphangitis, nor fever is seen. Examination of the hand by a trained specialist is always indicated in order to assess the extent of bone and joint injury and the presence of sensory or motor dysfunction. Hospitalization is usually indicated for formal wound exploration and debridement in the operating room. The unusual person who presents within the first 8 hr of injury and who does not demonstrate bone, joint capsule, or tendon involvement may be successfully managed in the outpatient area and treated with oral antimicrobial agents.[23] It must always be noted that this cohort of patients will often prove to be noncompliant and may be lost to outpatient follow-up in at least 25% of instances.

Most authorities feel that antibiotics should be routinely employed in patients with human bite wounds.[3,5,6,9] Choice should be based on the extent of injury, allergic history of the patient, and suspected pathogens. Despite the fact that patients seen early in the course of injury may have no clinical evidence of infection, the use of antibiotics should always be considered "therapeutic" (i.e., treatment of subclinical infection) rather than "prophylactic." No consensus exists with regard to optimal antibiotic choice; however, many investigators have recommended the combination of penicillin VK plus an antistaphylococcal penicillin such as dicloxacillin in patients with mild injury capable of outpatient treatment.[3] This regimen provides excellent coverage for the usually encountered oral anaerobes as well as species of *S. aureus,* viridans streptococci, and *E. corrodens.* However, some data exist that demonstrate that up to 21% of *Bacteroides* spp. isolated from bite wounds are penicillin-resistant.[24] Usual dosage is 250–500 mg four times daily for each drug. More recently, amoxicillin/clavulanic acid (Augmentin®) in a dose of 250–500 mg thrice daily has been demonstrated to be as effective as the combination of penicillin VK plus dicloxacillin[25] and allows treatment with a single agent. Some investigators now consider this to be the drug of choice for mammalian bites.[21,26]

Agents such as clindamycin and "first-generation" cephalosporins [cephalexin (Keflex®) or cefadroxil (Duracef®, Ultracef®) have frequently been employed for human bites but lack activity against *E. corrodens.*[24] It is the author's opinion that unless definitive absence of this pathogen has been proven, these antimicrobials should not be routinely employed for mammalian bites. The penicillin-intolerant patient is probably best treated with a tetracycline, although some strains of *S. aureus* will be resistant to this agent. Patients who require hospitalization will usually be started on intravenous antibiotics. No scientifically valid data are available that compare different parenteral regimens; however, some recommendations for the combination of aqueous penicillin G plus either nafcillin/oxacillin or a first-generation cephalosporin exist.[13] Penicillin G will usually be administered in doses of 2–3 million units every 4 hr, but 1–2 g every 4–6 hr for the semisynthetic penicillin or cephalosporin should suffice. Dose will depend in part on the extent of injury and the presence of bone or joint involvement. Alternatively, the use of ticarcillin/clavulanic acid (Timentin®) as monotherapy has proven reliable in several cases of infected mammalian bite wounds.[27,28]

Length of antibiotic therapy will be contingent on the extent of infection and clinical response. Patients with minor, clinically noninfected bites can be successfully managed with approximately 5 days of antibiotics. If infection is present, a minimum of 10–14 days of treatment is usually necessary. Therapy should be continued until significant clinical improvement is noted. Those unfortunate individuals with septic arthritis, osteomyelitis, or deep tendon infections may require parenteral therapy for 4–6 weeks. Much of this may now take the form of home i.v. therapy, which allows many such patients to be managed outside of the hospital.

The use of hyperbaric oxygen for severe human bite wound infections of the hand has recently been assessed. In a population of patients admitted to a large general hospital, use of hyperbaric oxygen administered via a portable bedside unit resulted in significant shortening of hospital stay for patients with severe injuries.[29] Further studies are needed to support this contention.

Time to functional recovery will vary with the extent of the injury. With minor injuries, several days will suffice. However, for cases of osteomyelitis or septic arthritis, months may be necessary for full functional recovery. Severe cases that either are mismanaged or are treated after prolonged presence of infection may result in permanent loss of function or may require amputation for cure of infection.

DOG BITES

Dog bites have justifiably been referred to as "an unrecognized epidemic."[30] Between 1965 and 1972, the number of reported injuries increased from 27,700 to 37,900,[30] and 13 states listed approximately 135,000 animal bites (mostly dog bites) in 1976.[31] Best estimates are that a minimum of one million dog-bite injuries occur in the United States each year.[3] Up to 20 deaths per year are directly attributable to this injury.[32] Fifty percent of dog bites occur in persons under the age of 20, almost 60% occur in males, and most are demonstrated during the summer.[33] Seventy percent of injuries occur on the extremities. Twenty percent occur on the right upper extremity, 30% are equally distributed between the lower extremities, and 12% occur on the left upper extremity. Almost 11% of injuries were about the face. The latter bites are most commonly seen in children under 4 years old, where annual rates of dog bites may be as high as 152/100,000 population.[34] Thus, up to 44,000 significant facial bites may occur annually in the United States. Multiple bites occurred in 5% of patients.

Most commonly the owner of the dog is known by the victim. In most instances the biting dog is considered "large" and weighs at least 50 lb. German shepards are often implicated. Such animals are capable of generating jaw pressures in excess of 200–450 pounds/sq inch,[35] which in turn can cause major crush injuries. Severe attacks, characterized as repetitive and uninhibited biting by a dog that is unresponsive to human intervention, comprise a small percentage of total dog bites but are most commonly noted in reproductively intact young males with known owners.[32] "Pit bull" terriers have been most commonly implicated.

Although the general principles regarding bite wound management apply to injuries from dogs, several important specifics must be addressed. The bacteriology of the canine mouth is subtly different from that of the human. Up to 30 separate genera of aerobic organisms have been isolated and include a wide variety of gram-negative cocci and bacilli and a large number of different gram-positive cocci and rods.[36] Numerous species of anaerobic organisms have similarly been noted.[31] *Pasteurella multocida,* a gram-negative bacillus, is isolated from canines in up to 60% of instances[36] and appears to be far more common in the mouths of canines and felines than in humans. Unlike most enteric gram-negative bacilli, this organism is penicillin-sensitive and may be associated with up to 20–50% of dog bite infections.[3,21,31,37] Other bacteria that are routinely encountered in the canine mouth include *S. aureus* and *S. epidermidis,* anaerobic gram-positive and gram-negative organisms, and some rather unusual bacteria identified only by CDC alphanumeric designations.[31,36] Some of these, especially DF-2 (dysgonic fermenter 2), have been associated with lethal infectious complications.[38,39] This organism is a slow-growing gram-negative bacillus that is penicillin-sensitive but aminoglycoside-resistant and not easily grown on standard media. Splenectomized persons are especially suceptible to fulminant sepsis caused by this organism.[39] Presentation is usually accompanied by disseminated intravascular coagulation and peripheral gangrene, and diagnosis can be suspected by evaluation of buffy coat smears of blood.[39] As with human bites, mixed infections caused by a variety of organisms are most commonly identified.

Prospective studies of clinically noninfected wounds demonstrate that 10% had positive Gram stains on initial presentation, often demonstrating multiple morphologies.[40] Up to 67% harbored potential pathogens when routinely cultured.[31] Gram stains often failed to predict the presence of organisms identifiable by culture but can be useful if positive. Thus, neither routine smears nor cultures of clinically noninfected wounds are indicated. Use of prophylactic antibiotics in dog bites remains controversial. Many authorities recommend that all but the most trivial and early dog bites be treated with antimicrobial agents.[3,5,9] A recent investigation demonstrated a reduction of infection from 25% to 10% following dog bites with the use of prophylactic penicillin VK.[41] However, these results failed to achieve statistical significance. Another recent study failed to demonstrate an advantage for antibiotic use in dog-bite injuries managed within the first 8 hr.[42] Other investigators cite the lower risk of infection following dog bites when compared to those from felines or humans and list specific indications for the use of antimicrobial agents following this type of wound. These include (1) dog bites older than 8 hr, (2) all hand bites, (3) deep puncture wounds where debridement is difficult, (4) bites in immunocompromised patients, and (5) wounds that are candidates for delayed primary closure.[26]

A variety of agents have been studied, but there is presently little science to this subject. Penicillin, ampicillin, trimethoprim–sulfamethoxazole, and tetracycline offer good therapeutic alternatives for *P. multocida;* however, the latter agent has little anaerobic activity. Clindamycin, erythromycin, and first-generation cephalosporins are poor alternatives when *P. multocida* is considered a possible pathogen. Thus, therapeutic regimens similar to those utilized for human bites should be effective. The author's personal recommendation would be to utilize amoxicillin/clavulanic acid (Augmentin®) as monotherapy is a dose of 250–500 mg thrice daily. Length of therapy is determined by the extent of the injury and the presence of overt infection. Minimum treatment is for approximately 5 days, but therapy (usually initiated by parenteral routes in the hospital setting) for 4–6 weeks is indicated for osteomyelitis. Parenteral therapy, as outlined previously in this chapter, may be necessary.

CAT BITES

Cats are thought to represent the second most common cause of mammalian bites and may be associated with 5–20% of all cases.[21,43] Cat bites are unique primarily because of the sharpness of the teeth and their propensity to cause puncture wounds that may penetrate bones and joint capsules. Thus, the potential for significant deep-space infections must always be assessed in the evaluation of feline wounds, and this may help explain the higher incidence of clinical infection seen with felines compared to canines.

Approximatley 40% of cat bites become infected.[44] *P. multocida* has been demonstrated in the mouths of up to 75% of healthy cats and is arguably the most frequently implicated organism in infections following cat bites.[45] Management strategies for cat bites follow those utilized for dogs and humans. Most authorities recommend the empirical use of antibiotics following cat bites. Although a small study demonstrated decreased likelihood of infection with oxacillin when compared to placebo,[45] this agent has little activity against *P. multocida* or common mouth anaerobes. Thus, most clinicians recommend either the combination of penicillin or ampicillin or amoxicillin plus dicloxacillin or amoxicillin/clavulanic acid. Therapy for clinically noninfected wounds is for approximately 5 days.

ASSESSMENT FOR RABIES AND TETANUS

An in-depth discussion of these issues is given in other chapters that deal with immunization. It is imperative that the physician evaluating bite wound injuries make inquiry about the immunization status of the patient and the biting animal. Although tetanus following mammalian bite injuries must be an exceedingly rare event, the presence of *C. tetani* in the mouths of canines, felines, and humans make this a potential adverse occurrence. Diligent debridement of the wound is of paramount importance for the prevention of anaerobic infections such as tetanus. All antibiotic regimens that have been recommended will be active against this pathogen; however, it must be stressed that antibiotics play a minor role in the prevention of this disease.

Although human rabies is a rare event in the United States, the resultant, almost uniformly fatal illness, and the fact that it can be prevented, necessitate a consideration of it in appropriate animal injuries. Rabies in cats and dogs is exceedingly unusual in developed areas of this country; however, local areas have had occasional outbreaks of rabies in wild canine populations. The examining physician should ascertain the rabies immunization status of biting canines and felines and document this information in the medical record. In clinical situations where rabies immunization status cannot be obtained, the clinician must individualize the need for rabies prophylactic measures based on the likelihood of rabies in the biting animal and the provocative circumstances surrounding the bite.

SUMMARY AND CONCLUSIONS

Bite injuries suffered from mammals are common and are often not trivial. The clinician must carefully assess each bite with regard to potential for bacterial infections, rabies, and tetanus. Compulsive management of all but the most trivial of wounds must include careful history and physical examination to define the extent of the injury. Often the initial site does not define the true extent of injury. Although infection may occur despite optimal management, diligent irrigation, drainage, and debridement of the bite site will help reduce the likelihood of this significant complication. In all but the most trivial injuries, oral antibiotics are indicated to treat early or subclinical infection. Choice of drug is based on the likely pathogens and must recognize the important role of the mouth flora of the biting animal. With regard for the need for hospitalization, the physician should exercise conservative judgment and reserve outpatient management for the most trivial of injuries that are unaccompanied by clinical infection and that do not extend into vital deep structures.

REFERENCES

1. Callaham M: Dog bite wounds. *JAMA* 1980; 244:2327–2328.
2. Douglas L: Bite wounds. *Am Fam Physician* 1975; 11:93–99.
3. Goldstein E: Bites. In: Mandell GL, Douglas RG Jr, Bennett JE, eds. *Principles and Practice of Infectious Disease,* ed 2. New York, John Wiley & Sons, 1985:632–635.
4. Kaplan K: Animal bites and infection. *Infect Dis Pract* 1986; 9(7):1–8.
5. Rest JG, Goldstein EJC: Management of human and animal bite wounds. *Emerg Med Clin North Am* 1985; 3:117–126.
6. Kizer KW: Epidemiologic and clinical aspects of animal bite injuries. *J Am Coll Emerg Physicians* 1979; 8:134–139.
7. Goldstein EJC: Clenched-fist injury infections. *Infect Surg* 1986; 5:384–390.
8. Stevenson TR, Thacker JG, Rodeheaver GT, *et al:* Cleansing traumatic wounds by high-pressure syringe irrigation. *J Am Coll Emerg Physicians* 1976; 5:17–21.

9. Edlich RF, Spengler MD, Rodeheaver GT, *et al:* Emergency department management of mammalian bites. *Emerg Clin North Am* 1986; 4:595–604.
10. Marr JS, Beck AM, Lugo JA Jr: An epidemiologic study of the human bite. *Public Health Rep* 1979; 94:514–521.
11. Shields C, Patzakis MJ, Meyers MH, *et al:* Hand infections secondary to human bites. *J Trauma* 1975; 15:35–36.
12. Goldstein EJC, Citron DM, Finegold SM: Role of anaerobic bacteria in bite-wound infections. *Rev Infect Dis* 1984; 6(suppl):177–183.
13. Goldstein EJC: Infections following human bites. *Infect Surg* 1985; 4:849–859.
14. Mann RJ, Hoffeld TA, Farmer CB: Human bites of the hand: Twenty years of experience. *J Hand Surg* 1977; 2:97–104.
15. Peeples E, Bostwick JA Jr, Scott FA: Wounds of the hand contaminated by human or animal saliva. *J Trauma* 1980; 20:383–389.
16. Narsete TA, Omer GE, Moneim MS: Hand Infections from human saliva. *Orthop Rev* 1983; 12:81–85.
17. Chuinard RG, ĎAmbrosia RD: Human bite infections of the hand. *J Bone Joint Surg* 1977; 59A:416–418.
18. Dreyfuss UY, Singer M: Human bites of the hand: A study of one hundred six patients. *J Hand Surg* 1985; 10A:884–889.
19. Schmidt DR, Heckman JD: *Eikenella corrodens* in human bite infections of the hand. *J Trauma* 1983; 23:478–482.
20. Goldstein EJC, Citron DM, Wield B, *et al:* Bacteriology of human and animal bite wounds. *J Clin Microbiol* 1978; 8:667–672.
21. Brook I: Microbiology of human and animal bite wounds in children. *Pediatr Infect Dis* 1987; 6:29–32.
22. Goldstein EJC, Barones MF, Miller TA: *Eikenella corrodens* in hand infections. *J Hand Surg* 1983; 8:563–567.
23. Malinowski RW, Strate RG, Perry JF, *et al:* The management of human bite injuries of the hand. *J Trauma* 1979; 19:655–659.
24. Goldstein EJC, Citron DM, Vagvolgyi AE, *et al:* Susceptibility of bite wound bacteria to seven oral antimicrobial agents, including RU-985, a new erythromycin: Considerations in choosing empiric therapy. *Antimicrob Agents Chemother* 1986; 29:556–559.
25. Goldstein EJC, Reingardt JR, Murray PM, *et al:* Animal and human bite wounds: A comparative study, Augmentin vs penicillin +/− dicloxacillin. *Postgrad Med* 1984; Custom Commun: 105–110.
26. Trott A: Care of mammalian bites. *Pediatr Infect Dis* 1987; 6:8–10.
27. Johnson CC, Reinhardt JF, Wallace SL, *et al:* Safety and efficacy of ticarcillin plus clavulanic acid in the treatment of infections of soft tissue, bone, and joint. *Am J Med* 1985; 79(suppl 5B):136–140.
28. LeFrock JL, Johnson ES, Smith LG, *et al:* Noncomparative trial of ticarcillin plus clavulanic acid in skin and soft tissue infections. *Am J Med.* 1985; 79(suppl 5B):122–125.
29. Lehman WL Jr, Allo MD, Jones WW, *et al:* Human bite infections of the hand: Adjunct treatment with hyperbaric oxygen. *Infect Surg* 1985; 4:460–465.
30. Harris D, Imperato PJ, Oken B: Dog bites—an unrecognized epidemic. *Bull NY Acad Med* 1974; 50:981–1000.
31. Goldstein EJC, Citron DM, Finegold SM: Dog bite wounds and infection: A prospective clinical study. *Ann Emerg Med* 1980; 9:508–512.
32. Wright JC: Severe attacks by dogs: Characteristics of the dogs, victims, and the attack settings. *Public Health Rep* 1985; 100:55–61.
33. Boenning DA, Fleisher GR, Campos JM: Dog bites in children: Epidemiology, microbiology, and penicillin prophylactic therapy. *Am J Emerg Med* 1983; 1:17–21.

34. Karlson TA: The incidence of facial injuries from dog bites. *JAMA* 1984; 251:3265–3267.
35. Chambers GH, Payne JF: Treatment of dog bite wounds. *Minn Med* 1969; 52:427–430.
36. Bailie WE, Stowe EC, Schmitt AM: Aerobic bacterial flora of oral and nasal fluids of canines with reference to bacteria associated with bites. *J Clin Microbiol* 1978; 7:223–231.
37. Feder HM, Shanley JD, Barbera JA: Review of 59 patients hospitalized with animal bites. *Pediatr Infect Dis* 1987; 6:24–28.
38. Newton NL, Sharma B: Acute mycoardial infarction associated with DF-2 bacteremia after a dog bite. *Am J Med Sci* 1986; 291:352–354.
39. Hicklin H, Verghese A, Alvarez S: Dysgonic fermenter 2 septicemia. *Rev Infect Dis* 1987; 9:884–890.
40. Ordog GJ: The bacteriology of dog bite wounds on initial presentation. *Ann Emerg Med* 1986; 15:1324–1329.
41. Callaham M: Prophylactic antibiotics in common dog bite wounds: A controlled study. *Ann Emerg Med* 1980; 9:410–414.
42. Rosen RA: The use of antibiotics in the initial management of recent dog-bite wounds. *Am J Emerg Med* 1985; 3:19–23.
43. Strassburg MA, Greenland S, Marron JA, *et al:* Animal bites: Patterns of treatment. *Ann Emerg Med* 1981; 10:193–197.
44. Francis DP, Holmes MA, Brandon G: *Pasteurella multocida* infections after domestic animal bites and scratches. *JAMA* 1975; 233:42–45.
45. Elenbaas RM, McNabney WK, Robinson WA: Evaluation of prophylactic oxacillin in cat bite wounds. *Ann Emerg Med* 1984; 13:155–157.

16

Endocarditis Prophylaxis

Nelson M. Gantz

INTRODUCTION

The subject of endocarditis prophylaxis continues to stir controversy. Despite recommendations for prevention of endocarditis from committees of the American Heart Association,[1] Working Party of the British Society for Antimicrobial Chemotherapy,[2] and the *Medical Letter,*[3] these guidelines are not based on controlled clinical studies. No such studies have been published or are likely to be forthcoming.

A number of questions regarding prophylaxis remain unanswered, such as: Can endocarditis be prevented by giving prophylactic antibiotics? What is the risk of developing endocarditis following procedures such as dental extraction associated with transient bacteremia? Which antibiotic regimens for prophylaxis are the best? Are parenteral antibiotics more effective than oral drugs? Is it necessary to use a bactericidal drug for prophylaxis? Are the data derived from the animal models of experimental endocarditis relevant to prophylaxis in humans? Which procedures merit the use of prophylactic antibiotics to prevent endocarditis? How should patients with mitral valve prolapse who are to undergo various diagnostic or therapeutic manipulations be managed? Should patients with arterial grafts or orthopedic devices (e.g., prosthetic hip) receive prophylactic antibiotics for special clinical situations associated with a transient bacteremia? This is only a partial list of questions which the clinician faces daily in caring for patients at risk for endocarditis. Despite the widespread availability of antibiotics, the incidence of endocarditis has not declined in recent years.[4]

Infective endocarditis has major morbidity and mortality despite the availability of antimicrobial agents. Patients who have underlying valvular heart disease are at risk for the development of infective endocarditis when organisms invade the bloodstream. A key factor in the pathogenesis of infective endocarditis is the occurrence of a transient bacteremia.[5] The AHA recommends that patients with rheumatic, congenital, or other cardiovascular diseases, as well as those with a prosthetic heart valve, receive prophylactic antibiotics when they have a procedure associated with a transient bacteremia.[1,6,7]

In this chapter I discuss the procedures associated with transient bacteremia, the types of underlying cardiovascular diseases that predispose a patient to infective endocarditis, and the antibiotic regimens recommended for prevention of endocarditis in predisposed patients.

Most cases of endocarditis are not preventable by the administration of prophylactic antibiotics. Only half of the patients who develop endocarditis have a recognized cardiac lesion for which prophylaxis would be a consideration. Furthermore, fewer than 25% of patients with endocarditis caused by viridans streptococci and about 40% of cases of endocarditis caused by enterococci have an indentified portal of entry for which prophylaxis could be given. In addition, the usually recommended antibiotics are likely to be effective in only 67% of cases of endocarditis. Therefore, it is estimated that only 8–10% of cases of endocarditis are potentially preventable.

TRANSIENT BACTEREMIA

Transient bacteremias occur commonly.[5] They may occur spontaneously, such as with chewing food or with defecation. They may result from many procedures that traumatize mucous membranes with an indigenous microbial flora such as a dental extraction or urethral catheterization. Bacteremias following procedures resulting in mucosal trauma are asymptomatic, usually occur about 1 to 5 min following the procedures, and generally last less than 15 min. Blood cultures are usually sterile 30 min after the procedure. Quantitative blood cultures usually reveal colony counts of less than 10 organisms per milliliter of blood. Transient bacteremias also occur with local infections such as those occurring with incision and drainage of an abscess or manipulation of the urinary tract in a patient with asymptomatic bacteriuria. The organisms associated with these bacteremias reflect either the normal flora at the manipulated site or the pathogen causing the local infection.

A history of a predisposing event can at times be elicited from patients with endocarditis. A preceding dental procedure has been noted in 15–20% of patients with nonenterococcal streptococcal endocarditis. A preceding genitourinary tract procedure has been reported in 40% of patients with enterococcal endocarditis. A preceding infection of the skin or soft tissue has been noted in 35% of patients with staphylococcal endocarditis.[8]

The oropharynx is a frequent portal of entry for organisms into the bloodstream. Blood cultures are positive in 18–85% of patients after a dental extraction.[5] The frequency of bacteremia correlates with the severity of gingival infection and the extent of tissue trauma. The organisms isolated reflect the normal mouth flora. Viridans streptococci are isolated most frequently, but anaerobic streptococci, coagulase-negative staphylococci, diphtheroids, and fusobacteria are also seen. Strains of viridans streptococci account for 50–75% of cases of endocarditis and are usually penicillin-sensitive. Streptococci that are relatively resistant to penicillin are found in patients receiving prophylactic penicillin for rheumatic fever and in those starting antibiotic prophylaxis 1 to 2 days before a procedure.[9]

Prophylaxis should begin 1 to 2 hr prior to a procedure so that serum levels of the antibiotic are adequate at the time of anticipated bacteremia. Penicillin given just prior to a dental extraction decreases the incidence of positive blood cultures after the procedure. Gingival degerming agents (compared with placebo), such as povidone-iodine mouthwash, also reduce the incidence of bacteremia associated with dental procedures. Topical antiseptic agents, however, should never be given without concomitant systemic antibiotic therapy.

Other dental procedures that may result in a transient bacteremia include periodontal operations such as gingivectomy, root canal surgery, and dental cleaning. Blood cultures are positive in up to 88% of patients, depending on the severity of gum disease.[5] The predominant organisms are the same as following dental extraction. Positive blood cultures are also seen after tooth brushing (0–26%), the use of oral irrigation devices (7–50%), the use of dental floss (20%), and gum cleaning or eating hard candy (0–22%). Antibiotic prophylaxis obviously is impractical for preventing a transient bacteremia secondary to these common daily activities. The cumulative risk of transient bacteremia is far greater for the usual daily events of living such as eating, brushing the teeth, or defecation than for that from an occasional surgical procedure.[10] Maintenance of good oral hygiene decreases the amount of gum disease, which is a key determinant of the frequency of a transient bacteremia following any dental manipulation.

Other procedures involving the oropharynx and respiratory tract may result in bacteremia; these include tonsillectomy, nasotracheal intubation, and rigid-tube bronchoscopy. Positive blood cultures, however, rarely occur in association with flexible fiberoptic bronchoscopy and lung biopsy. This contrasts with the rate of bacteremia of 15% associated with the use of a rigid bronchoscope.[5]

Diagnostic procedures involving the gastrointestinal tract are another source of transient bacteremias.[5,11] Positive blood cultures are found in 0–10% (4% overall) of patients having fiberoptic gastrointestinal endoscopy, 0–9.5% (5% overall) of patients following rigid sigmoidoscopy, 3–14% of patients undergoing a liver biopsy, 11% of patients having a barium enema, and 0–27% (5% overall) of patients undergoing colonoscopy.[11] The predominant organisms isolated with these procedures are enterococci, which are frequent causes of endocarditis, and gram-negative bacilli, organisms rarely involved in endocarditis.

Transient bacteremia and infective endocarditis can occur following urinary tract, obstetric, and gynecological procedures.[5] The urinary tract is the portal of entry in 20–50% of patients with enterococcal endocarditis, and 20% of cases caused by this organism are related to obstetric and gynecological procedures. A genitourinary tract source is implicated in about 15% of all patients with endocarditis. A transient bacteremia occurs in 8% of patients undergoing urethral catheterization, 24% of those undergoing urethral dilation, 17% of those have cystoscopy, and 12–31% of those having transurethral prosthetic resection. The frequency of positive blood cultures increases severalfold in patients with infection at the instrumented site.[12] One example of such an infection is that of the urinary tract.

Transient bacteremia also occurs in 0–5% of patients after vaginal delivery, cesarean section, dilatation and curettage of the uterus, and during insertion or removal of an intrauterine contraceptive device.[5]

Manipulation of an infected focus, such as massage of an infected prostate or incision and drainage of an abscess, is associated with bacteremia and the risk of endocarditis. Transient bacteremia, however, is rare with cardiac catheterization and angiographic procedures.

Table 16.1 lists the procedures associated with transient bacteremia and the indications for antibiotic prophylaxis.

CARDIAC LESIONS PREDISPOSING TO ENDOCARDITIS

Prevention of endocarditis requires a knowledge both of the events likely to produce bacteremia and of patients with predisposing cardiac lesion. Unfortunately, half the patients with endocarditis have no recognized underlying heart disease, making antibiotic prophylaxis impossible for this group.[8] Rheumatic valvular disease still remains the most common form of underlying cardiac disease in patients in whom endocarditis develops. The frequency has declined in recent years, however, because of the decreasing incidence of rheumatic fever. Patients with a bicuspid aortic valve are predisposed to endocarditis, as are patients with calcific or atherosclerotic changes in the aortic and mitral valves or anulus.

Patients with mitral valve prolapse—click murmur syndrome—have been reported to be at increased risk of endocarditis. In a case-controlled study, the risk of endocarditis in patients with mitral valve prolapse was approximately 8 times higher than that for matched controls.[13] In a study of endocarditis prophylaxis failures, mitral valve prolapse was the most frequent cardiac abnormality identified, accounting for 33% of the cases of endocarditis.[14] Bor and Himmelstein estimated the risks and benefits of antibiotic prophylaxis for patients with mitral valve prolapse undergoing a dental procedure. For such patients, their analysis suggested that the risk of fatal penicillin reactions far outweighed its benefits in preventing endocarditis.[15] They suggested either no prophylaxis or using erythromycin rather than penicillin for prophylaxis. This is only a theoretical analysis, however, and not a controlled clinical trial. Prophylaxis in all

Table 16.1
Indications for Antibiotic Prophylaxis in Procedures Associated with Transient Bacteremia

- Antibiotic prophylaxis recommended for all patients with valvular heart disease
  - Dental procedures with gingival bleeding
    - Dental extraction
    - Dental cleaning
    - Periodontal surgery (e.g., gingivectomy)
  - Procedures involving the airways
    - Tonsillectomy or adenoidectomy
    - Bronchoscopy with a rigid bronchoscope
  - Genitourinary manipulations
    - Cystoscopy
    - Transurethral prostatic resection
    - Urethral dilation
  - Gastrointestinal tract
    - Cholecystectomy
    - Intestinal surgery
  - Gynecological and obstetric conditions
    - Dilation and curettage of uterus
    - Vaginal hysterectomy
    - Vaginal delivery (complicated)
    - Cesarean section
  - Manipulation of septic foci
    - Incision and drainage of abscesses
- Antibiotic prophylaxis recommended only for patients at high risk, i.e., presence of prosthetic or bioprosthetic heart valves
  - All procedures listed above
  - Procedures involving the airway
    - Nasotracheal intubation
    - Fiberoptic bronchoscopy (?)
  - Gastrointestinal procedures
    - Sigmoidoscopy
    - Barium enema
    - Colonoscopy
    - Liver biopsy
    - Upper gastrointestinal endoscopy with biopsy
    - Endoscopic retrograde cholangiopancreatography
- Procedures for which antibiotic prophylaxis is not indicated for patients with valvular heart disease
  - Procedures involving the airway
    - Orotracheal intubation
    - Nasotracheal suctioning
  - Gynecological procedures
    - Insertion or removal of intrauterine device
    - Vaginal delivery (uncomplicated)
  - Other procedures
    - Cardiac catheterization and angiographic procedures
    - Pacemaker insertion
    - Peritoneal dialysis

such patients would be difficult because of the high incidence of mitral valve prolapse: 5% to 6% of the American population is affected. I therefore recommend that antibiotic prophylaxis be given only to those with associated mitral insufficiency documented by a holosystolic murmur and not to those who have only a systolic click.

Patients with a previous episode of endocarditis should also receive prophylaxis for predisposing events. Finally, patients with prosthetic or bioprosthetic heart valves are also predisposed to endocarditis. Because infection of a prosthesis is often difficult to eradicate and carries a high mortality, antibiotic prophylaxis is recommended both for the usual predisposing events and for additional procedures that are associated with a transient bacteremia but with a lower risk of infection, such as sigmoidoscopy (see Table 16.1).[1,5]

Although there are no controlled studies to establish the effectiveness of prophylactic antibiotics in patients with these predisposing carciac lesions, prophylaxis is generally recommended. The value of prophylaxis for procedures that may be associated with a transient bacteremia is unclear in patients with transvenous pacemakers, arteriovenous shunts for hemodialysis, and ventriculoatrial shunts. The risk in the last situation is probably low, and the majority of experts do not recommend prophylaxis in such cases.

RISK OF ENDOCARDITIS

Only rough estimates are available for the incidence of endocarditis in susceptible persons after exposure to an event associated with transient bacteremia. The incidence is clearly low, because bacteremias often occur after operative procedures, and resultant endocarditis is relatively rare. One report noted no instance of endocarditis after 403 tooth extractions among 98 patients with rheumatic heart disease.[16] In another report, there were four cases of endocarditis among 350 children with rheumatic heart disease who had a recent tooth extraction without antibiotic prophylaxis.[17]

Similarly, the effectiveness of antibiotic prophylaxis for infective endocarditis remains undetermined. Because a carefully controlled study with a large number of patients would be required to answer some of the questions surrounding this issue, animals have been used to study the pathogenesis and efficacy of antibiotic prophylaxis on infective endocarditis.

In the rabbit model of Garrison and Freedman, a polyethylene catheter is inserted across the tricuspid or aortic valve, resulting in sterile vegetations.[18] A suitable organism is injected intravenously 24 to 48 hr later, causing endocarditis. The efficacy of various antibiotic regimens is tested by giving the drugs 30 min before the injection of the bacteria. The animal is later sacrificed, and cultures of the vegetations are obtained. A major criticism of this model is the high inoculum (e.g., 10^5) of organisms per milliliter used to produce infection compared with 100 organisms per milliliter in the blood following a dental extraction; therefore, the animal models tend to overestimate the margin of safety of any antimicrobial regimen.

PRINCIPLES OF ANTIBIOTIC PROPHYLAXIS

Effective use of prophylactic antibiotics requires that adequate drug levels be present at the appropriate site at the time of the event posing the risk of transient bacteremia. According to data from the rabbit model of experimental endocarditis, it is necessary to have bactericidal activity in the serum for 9 hr after the bacterial challenge.[19] The 3-g amoxicillin prophylactic regimen advocated by the British provides 10 hr of serum inhibitory activity.[2,20] To accomplish this goal, the antimicrobial should be given initially 1 to 2 hr prior to the procedure and continued for 12 to 24 hr. Increasing the duration of treatment beyond one dose after the initial loading dose only raises the cost and increases the possibility of an adverse drug reaction.

For dental procedures and other procedures involving the airway, the antibiotic selected should be directed against viridans streptococci. Genitourinary manipulations and gastrointestinal, gynecological and obstetric procedures require that the antibiotic prophylaxis be adequate for enterococci. Antibiotics should be directed against penicillinase-producing staphylococci in a predisposed person having incision and drainage of an abscess. A urine culture should be obtained prior to a genitourinary procedure, so that any infection can be identified and treated before the instrumentation. Bactericidal antibiotics should be used if possible, because in the animal model, all the bacteriostatic agents tested were ineffective.

Table 16.2 lists the regimens of antibiotic prophylaxis preceding dental and surgical procedures.[1]

The recommendations for prophylaxis for the various procedures are empiricial. It is useful to classify procedures into those that are low risk, such as a barium enema, and those at higher risk, such as a dental extraction.[21] The classification of the various procedures into risk group is arbitrary. Similarly, one can categorize patients into risk groups based on the underlying cardiac lesion. Patients with a prosthetic heart valve or arterial graft would be at high risk, and those with rheumatic valve disease at lower risk. The consequences and difficulty in eradicating infection from a prosthetic heart valve are far greater than infection of a native heart valve. If both risks are high, then prophylaxis is indicated: for example, endoscopy with biopsy in a patient with a prosthetic heart valve. If a patient has underlying rheumatic valvular heart disease, then prophylaxis would be indicated for a dental extraction but not for a low-risk procedure such as a barium enema. If neither risk is high, then prophylaxis is

Table 16.2
Antibiotic Prophylactic Regimens[a]

For dental procedures and upper respiratory tract surgical procedures:
- Penicillin V, 2 g p.o. 1 hr prior to procedure, then 1 g q6h for one dose
- Aqueous crystalline penicillin G, 2 million units i.m. or i.v. ½–1 hr before procedure, then 1 million units 6 hr later
- Ampicillin, 1–2 g i.v. or i.m., plus gentamicin, 1.5 mg/kg i.m. or i.v., not to exceed 80 mg, ½–1 hr before procedure; repeat once 8 hr later
- Amoxicillin, 3 g p.o. 1 hr prior, then amoxicillin, 1.5 g p.o. 6 hr later

If patient is allergic to penicillin or receiving continuous oral penicillin for prevention of rheumatic fever:
- Erythromycin, 1 g p.o. 1½ hr prior to procedure, then 500 mg p.o. q6h for one dose
- Vancomycin, 1 g i.v. administered over 30 min; start infusion ½–1 hr prior to procedure; then give erythromycin, 500 mg p.o. q6h for one dose after instrumentation

For urinary, gynecological, and gastrointestinal procedures:
- Ampicillin, 2 g i.m. or i.v., plus gentamicin, 1.5 mg/kg i.m. or i.v., not to exceed 80 mg; give the two drugs ½–1 hr prior to procedure, then repeat in 8 hr as one additional dose
- Amoxicillin, 3 g p.o. 1 hr prior, then amoxicillin, 1.5 g p.o. 6 hr later

If patient is allergic to penicillin:
- Vancomycin, 1 g i.v. over 30 min, plus gentamicin, 1.5. mg/kg i.m. or i.v., not to exceed 80 mg; give drugs 1 hr prior to procedure and repeat in 8 hr as one additional dose

For incision and drainage of skin abscesses caused by coagulase-positive staphylococci[b]:
- Nafcillin or oxacillin, 2 g i.v. ½–1 hr prior to procedure, then 2 g i.v. q4h
- Dicloxacillin, 500 mg p.o. 1 hr prior to procedure, then 500 mg q6h

If patient is allergic to penicillin:
- Cephalothin, 2 g i.v. ½–1 hr prior to procedure, then 2 g i.v. q4h
- Cefazolin, 1 g i.m. 1 hr prior to procedure, then 500 mg i.m. q6h
- Vancomycin, 1 g i.v. over 30 min: start infusion ½–1 hr prior to procedure, then 500 mg i.v. q6h

[a]Parenteral regimens are recommended for patients with prosthetic or biosynthetic heart valves.[2]
[b]Route and duration of therapy depend on the severity of the infection and whether or not the predisposed person is at high risk (e.g., prosthetic heart valve). Results of Gram stains and cultures should also guide antibiotic selection.

optional. I do not recommend prophylaxis for patients with prosthetic joints who are to undergo various diagnostic or therapeutic manipulations, although this is controversial.

REFERENCES

1. Shulman ST, Amren DP, Bisno AL, *et al:* Prevention of bacterial endocarditis. *Circulation* 1984; 70:1123A–1127A.
2. Working Party of the British Society for Antimicrobial Chemotherapy: The antibiotic prophylaxis of infective endocarditis. *Lancet* 1982; 2:1323–1326.
3. *Medical Letter:* Prevention of bacterial endocarditis. *Med Lett* 1986; 28:22–25.
4. Bayliss R, Clarke C, Oakley C, *et al:* The teeth and infective endocarditis. *Br Heart J* 1983; 50:506–512.

5. Everett ED, Hirschmann JV: Transient bacteremia and endocarditis prophylaxis. A review. *Medicine (Baltimore)* 1977; 56:61–77.
6. Sipes JN, Thompson RL, Hook EW: Prophylaxis of infective endocarditis: A reevaluation. *Annu Rev Med* 1977; 28:371–391.
7. Lowy F, Steigbigel NH: Infective endocarditis. Part III. Prevention of bacterial endocarditis. *Am Heart J* 1978; 96:689–695.
8. Kaye D: Prophylaxis against bacterial endocarditis: A dilemma in infective endocarditis. In: Kaplan EL, Taranta AV, eds. *Infective Endocarditis. American Heart Association Monograph Series, No. 52.* Dallas, American Heart Association, 1977:67–69.
9. Garrod LP, Waterworth PM: The risks of dental extraction during penicillin therapy. *Br Heart J* 1962; 24:39–46.
10. Guntheroth WG: How important are dental procedures as a cause of infective endocarditis? *Am J Cardiol* 1984; 54:797–801.
11. Shorvan PJ, Eykyn SJ, Cotton PB: Gastrointestinal instrumentation, bacteremia, and endocarditis. *Gut* 1983; 24:1078–1093.
12. Sullivan NM, Sutter VL, Mims MM, *et al:* Clinical aspects of bacteremia after manipulation of the genitourinary tract. *J Infect Dis* 1973; 127:49–55.
13. Clemens JD, Horowitz RI, Jaffe CC, *et al:* A controlled evaluation of the risk of bacterial endocarditis in persons with mitral-valve prolapse. *N Engl J Med* 1982; 307:776–781.
14. Durack DT, Bisno AL, Kaplan EL: Apparent failures of endocarditis prophylaxis. Analysis of 52 cases submitted to a national registry. *JAMA* 1983; 250:2318–2322.
15. Bor DH, Himmelstein DU: Endocarditis prophylaxis for patients with mitral valve prolapse. A quantitative analysis. *Am J Med* 1984; 76:711–717.
16. Schwartz SP, Salman I: The effect of oral surgery on the course of patients with disease of the heart. *Am J Orthodont* 1942; 28:331–345.
17. Taran LM: Rheumatic fever in relation to dental disease. *NY J Dent* 1944; 14:107–113.
18. Garrison PK, Freedman LR: Experimental endocarditis I: Staphylococcal endocarditis resulting from placement of a polyethylene catheter in the right side of the heart. *Yale J Biol Med* 1970; 42:394–410.
19. Durack DT, Petersdorf RG: Chemotherapy of experimental streptococcal endocarditis: I. Comparison of commonly recommended prophylactic regimens. *J Clin Invest* 1973; 52:592–598.
20. Kaye D: Prophylaxis for infective endocarditis: An update. *Ann Intern Med* 1986; 104:419–423.
21. Durack DT: Current issues in prevention of infective endocarditis. *Am J Med* 1985; 78(Suppl. 6B):149–156.

17

Tuberculin Skin Testing and Managing a Positive Tuberculin Reactor

Nelson M. Gantz

INTRODUCTION

Tuberculosis continues to be a serious problem in the United States. It is imported regularly from the Third World, and it is often seen in the elderly.[1] There is also an increase in tuberculosis infections caused by *Mycobacterium tuberculosis* and *M. avium-intracellulare* complex in patients with diagnosed AIDS.

The tuberculin skin test has been available since the turn of the century. Although it was intended primarily as an epidemiologic tool for identifying persons at risk in the general population, the tuberculin skin test remains an inexpensive and useful adjunct in diagnosing individual cases. This chapter focuses on the use and interpretation of the tuberculin skin test as well as preventive therapy with isoniazid.

TUBERCULIN PREPARATIONS

Two preparations of tuberculin are licensed for use in the United States: old tuberculin (OT) and purified protein derivative (PPD).[2,3] Old tuberculin is a sterilized solution prepared by filtration from cultures of tubercle bacilli. Purified protein derivative also is a sterile solution, produced by heating and precipitating the protein from tubercle cultures. Purified protein derivative contains several antigens and is neither pure nor solely protein. Both OT and PPD are crude preparations, and cross reactions caused by sensitization by other mycobacterial species occur frequently. However, PPD is more specific than OT for *M. tuberculosis*.

Purified protein derivative was produced in 1939 by Florence Seibert and is designated as PPD-S. It is the reference standard for all tuberculin materials. Because PPD is adsorbed to some extent by glass or plastic, a detergent is added to the solution to reduce adsorption. Nevertheless, PPD test material should not be stored in a syringe but used as soon as the syringe is filled. After the PPD test solution is removed aseptically from the vial, the remaining solution should be refrigerated in the dark, and the vial should be dated.

The PPD test material is available in three strengths: 1 tuberculin unit (1 TU), or first strength; 5 TU, intermediate strength; and 250 TU, second strength. The standard test is the 5-TU dose. The 1-TU dose has been advocated for patients who may be hypersensitive and thus may develop a severe ulcerating local reaction with a 5-TU test dose. The 1-TU test is not standardized, however, and should be used only as a precaution against excessive reactivity.

The 250-TU dose is of limited value in the diagnosis of tuberculosis and can provoke severe necrotizing skin reactions in persons who have active cellular immunity. When necrotizing reactions occur, topical application of a potent corticosteroid ointment or even a short course of systemic steroid therapy may be indicated. In one study, false-positive reactions with 250 TU occurred with a frequency of 36%; this probably represented cross sensitivity to atypical mycobacteria. In the same study, a positive skin test to another antigen used for delayed hypersensitivity skin testing and selective anergy to the 250-TU dose occurred in only 5% of patients. This means that a negative second-strength tuberculin test in a patient who is not anergic is powerful evidence against the diagnosis. The second-strength tests should therefore be used in only a few specific situations.[4]

The nomenclature of the skin test strengths—first, intermediate, and second—can cause confusion, with the result that the second-strength skin test material is used instead of the standard 5-TU intermediate strength. A false-positive reaction to the 250 TU is not unusual; in a patient with a reported positive skin test, it is important to verify that a 5-TU test dose was applied.

TEST METHODS

Two methods are available for the administration of the tuberculin skin test: the multipuncture technique and the intradermal Mantoux test. The multiple-puncture test introduces either dried or liquid tuberculin by puncturing the skin with an applicator. Examples of the multiple-puncture test are the tine test, which has four metal prongs coated with either dried OT or PPD, and the Mono-Vacc test, which consists of nine prongs and uses a solution of OT. Although they are inexpensive and easy to administer, particularly in children, the 10% to 15% incidence of false-negative reactions limits their usefulness in screening studies. The incidence of false-negative reactions to the Mono-Vacc test was about 1% in one study, making it the preferred multiple-puncture test. The Mantoux test remains the procedure of choice for assessing tuberculin delayed hypersensitivity. The test is performed by injecting 0.1 ml of PPD intradermally on the volar surface of the forearm.

The tuberculin skin test can be a valuable tool in diagnosing active tuberculosis, assessing the presence of disease in contacts of infected patients, and determining past inactive tuberculous infection in patients about to receive immunosuppressive therapy. The tuberculin skin test can also be used in institutions where there is a risk of acquiring tuberculosis, e.g., health care facilities and correctional institutions. Routine tuberculin skin testing is warranted in selected populations with high infection rates. Finally, tuberculin skin testing can be used for surveillance to accumulate epidemiologic data (see Table 17.1).

Tuberculin skin tests should be read at 48 to 72 hr after administration. Only induration, not erythema, should be measured, in millimeters. For the Mantoux test, the extent of induration should be measured in two directions and recorded. Multiple-puncture tests should be measured for the extent of induration and the presence or absence of vesiculation.

The two methods of reading skin tests are palpation and the ballpoint pen technique described by J. E. Sokal.[5] With the ballpoint method, four lines (two vertical, two horizontal) are drawn toward the margins of induration starting 1 to 2 cm from the edges. When the ballpoint reaches the edge of the induration, resistance is noted and movement of the pen is more difficult. The distance between the lines at the exact edge of induration in the four quadrants is recorded. If the diameter of the lesion between either set of lines is greater than 1 cm, the test is considered positive. There is some variability in the size of tuberculin reactions even when paired PPD skin tests administered at the same time are compared.

Table 17.1
Indications for Tuberculin Skin Testing

Diagnosis of active infection
Diagnosis of present or remote inactive infection
Diagnosis of infection in contacts of newly diagnosed cases
Diagnosis of past infection before initiation of immunosuppressive therapy
Screening of high-risk groups
Accumulation of epidemiologic data

INTERPRETATION OF TESTS

Approximately 75% of patients with active tuberculosis will have a positive intermediate-strength (5-TU) skin test at the time of presentation. Further testing with a 250-TU PPD of patients with negative 5-TU tests will increase the proportion of positive reactions to 90% to 95%. Thus, a negative 250-TU PPD skin test in a patient who is not anergic makes the diagnosis of tuberculosis very unlikely.

Interpretation of what constitutes a positive skin test is not always simple and is complicated by cross reactivity to the tuberculin induced by atypical mycobacteria. Generally, 10 mm or more of induration is considered a positive reaction to a Mantoux skin test. Induration of 5 to 9 mm may or may not indicate a positive test, depending on the clinical setting. In Georgia, a 7-mm skin test reaction probably represents infection with atypical mycobacteria. In Alaska, the same-size reaction probably indicates infection with *M. tuberculosis,* since atypical mycobacteria generally are not found in that area. In geographic areas where infection with atypical mycobacteria is common, 15 mm of induration is considered positive for tuberculosis.

For close contacts of patients with active tuberculosis and for persons with abnormal chest x rays consistent with tuberculosis, 5 mm of induration can be considered a positive skin test; reactions of less than 5 mm of induration are considered negative. Most persons who are infected, and especially those who have active disease, will have skin tests showing 14 to 16 mm of induration unless disseminated or severe infection produces relative or absolute anergy.

A positive multiple-puncture skin test consists of 2 mm or more of induration, coalescence of two puncture sites, or vesiculation. Except for a vesicular reaction, positive reactions should be confirmed with a Mantoux test.

Someone whose skin test changes from negative to positive on retesting is referred to as a converter. If the change occurs within a 2-year period, the patient is a "recent converter" and is at risk of active disease in the next few years. Conversion of a Mantoux skin test is defined as an increase in size of the induration of 6 mm or more, from less than 10 mm to more than 10 mm.

The form of tuberculin that was used for testing before 1970 was not stabilized with detergent, and it yielded false-negative results in many patients. When those previously "negative" patients were rechallenged with the more reliable stabilized antigen, many conversions were identified. Obviously, those patients were not converters but had simply been tested inadequately. Thus, a conversion in a person whose last skin test was in the 1960s may not be a conversion at all.

THE BOOSTER EFFECT

Another issue to consider in classifying individuals as recent converters is the booster effect.[6–8] This phenomenon refers to an increase in skin-test reactivity within a week to a year after the initial skin test because of immunologic recall or an enhanced cross reaction resulting from infection with other mycobacteria. An individual could incorrectly be considered a recent skin test converter as a result of the boosting effect.

The Centers for Disease Control recommend that when an individual has an initial Mantoux skin test of less than 10 mm, a second test should be done at least 1 week but no more than 3 weeks later. Approximately 6% of persons who have a repeat tuberculin test within 1 week will have a larger reaction to the second test. Because of the short interval between skin tests, boosting rather than a recent conversion following new infection is the most likely explanation. The dual skin testing technique will eliminate false recent converters and thus prevent unnecessary isoniazid therapy. The decision to administer isoniazid to a converter who exhibits the boosting effect should be based on the usual clinical indications for the therapy, and the person should not be considered a recent converter.

ANERGY

A positive tuberculin skin test can provide valuable supportive evidence for the diagnosis of active or past tuberculosis infection, but approximately 25% of patients with active pulmonary tuberculosis fail to respond to a 5-TU skin test.[10] The absence of delayed hypersensitivity can be generalized or specific for a single antigen. As noted, a positive 250-TU skin test also can be misleading, since it may reflect a sensitivity to cross-reacting tuberculosis antigens that results in a false-positive skin test. The value of the 250-TU skin test, then, is the virtual exclusion of the diagnosis of tuberculosis by a negative result, especially in patients who respond to other antigens such as *Candida* or mumps. Specific anergy to a PPD skin test occurs in fewer than 5% of patients with active tuberculosis.

Skin test anergy has various explanations, including problems with the skin test used, errors in administration of the tuberculin antigen, and misreading of the skin test. Suppression of tuberculin skin reactivity can also result from an acute viral infection (such as rubella), but reactivity is usually restored within 30 days after onset of the infection (see Table 17.2).

False-positive tuberculin skin tests have been reported rarely and should be suspected if a marked increase in positive PPD skin tests is noted at an institution. This may be caused by the tuberculin antigen used. This problem relates to the brand of tuberculin use and has been described with Parke Davis's Aplisol® as compared with another preparation, Tubersol®, prepared by Connaught.[9] Retesting of tuberculin-positive individuals with a different test brand is recommended to prevent unnecessary administration of isoniazid.

Delayed hypersensitivity to tuberculin generally develops 6 to 8 weeks after the initial infection. Corticosteroids, immunosuppressive drugs, and cytotoxic

Table 17.2
Causes of False-Negative Tuberculin Reactions

Technical errors
Inaccurate reaction measurement
Faulty antigen or administration
Reaction read too early (test conversion requires 6–8 weeks)
Impaired cellular immunity
Nonspecific
Hypoalbuminemia (<2 g/dl)
Old age (>70 years)
Anemia
Fever
Azotemia
Drugs and other therapy
Immunosuppressants
Irradiation
Antiviral vaccines
Specific diseases
Viral infection (e.g., rubella, infectious mononucleosis, mumps, influenza)
Overwhelming bacterial infections
Hodgkin's disease
Leukemia

agents induce anergy; therefore, patients should be skin-tested before these drugs are administered in order to avoid error in interpreting the test results.

Conversely, those who have received a bacillus Calmette–Guerin (BCG) vaccination usually have a skin test reaction of less than 15 mm of induration. A reaction of greater than 15 mm of induration suggests infection with *M. tuberculosis* or allergy to the vaccine. If infection is likely on the basis of a family history of tuberculosis or recent close contact with a patient with tuberculosis, the positive skin test should be attributed to *M. tuberculosis* infection and not the BCG vaccination.[11]

DIAGNOSIS

Tuberculosis remains one of the most difficult diagnostic problems for clinicians. The incidence of tuberculosis is high in some sectors of our population (notably, recent immigrants from Third World countries), and the disease has a persistent reservoir in the population of elderly Americans. When the diagnosis is unsuspected, the consequences can be disastrous for the patient and those in close contact with the patient. If employed appropriately and interpreted wisely, tuberculin skin testing is an inexpensive, useful adjunct in the diagnosis of an insidious, contagious, and potentially lethal disease if untreated.

A positive skin test using intermediate PPD-S (5-TU as noted above) of 10 mm of induration indicates a recent or remote infection, usually with *M. tuberculosis*. In the absence of evidence of active disease, a positive delayed hypersensitivity reacton to tuberculin means that the primary infection has been arrested by the host. Thus, the tuberculin-positive person contains viable tubercle bacilli that, although contained by acquired cellular immunity, may multiply in subsequent years with alterations in host resistance factors. In fact, 92% of all new cases of active pulmonary tuberculosis are reactivation disease. The term isoniazid chemoprophylaxis is not in fact prophylaxis but actual treatment to prevent the development of active tuberculosis. Single-drug therapy is effective since the number of organisms is small, and thus there is little chance of selecting out resistant mycobacteria.

When recent converters have daily cultures of an early morning gastric aspirate, urine, and induced sputum, in most, a few colonies of mycobacteria can be isolated.[12] The risk that this primary infection with few tubercle bacilli will progress to active disease varies with different groups.[13,14] The highest risk occurs in recent tuberculin converters. Those with a positive skin test within the past 2 years have a 3.3% chance of the development of active disease within the first year. The risks in other groups of tuberculin reactors are as follows: household contacts of patients with active disease, if tuberculin-positive, a 2.7% risk, or tuberculin-negative, a 0.5% risk; patients with a history of tuberculosis, now inactive, but inadequately treated, a 1.3% risk; tuberculin reactors with a chest x ray consistent with healed adult-type tuberculosis, i.e., apical scaring and calcifications, a 0.8% risk; tuberculin reactors under the age of 35 years, especially children and adolescents, with a normal or abnormal chest x ray, a 0.2% risk; tuberculin-positive adults over 35 years of age with a normal chest film, a 0.08% risk; and tuberculin reactors with certain underlying diseases or conditions such as hematological or reticuloendothelial malignancy, acquired immune deficiency syndrome, diabetes, and silicosis, or patients who have had a gastrectomy or who are receiving corticosteroids, immunosuppressive drugs, or other cytotoxic agents. The risk of reactivation in patients with various underlying illnesses listed above is unknown, but establishing the tuberculin status at the time of disease onset or immunosuppressive therapy is valuable.[15–18]

TREATMENT

Numerous controlled studies have shown that 12 months of isoniazid therapy is effective in reducing the number of cases of active disease in tuberculin reactors.[19,20] The risk of active disease in a placebo group was found to be as much as 61 times that seen in patients treated with isoniazid. It was shown that 80% of the active cases in a placebo group occurred in the first year after diagnosis, but the onset of active disease may be delayed as long as 8 years.

Since isoniazid chemoprophylaxis was found so effective in reducing the risk of development of active disease, it was recommended to all persons whose tuberculin skin test was positive. However, since reports of isoniazid hepatitis have appeared, its use has been restricted to the high-risk groups discussed previously.

The management of adults with a positive tuberculin skin test and a negative chest x ray who are not in another high-risk group or are recent converters is controversial.[21–24] For those persons under age 35 years, isoniazid chemoprophylaxis is advised by the American Thoracic Society and the Centers for Disease Control. For individuals above 35 years of age, the risk of isoniazid hepatitis is felt by some experts to exceed the benefits of isoniazid chemoprophylaxis. Various reports using decision analysis for low-risk tuberculin reactors have come to conflicting conclusions.[21–24] In a recent analysis using four outcome measurements—life expectancy, likelihood of isoniazid hepatitis, likelihood of active tuberculosis, and risk of fatal illness—the authors concluded that for all low-risk tuberculin reactors from ages 35 to 80 years, the benefits of isoniazid chemoprophylaxis outweighed the risks.[24] In another large study of nursing home residents over age 50 years, the authors demonstrated that persons whose tuberculin skin test has shown a conversion with an increase of at least 12 mm of induration from the last negative reaction would also clearly benefit from isoniazid chemoprophylaxis.[25] In this group of converters, the risk for active tuberculosis in those not given isoniazid was 7.6% for women and 11.7% for men. It should be noted that these elderly persons were not recent converters, a group that clearly needs to be treated with isoniazid. When a comparable group of tuberculin converters was given isoniazid, only 0.1 to 0.2% developed active tuberculosis.[25] The risk of hepatic toxicity was 3.4 to 4.9%, and there were no isoniazid-related deaths. In those persons given isoniazid, the risk of developing clinical tuberculosis was only 0.2%.

Another controversial issue is the 12-month duration of isoniazid chemoprophylaxis compared with only 6 to 9 months to treat active disease.[26] In a trial conducted in Eastern Europe, persons with a positive tuberculin skin test and fibrotic lesions on chest x ray were given isoniazid for 12, 24, and 52 weeks' duration.[27] The 24-week regimen appeared to be superior to either the 12- or the 52-week course in terms of effectiveness and toxicity. The 12-week course of isoniazid was not very efficacious, and concern was raised in the article that if the drug were prescribed for 24 weeks, some patients might take the drug for only 12 weeks. Although a 12-month course is effective, future studies should look at 6-month regimens, which appear to be effective, and to have less associated toxicity and cost than the standard 12-month course of therapy.

Another controversial area concerns the use of alternative regimens if isoniazid resistance is suspected or if a patient cannot tolerate isoniazid. Isoniazid resistance occurs in 0 to 41% of *Mycobacterium tuberculosis* isolates from patients from Southeast Asia.[28] No other drugs have been studied, but rifampin in a dosage of 600 mg/day for 6 to 12 months should be effective.

Although the exact pathogenic mechanism of isoniazid-associated hepatitis is unknown, certain features seem clear.[29,30] Elevations in the liver enzymes with or without symptoms will develop in about 10–20% of those taking isoniazid. A small percentage of patients will have jaundice and fatal hepatitis. The onset of the liver function abnormalities varies widely from 1 week to 11 months after starting treatment. Half the reactions occur within the initial 2 months, especially during the second month. Fatal hepatitis has been more common in patients taking isoniazid for at least 8 weeks than in those on therapy for a shorter period, and it has often occurred in patients who were continued on therapy even after symptoms developed. Symptoms of liver disease—anorexia, malaise, nausea, and vomiting—are insensitive predictors of isoniazid liver toxicity, and biochemical monitoring is required. The incidence of isoniazid hepatitis is age related, being rare under the age of 20 years and increasing progressively with age. The incidence is 0.3% in the age group 20 to 34 years and 1.2% in those 35 to 49 years of age. In patients 50 or more years of age, the incidence rises to 2.3%. Clinically, biochemically, and histologically, the liver injury is indistinguishable from viral hepatitis.

Thus, the decision to treat a tuberculin reactor with isoniazid is not easy and should be individualized. Active tuberculosis should be excluded, since two or more drugs will be required if it is present. An alternative approach to isoniazid administration is careful observation of reactors and institution of therapy for active tuberculosis if it occurs. On the other hand, if isoniazid is selected, its benefits must be weighed carefully against the risk of toxicity. The high-risk groups with positive skin tests deserve strong consideration, especially if they are children or adolescents. Monthly monitoring of hepatic function tests is suggested, and the drug must be discontinued if the SGOT or SGPT values exceed four to five times the normal value. Although transient enzyme elevations can occur in patients 35 years of age, close surveillance is required. Discontinuation of isoniazid is necessary in 5–7% of patients. Future studies may provide alternative agents or short-course regimens with greater benefit–risk ratios than exist at present.

REFERENCES

1. Stead WW, Lofgren JP, Warren E, *et al:* Tuberculosis as an endemic and nosocomial infection among the elderly in nursing homes. *N Engl J Med* 1985; 312:1483–1487.
2. American Thoracic Society: The tuberculin skin test. *Am Rev Respir Dis* 1981; 124:356–363.
3. Snider DE Jr: The tuberculin skin test. *Am Rev Respir Dis* 1982; 125:108–118.
4. Nash DR, Douglass JE: Anergy in active pulmonary tuberculosis: A comparison between

positive and negative reactors and an evaluation of 5 TU and 250 TU skin test doses. *Chest* 1980; 77:32–37.
5. Sokal JE: Measurement of delayed skin-test responses. *N Engl J Med* 1975; 293:501–502.
6. Thompson NJ, Glassroth, JL, Snider DE Jr, *et al:* The booster phenomenon in serial tuberculin testing. *Am Rev Respir Dis* 1979; 119:5O7–597.
7. Simon JA, McVicker SJ, Ferrell CR, *et al:* Two-step tuberculin testing in a veterans domiciliary population. *South Med J* 1983; 76:866–869.
8. Snider DE, Cauthen GM: Tuberculin skin testing of hospital employees: Infection, ''boosting,'' and two-step testing. *Am J Infect Control* 1984; 12:305–311.
9. Kallay MC, Bell KM, Montalbano B: False positive reactions to Aplisol (Parke-Davis) with serial PPD skin testing (abstract). *Am Rev Respir Dis* 1987; 135(Suppl):A45.
10. Johnston WW, Saltzman HA, Bufkin JH, *et al:* The tuberculin test and the diagnosis of clinical tuberculosis. *Am Rev Respir Dis* 1960; 81:189–195.
11. Snider DE Jr. Bacille Calmette–Guerin vaccination and tuberculin skin test. *JAMA* 1985; 253:3438–3439.
12. Kent DC, Reid D, Sokolowski JW, *et al:* Tuberculin conversion. The iceberg of tuberculosis pathogenesis. *Arch Environ Health* 1967; 14:580–584.
13. Moulding T: Chemoprophylaxis of tuberculosis: When is the benefit worth the risk and cost? *Ann Intern Med* 1971; 74:761–770.
14. American Thoracic Society, American Lung Association, and Centers for Disease Control: Preventive therapy for tuberculosis infection. *Am Rev Respir Dis* 1974; 110:371–374.
15. Sahn SA, Lakshminarayan S: Tuberculosis after corticosteroid therapy. *Br J Dis Chest* 1976; 70:195–205.
16. Kaplan MH, Armstrong D, Rosen P: Tuberculosis complicating neoplastic disease: A review of 201 cases. *Cancer* 1974; 33:850–858.
17. Befeler B, Baum GL: Active pulmonary tuberculosis after upper gastrointestinal surgery. *Am Rev Respir Dis* 1967; 96:977–980.
18. Rose DN, Silver AL, Schechter CB: Tuberculosis chemoprophylaxis for diabetics: Are the benefits of isoniazid worth the risk? *Mt Sinai J Med* 1985; 52:253–258.
19. Curry FJ: Prophylactic effect of isoniazid in young tuberculin reactors. *N Engl J Med* 1967; 277:562–567.
20. Hsu KHK: Isoniazid in the prevention and treatment of tuberculosis. A 20-year study of the effectiveness in children. *JAMA* 1974; 229:528–533.
21. Comstock GW, Edwards PQ: The competing risks of tuberculosis and hepatitis for adult tuberculin reactors. *Am Rev Respir Dis* 1975; 111:573–577.
22. Taylor WC, Aronson MD, Delbanco TL: Should young adults with a positive tuberculin test take isoniazid? *Ann Intern Med* 1981; 94:808–813.
23. Comstock GW: Evaluating isoniazid preventive therapy: The need for more data. *Ann Intern Med* 1981; 94:817–819.
24. Rose DN, Schechter CB, Silver AL: The age threshold for isoniazid chemoprophylaxis. *JAMA* 1986; 256:2709–2713.
25. Stead WW, To T, Harrison RW, *et al:* Benefit–risk considerations in preventive treatment for tuberculosis in elderly persons. *Ann Intern Med* 1987; 107:843–845.
26. Snider DE, Caras, GJ, Koplan JP: Preventive therapy with isoniazid. Cost-effectiveness of different durations of therapy. *JAMA* 1986; 255:1579–1583.
27. Thompson NJ: Efficacy of various durations of isoniazid preventive therapy for tuberculosis: Five years of followup in the IUAT trial. *Bull WHO* 1982; 60:555–564.
28. Centers for Disease Control: Drug resistance among Indochinese refugees with tuberculosis. *Morbid Mortal Week Rep* 1981; 30:273–274.

29. Mitchell JR, Zimmerman HJ, Ishak KG, *et al:* Isoniazid liver injury: Clinical spectrum, pathology and probable pathogenesis. *Ann Intern Med* 1976; 84:181–192.
30. Black M, Mitchell JR, Zimmerman HJ, *et al:* Isoniazid-associated hepatitis in 114 patients. *Gastroenterology* 1975; 69:289–302.

ADDITIONAL READINGS

Snider DE Jr: Decision analysis for isoniazid preventive therapy: Take it or leave it? *Am Rev Respir Dis* 1988; 137:2–3.

Snider DE, Farer LS: Preventive therapy for tuberculosis infection: An intervention in need of improvement. *Am Rev Respir Dis* 1984; 130:355–356.

Tsevat J, Taylor WC, Wong JB, *et al:* Isoniazid for the tuberculin reactor: Take it or leave it. *Am Rev Respir Dis* 1988; 137:215–220.

18

Selective Laboratory Studies

Richard A. Gleckman and John S. Czachor

BLOOD CULTURES

Bacteremia occurs in the course of both localized and systemic infections. Bacteremia can be transient, as when colonized mucosal surfaces are instrumented; intermittent, a characteristic of undrained abscess and gram-negative bacteremia; or continuous, the hallmark of an intravascular infection, particularly endocarditis and septic thrombophlebitis. There should be no hesitation to obtain blood cultures in selected outpatients, such as patients with persistent fever who have no obvious explanation for this abnormality and do not appear so ill that they require hospital admission, patients with known rheumatic heart disease or with prosthetic heart valves who appear to have a febrile, flulike illness, and patients with fever and bleeding into the skin (petechiae, ecchymoses) or fever with pustular lesions.

Table 18.1 details the value of blood cultures. In addition to the merits of blood cultures depicted in the table, blood cultures also serve an additional dimension (objective criterion), to gauge the adequacy of therapy.

Virtually all bacteremias will be detected if adequate amounts of blood are obtained (>10 cc/bottle of 90 cc medium), multiple blood cultures are performed (at least two, and preferably three), and the patient has not recently received an antimicrobial agent.[1] The recovery of pneumococci, *Haemophilus influenzae, Neisseria gonorrhoeae,* group A or B β-hemolytic streptococci, *Listeria* sp., and gram-negative aerobic bacilli (Enterobacteriaceae and *Pseudomonas* sp.) is consistent with the isolation of a pathogen, not a contaminant.[2] Alternatively, when *Staphylococcus* non-*aureus, Bacillus* sp., diphtheroids and α-hemolytic streptococci are isolated, they can usually be regarded as "contaminants." However, in selected high-risk patients (those with rheumatic heart disease or prosthetic heart valves; those with intravascular Hickman or Broviac catheters; those who are intravenous drug addicts) and immunocompromised

Table 18.1
Value of Blood Cultures

1.	Confirm the fact that the patient's clinical features are caused by an infection
2.	Support the clinical impression (e.g., prosthetic valve endocarditis, disseminated gonococcemia, chronic meningococcemia)
3.	Establish the etiology of an infection not readily accessible to direct bacteriological analysis (e.g., endocarditis, acute osteomyelitis)
4.	Provide direction for the diagnostic work-up in identifying the tissue source of an infection
5.	Reveal occult life-endangering processes (association of α-hemolytic *Streptococcus* with endocarditis, *Streptococcus bovis* with colon cancer, *Clostridium septicum* with hematological malignancy)
6.	Offer a guideline for initial antibiotic therapy while awaiting definitive susceptibility data

hosts (granulocytopenic individuals), these organisms can represent true pathogens. As a general rule, the infrequent or isolated recovery of these organisms that are often considered "contaminants," combined with a delay before they are detected in the blood culture bottles (>4 days), reaffirms the suspicion that the isolates represent contamination, not real pathogens.

When the patient has previously received an antibiotic, the clinician might consider using the antimicrobial removal device (ARD, Marion Laboratories). This system contains antibiotic-adsorbent resins and, on occasion, will be advantageous to increase the yield of some bacteria, particularly *Staphylococcus aureus*.[3] Another approach is to use the technique of lysis centrifugation, a system known as the isolator (DuPont). The isolator detects more bacteremias and accomplishes this more rapidly. An additional advantage of the isolator is the earlier availability of colonies for identification and susceptibility testing. The isolator is considered the single best blood culture technique for the recovery of atypical mycobacteria and fungi in immunocompromised hosts.[4] However, the isolator is inferior to traditional systems to recover anaerobes and pneumococci, and this new system is not only more expensive but also rather frequently associated with the recovery of "contaminants."

SERUM ANTIBIOTIC CONCENTRATIONS

There is a national trend to complete antibiotic treatment at home for those hospitalized patients who appear to be entering the resolution phase of their infectious disease. Particularly for those patients who are elderly and have evidence of renal insufficiency and/or eighth nerve damage, sequential assays of antimicrobial activity in the serum are essential when prolonged treatment with an aminoglycoside antibiotic (gentamicin, tobramycin, amikacin, netilmicin) or vancomycin is contemplated. Therapeutic drug monitoring is designed to confirm the achievement of therapeutic concentrations of these antibiotics and to preclude antibiotic-related toxicities attributable to excessive serum drug levels. Nomograms have been consistently unreliable as guides for aminoglycoside prescribing, because the pharmacokinetic parameters of these compounds vary greatly from individual to individual, such that the plasma concentrations produced by the same absolute or relative dose of these drugs vary severalfold between patients.

Desirable peak and trough plasma concentrations for outpatients receiving the aminoglycoside antibiotics or vancomycin could consist of the following: for gentamicin and tobramycin, peaks of 5–7 μg/ml, with trough <2 μg/ml; for amikacin, a peak of 25 μg/ml, with trough of <8 μg/ml; and for vancomycin, a peak of 30 μg/ml, with a trough of <10 μg/ml. The aminoglycosides are prescribed as an intravenous infusion administered over 30 to 60 min. Vancomycin infusions are administered over 60 to 90 min to prevent acute histamine-mediated flushing (the red-man syndrome) as well as potentially life-threatening cardiac arrhythmias.

The essential element in the performance of antibiotic assays is appropriate timing of the specimen collections.[5] Patients receiving out-of-hospital aminoglycoside or vancomycin should have monitoring of renal function (serum creatinine measurements) and antibiotic assays performed at least once a week. These measurements should be obtained more often if desired plasma drug concentrations have not been achieved or the patient has impaired hearing or renal insufficiency.

TESTS FOR SEXUALLY TRANSMITTED DISEASES

Gonorrhea

For men with symptomatic gonococcal urethritis, the Gram stain can be regarded as a highly sensitive and specific test. The Gram stain is very specific but not very sensitive for symptomatic women. For asymptomatic men and women, culture is the traditional technique to establish the diagnosis of gonorrhea. A number of potential problems with cultures have been recognized, however. The technique requires 24 to 72 hr for the isolation and identification of *Neisseria gonorrhoeae*. In addition, some gonococci will not grow on the selective media because the organisms are suppressed by the vancomycin or trimethoprim added to the medium. Ideally there should be immediate plating of the specimen. If this is not possible, inoculate selective media and transport the specimen in a plastic bag containing a CO_2-generating tablet.[6]

An immunologic method, known as Gonozyme, has been developed as an alternative to the culture technique.[7] The Gonozyme test detects gonococcal antigens contained in urethral and endocervical secretions. This immunologic procedure can provide results within 3 hr of collection of the specimen, and it can potentially detect organisms that fail to grow because of mishandling of the culture system or inhibition of the bacterium by antimicrobial agents incorporated into the culture media. The test has a number of limitations, however: it cannot be used to test rectal or pharyngeal specimens; it cannot be used as a test of cure for women; and it has been associated with an unacceptable number of false-negative results when evaluated in a population of women with a low prevalence of disease.[8,9] As importantly, this test does not lend itself to the performance of β-lactamase or susceptibility testing, an important consideration in light of the recognition of the increasing emergence of antimicrobial-resistant strains.

Chlamydia trachomatis

Genital infection caused by *Chlamydia trachomatis* is the most common bacterial sexually transmitted disease in the United States. The organism can cause symptomatic cervicitis, salpingitis, postpartum endometritis, perihepatitis, and the urethral syndrome in women and symptomatic urethritis, epididymitis, proctitis, and trigger Reiter's syndrome in men.[10] The organism can exist in an asymptomatic state in both men and women. Asymptomatic disease in men can be transmitted to women, and vice versa. In women asymptomatic disease can cause pelvic inflammatory disease, with its potential sequelae of involuntary infertility, as well as ectopic pregnancy. Asymptomatic disease in the pregnant woman can result in neonatal conjunctivitis and pneumonia.

The diverse manifestations of disease caused by *Chlamydia trachomatis* and the potentially serious nature of infection caused by this organism have stimulated efforts to devise techniques to screen for this bacterium. Groups for whom screening would be desirable include the following: pregnant women; family planning clinic attendees; persons attending sexually transmitted disease clinics; and women with mucopurulent cervicitis, sterile pyuria with dysuria, and pelvic inflammatory disease.

Cell culture isolation has traditionally been regarded as the "gold standard" or definitive means of diagnosing *Chlamydia* infection. However, there are numerous factors that influence the recovery of *Chlamydia* (number of samples obtained; number of body sites sampled; acquisition, transport, and storage of the sample; and serial tissue-culture passages), so that even a negative culture result does not absolutely exclude the possibility of a chlamydial infection.[11]

The insensitivity of the culture technique, particularly when the patient is asymptomatic or blind passage is not performed, coupled with the cost, technical difficulty, rigid transport requirements, and delay in interpretation, has encouraged the development of two alternative antigen tests for the detection of *Chlamydia* in clinical specimens.

The direct detection immunologic method marketed as Micro Trak (Syva, Palo Alto, CA) uses fluorescein-conjugated monoclonal antibodies directed against *Chlamydia trachomatis* to identify elementary bodies in genital secretions.[12] This test has been found to be uniformly specific, that is, smear negative when simultaneous culture was negative, in all populations studied. There are three distinct limitations of this test, however. Performance of the test requires skilled personnel, individuals very experienced in fluorescence microscopy. There are no standards, relative to the number of columnar cells in the specimen or number of elementary bodies, that constitute a positive test. In addition, the direct fluorescent antibody test is not very sensitive, particularly for patients such as those asymptomatic individuals attending a family planning clinic or a private physician's office when small numbers of organisms exist.[13]

An enzyme-linked immunoassay, known as Chlamydiazyme (Abbott Laboratories), consists of antiserum that reacts with chlamydial lipopolysaccharide in urethral and cervical secretions. This test requires only 4 hr, is less labor intensive than the direct fluorescein-labeled monoclonal antibody procedure, necessitates less skill for interpretation, and accommodates large-volume testing. Chlamydiazyme has consistently demonstrated a high level of specificity.[14] However, when this enzyme immunoassay is applied to a population with a low prevalence of chlamydial infections, such as asymptomatic women presenting for routine antepartum or gynecological care, the test will not be very sensitive.[13,15]

It appears that the nonculture antigen detection tests will fail to detect a modest number of chlamydial isolates. In addition, on occasion, these tests will provide a positive result that will not be confirmed by the culture technique. In essence, if clinicians seek a less expensive, more rapid test than culture, and if they are willing to accept the limitations of the antigen detection tests, the immunofluorescent procedure and the enzyme immunoassay offer alternatives. If, however, physicians seek a more precise but still not infallible test to detect *Chlamydia* (when there are issues regarding rape, suspected child abuse, social consequences of informing someone that he or she has a sexually transmissible disease), a culture should be performed.

ACUTE AND CONVALESCENT SERUM

Serological tests represent invaluable diagnostic tools for the microbiologist and the clinician. These studies measure the host's antibody response to infecting organisms. Currently, serological tests are available to detect evidence of infection from some bacteria, *Chlamydia,* rickettsiae, parasites, and viruses. Many of these organisms have fastidious growth requirements, necessitating special media or growth conditions, and are difficult for the microbiology laboratory to isolate and identify. The use of serological methods allows the clinician alternative means to diagnose these infections.

Although serological tests often provide exclusively retrospective information to confirm a diagnosis, there remain situations in which their use is beneficial, especially in selected acute infections. They also serve to determine immune status, as in the case of rubella.

Traditionally, two blood specimens are collected approximately 3 to 4 weeks apart. These are known as "paired sera" and constitute the acute and convalescent sera. The delay interposed between collections is necessary in order to allow the host significant time to generate an antibody response to microbial antigens. If the sera are drawn too close together, the rise of antibody titer will be missed; if they are drawn too far apart, then the timing of onset of an infection will be uninterpretable. The level of antibody titer should rise from lower to higher levels to reflect the appearance of antibody production. A fourfold rise in antibody titer is traditionally considered indicative of a "significant" change. Fourfold rises in antibody titers have been invaluable to establish the diagnosis of such disorders as Lyme disease, mycoplasma pneumonia, and *Legionella* sp.-related pneumonia. On occasion, a single high titer in the absence of a fourfold rise in antibody production is sufficient to diagnose some diseases, including cytomegalovirus, trichinosis, toxoplasmosis, tularemia, and brucellosis.

There are instances, however, in which specific antibody production to an infective process persists for a short period of time only, then disappears after the primary infection has remitted. In these situations, only one serological analysis is necessary to establish the diagnosis. The response of VCA IgM of Epstein–Barr virus is an example of a single specific serological response.

SERUM CIDAL TESTING

The serum bactericidal test (SBT) measures the ability of a patient's serum to demonstrate a bactericidal effect for the organism causing an infection. The test has been used by some physicians to monitor the antibiotic therapy of patients receiving treatment for endocarditis and osteomyelitis. There are a number of reasons, however, why there has not been universal acceptance of the SBT. The test is expensive and time consuming. Numerous variables, such as inoculum size, pH, cation concentration, composition of the medium, and temperature of incubation, influence the test results. In addition, little data exist to suggest that the test has clinical relevance.[16]

Using a standardized microdilution method, which in its own right has some inadequacies when compared to the traditional macrodilution method, researchers reported that a peak serum bactericidal titer of 1 : 64 or greater and trough titers of 1 : 32 or greater were associated with a 100% bacteriological cure of patients with endocarditis.[17] Lower titers were not useful in predicting bacteriological cure or bacteriological failure. However, it should be emphasized that the bactericidal titer was not a good predictor of clinical cure. The bottom line is that a consensus has emerged that the optimum, desired SBT (if one exists) to manage patients with endocarditis needs to be determined by multicenter clinical studies and that it is not appropriate for the clinician to administer excessive doses of antibiotics, with their inherent risk of toxicity, simply to achieve "desired" SBT results.[18]

The SBT has also been evaluated as a predictor of drug efficacy for patients subjected to surgical debridement for the management of chronic osteomyelitis. In the present DRG era, the lion's share of these patients will be managed in an outpatient setting. Using a microdilution technique, investigators noted a correlation between clinical cure and the achievement of peak serum bactericidal titers of 1 : 16 or greater and trough titers of 1 : 4 or greater.[19] If this observation is confirmed and the SBT technique becomes reproducible in additional laboratories, the clinician may want to employ the SBT to guide the antibiotic treatment of chronic osteomyelitis of adults.

SOFT TISSUE INFECTIONS

The final report issued by the laboratory on a specimen labeled "soft tissue" can, at times, be a source of frustration for the clinician. After collecting a specimen from a wound or alternative skin infection, the physician is often provided with a report that reads "normal flora." However, there are ways to obtain meaningful microbiological data.

Specimens from skin, soft tissues, wounds, and draining sinuses are subject to contamination with local skin bacteria, and the organisms isolated may not represent the actual pathogen responsible for the infection.[20] Appropriate antiseptic preparation of the skin is necessary prior to specimen collection, and it will enhance the opportunity to secure a valid result. Also, consideration must be given to obtaining deep cultures in wounds that have a sinus tract. This technique can help eliminate confusion with surface or colonizing bacteria. When concern exists for a bone or cartilage infection, histological evaluation, in addition to microbiological assessment, can be very helpful in supporting the presumptive clinical diagnosis of chronic infection.

Epidemiologic data should be provided by the clinician, as this extra information can alert the microbiology laboratory to the possibility of an unusual pathogen(s). Contact with sea water or fish tanks (*Mycobacterium marinum*), rose bushes (sporotrichosis), cats (*Pasteurella* sp.), or dogs (DF-2) exemplifies historical features that might assist in the isolation of a rare pathogen.

When considering soft tissue abscesses such as carbuncles, it is usually best to obtain specimens either through needle and syringe aspiration or incision with deep drainage collection, rather than trying to express the drainage through the skin, thereby resulting in contamination. If possible, prompt transport of the material in appropriate containers (capped syringe with needle properly disposed) will help to reduce the possibility of contamination and enhance the possibility of isolating fastidious organisms. A Gram stain and, on occasion, an acid-fast stain should supplement all culture requests.

Microbiological evaluation of cellulitits is accomplished by analyzing the aspirated material from the erythematous region beyond the indurated plateau ("the leading edge") or the center of the lesion. The preferred site has never been unequivocally determined. The use of nonbacteriostatic saline solution as a vehicle for recovery of organisms is recommended: 0.1 or 0.2 cc of this solution is injected, then back aspirated. The resultant material is examined via Gram stain and cultured. Aspiration of skin lesions or petechiae is performed in a similar fashion, but the procedure is directed at the base of the lesion.

Anaerobic infections appear to be increasing in frequency, either through greater physician awareness of the pathogenic potential of these microorganisms or improved microbiological isolation techniques. Signs that suggest potential anaerobic infection in soft tissues include foul-smelling discharge (although its absence does **not** rule out the possibility of anaerobic infection), an adjacent site harboring anaerobic bacteria, gas in the tissues, infection contained in necrotic tissues, Gram stain of purulent exudate revealing polymicrobic flora, and negative aerobic culture results despite organisms seen on Gram-stained smears.[21] Special anaerobic collection and transport media should be utilized once the specimen is recovered. As with any other specimens for culture, refrigeration or incubation should be avoided, and processing should be completed expeditiously.

INFECTIOUS DIARRHEA

Diarrhea is something everyone has intimate knowledge about, as most people average one to two episodes per year.[22] Younger children have the highest attack rates, and viral agents are the most frequently implicated offending pathogens. In industrialized countries, diarrhea is regarded as a nuisance, but in developing countries, it is responsible for significant morbidity and mortality. Diarrhea is second only to the common cold in terms of frequency of infectious disorders throughout the world, and as many as 10% of presenting chief complaints to primary care physicians are attributable to diarrheal diseases.[23]

In the past, indiscriminate use of stool cultures without regard to historical factors, plus testing for only a limited number of pathogens (*Salmonella* and *Shigella* species), resulted in only 1.5–2.5% of all specimens evaluated having a pathogen isolated, at a final cost of $900–1200 per positive culture.[22] By being more selective, that is, ordering cultures only in people with pertinent historical features, and by expanding the organisms tested/isolated, this cost has been drastically reduced from this original dollar amount.

Predisposing features that alert the physician to a process that requires a stool culture rather than a self-limiting disorder include fever, bloody diarrhea, persistent abdominal pain, travel, seafood ingestion, recent antibiotic use, receptive male homosexual activity, prolonged duration of illness, and outbreak of similar illness.

The fecal leukocyte test is a valuable screening tool for the evaluation of diarrhea. Stool is stained using methylene blue and examined under a microscope for the presence of neutrophils. However, the absence of leukocytes does not rule out an infectious diarrhea.

Stool cultures are able to isolate many enteric bacterial pathogens, routinely *Salmonella* sp., *Shigella* sp., and *Campylobacter* sp. Special cultures for *Yersinia, Vibrio, Aeromonas,* and *Plesiomonas* are available but must specifically be requested. Although *C. difficile* can be diagnosed through the use of sigmoidoscopy, with identification of pseudomembranes, the diagnosis can also be supported through the detection of the organism's cytotoxin in the stool. Currently, the only virus conventional laboratories are capable of identifying is the rotavirus, using one of a number of commercially available enzyme-linked immunosorbent assay tests (ELISA).

Diarrhea caused by parasites is evaluated by repetitive microscopic examination of stool samples for ova and parasites. Three stool samples, obtained from separate days, are the usual approach because of the intermittent nature of shedding of the ova or the adult parasite or an irregular migratory pattern of the parasite itself. Other sources of material from which parasites can be isolated include sigmoidoscopic aspirations, gastroduodenal contents, and, on rare occasions, abscesses.

Stool specimens can be examined in a number of ways. Wet-mount examination mixes the sample with physiological saline and is suitable for the detection of trophozoites and cysts. Concentration of stool samples is a valuable technique when low-grade infection exists. Cysts, ova, and larvae are recovered in greater amounts when concentrated, although trophozoites are unable to be identified using this method. Permanent staining of stool samples offers a number of advantages: a reproducible record of stool contents, the ability to have other microbiologists examine unusual findings, and the opportunity to maintain evidence of a parasitic infection. This method is especially useful when examining the stool for trophozoites and small organisms not detected by other means.

REFERENCES

1. Washington JA II: Blood cultures: Principles and techniques. *Mayo Clin Proc* 1975; 50:91–98.
2. Weinstein MP, Reller LB, Murphy JR, *et al:* The clinical significance of positive blood cultures: A comprehensive analysis of 500 episodes of bacteremia and fungemia in adults. *Rev Infect Dis* 1983; 5:35–53.
3. Washington JA II, Ilstrup DM: Blood cultures: Issues and controversies. *Rev Infect Dis* 1986; 5:792–802.

4. Henry NK, McLimans CA, Wright AJ, *et al:* Microbiological and clinical evaluation of the Isolator lysis-centrifugation blood culture tube. *J Clin Microbiol* 1983; 17:864–869.
5. Rosenblatt JE: Laboratory tests to guide antimicrobial therapy. *Mayo Clin Proc* 1987; 62:799–805.
6. Monif GRG, Jordan PA, Thompson JL, *et al:* Pragmatic factors influencing the detection of *Neisseria gonorrhoeae. Obstet Gynecol* 1982; 59:649–652.
7. Demetriou E, Sackett R, Welch DF, *et al:* Evaluation of an enzyme immunoassay for detection of *Neisseria gonorrhoeae* in an adolescent population. *JAMA* 1984; 252:247–250.
8. Granato PA, Roefaro M: Comparative evaluation of enzyme immunoassay and culture for the laboratory diagnosis of gonorrhea. *Am J Clin Pathol* 1985; 83:613–618.
9. Nachamkin I, Sondheimer SJ, Barbagallo S, *et al:* Detection of *Neisseria gonorrhoeae* in cervical swabs using the gonozyme enzyme immunoassay. *Am J Clin Pathol* 1984; 82:461–465.
10. Martin DH, Pollock S, Kuo CC, *et al: Chlamydia trachomatis* infections in men with Reiter's syndrome. *Ann Intern Med* 1984; 100:207–213.
11. Jones RB, Katz BP, VanderPol B, *et al:* Effect of blind passage and multiple sampling on recovery of *Chlamydia trachomatis* from urogenital specimens. *J Clin Microbiol* 1986; 24:1029–1033.
12. Stamm WE, Harrison HR, Alexander ER, *et al:* Diagnosis of *Chlamydia trachomatis* infections by direct immunofluorescence staining of genital secretions. *Ann Intern Med* 1984; 101:638–641.
13. Smith JW, Rogers RE, Katz PB, *et al:* Diagnosis of chlamydial infection in women attending antenatal and gynecologic clinics. *J Clin Microbiol* 1987; 25:868–872.
14. Howard LV, Coleman PF, England BJ, *et al:* Evaluation of Chlamydiazyme for the detection of genital infections caused by *Chlamydia trachomatis. J Clin Microbiol* 1986; 23:329–332.
15. Hipp SS, Han Y, Murphy D: Assessment of enzyme immunoassay and immunofluorescence tests for detection of *Chlamydia trachomatis. J Clin Microbiol* 1987; 25:1938–1943.
16. Wolfson JS, Swartz MN: Serum bactericidal activity as a monitor of antibody therapy. *N Engl J Med* 1985; 312:969–975.
17. Weinstein MP, Stratton CW, Ackley A, *et al:* Multicenter collaborative evaluation of a standardized serum bactericidal test as a prognostic indicator in infective endocarditis. *Am J Med* 1984; 78:262–269.
18. Reller LB: The serum bactericidal test. *Rev Infect Dis* 1986; 8:803–808.
19. Weinstein MP, Stratton CW, Hawley HB, *et al:* Multicenter collaborative evaluation of a standardized serum bactericidal test as a predictor of therapeutic efficacy in acute and chronic osteomyelitis. *Am J Med* 1987; 83:218–222.
20. Bartlett RC: Making optimum use of the microbiology laboratory. *JAMA* 1982; 247:1336–1338.
21. Lefrock JL, Molavi A: Necrotizing skin and subcutaneous infections. *J Antimicrob Chemother* 1982; 9:183–192.
22. Guerrant RL, Wallace CE, Barrett LJ, *et al:* A cost effective and effective approach to the diagnosis and management of acute infectious diarrhea. *Bull NY Acad Med* 1987; 63:484–499.
23. Guerrant RL, Shields DS, Thorson SM, *et al:* Evaluation and diagnosis of acute infectious diarrhea. *Am J Med* 1985; 78(suppl 6B):91–98.

19

Home Intravenous Antibiotic Therapy

Richard B. Brown

INTRODUCTION

The delivery of home therapy has become one of the most rapidly growing sectors of the health care industry.[1] Since 1971 Medicare expenditures for home health care have grown by 20% annually, while Medicaid costs in this area have risen from approximately $15 million to over $400 million.[2] Overall vists to patients at home have tripled.[2] Intravenous therapy constitutes the largest single portion of this market and consists of the delivery of home intravenous antibiotics, parenteral nutrition, cancer chemotherapy, and pain management.[1] This entire market is expected to experience a 34% rate of growth through at least 1990, and it is anticipated that the market will have a rise in revenues from $850 million in 1986 to at least $2.8 billion by 1990.[3] Of these, the delivery of intravenous antibiotics is expected to experience the most rapid growth over the next several years. This sector is anticipated to grow about tenfold from approximately $122 million in 1986 to over $1.3 billion in 1990 and by that time may account for 50% of the total home infusion market.[3]

Intravenous therapy has historically been utilized for a variety of reasons that include (1) need for reproducibly high serum levels of antibiotic, (2) lack of availability of a suitable oral agent, (3) failure to tolerate oral agents, and (4) need to ensure compliance with an antibiotic regimen. Classically, this mode of administration has required hospitalization with its attendant risks of nosocomial infection and the substantial costs, isolation from family, and lost time from work or school that accompany it. Recent pressures from many sources have forced the medical community to reassess the need and use of hospital-based intravenous antibiotic therapy and to develop alternative strategies to deal with patients who have historically needed this form of medical management. Although the problem has been complicated by a lack of scientifically valid knowledge concerning such basic issues as to how long to treat selected infections, who really needs parenteral therapy, and when one can safely switch from parenteral to oral therapy, many changes in therapeutic strategies are occurring nonetheless. These include earlier use of oral therapy for diseases traditionally treated parenterally[4] and attempts to devise criteria for management of selected infections outside of the hospital.[5] Perhaps most significant in this era of cost containment have been efforts to develop treatment strategies that allow for the out-of-hospital use of parenteral therapeutic modalities that include antimicrobial agents. The following discussion focuses on this issue.

RATIONALE FOR HOME INTRAVENOUS ANTIBIOTIC THERAPY

Although sound, scientifically valid data do not exist regarding the optimal management of many infectious diseases, historical precedent, medical textbooks, and some clinical data demonstrate that many infections should be treated with intravenous therapy. Several of these may require lengths of therapy of up to 6 weeks.[6–8] Table 19.1 details some infections for which long-term parenteral therapy has generally been recommended and those diagnoses that have been treated in the outpatient setting. In general, as physicians and health care providers have become increasingly comfortable with the concept of home intravenous antibiotic therapy, both the list of diseases and the agents that have been successfully administered outside of the hospital have increased. Anecdotal data now exist for the outpatient management of most infectious diseases that include

Table 19.1
Major Indications for Home Intravenous Antibiotic Therapy[a]

Infection	Percentage of total cases
Osteomyelitis	16–55
Septic arthritis	7–8
Pyelonephritis	7–20
Wound infection	7–20
Pelvic inflammatory disease	3
Infective endocarditis	2–7
Skin/soft tissue	5–26
Device-associated	3–24
Other	9–10

[a]Adopted from Poretz *et al.*,[13] Rehm,[23] and Sorbello *et al.*[24]

acute bacterial meningitis, once initial stability has been achieved within a hospital. Additionally, other clinical indications for home i.v. therapy now include selected patients unable to tolerate prolonged oral antibiotic therapy because of diarrhea, gastric upset, or intrinsic bowel disease.

Historically, such individuals have been managed with intravenous antibiotic therapy in hospitals. Two decades ago, it was not uncommon to note hospitalized patients whose sole reason for hospitalization was to receive parenteral antibiotic therapy.

Home intravenous antibiotic therapy was first utilized in 1974 for the treatment of patients with cystic fibrosis.[9] That pioneer study of 62 patients and 127 treatment courses demonstrated the efficacy of outpatient treatment, the lack of significant adverse reactions, and the successful avoidance of hospitalization and its accompanying cost. Studies published 4 years later demonstrated good clinical results in a small population of patients with bacteremia or osteomyelitis who were first stabilized in the hospital and then had their antibiotic courses completed as outpatients.[10] Satisfactory outcomes and adverse reactions no worse than those noted in an inpatient "control" group were reported. This investigation documented cost savings of approximately $3700.00 per patient. Another early investigation again demonstrated the efficacy and safety of outpatient antibiotic therapy after initial in-hospital stabilization.[11] In a study published in 1982, 150 patients were assessed for efficacy, safety, and cost savings from home i.v. antibiotic therapy.[12] Most individuals were managed for infections of bone or joint and were treated with a variety of antimicrobial agents. Outcomes and safety were excellent, and cost savings were estimated at $142.00 per day.

The current era of cost containment, most notably the institution of diagnostic related groups (DRGs), had made it increasingly important for hospitals to seek early discharge of patients once clinically stable. Under this plan, hospitals receive a fixed payment based on a predetermined length of hospital stay for a given discharge diagnosis regardless of the actual expenses incurred in the care for that patient. Individuals discharged in shorter periods of time become "DRG winners" for the institution, whereas those requiring prolonged hospitalization may become "DRG losers." The remuneration to the institution can be modified by the presence of comorbidities and old age. Table 19.2 presents allowable lengths of stay and hospital payments for several common infectious diseases that are now generally considered to be candidates for home intravenous antibiotic therapy. Thus, hospitals have an incentive to discharge patients in a timely fashion. Complicating this issue, however, is the unwillingness of several major health insurance carriers to reimburse adequately for home i.v. antibiotic therapy. This can force patients to remain hospitalized solely for economic reasons.

Cost savings resulting from home intravenous antibiotic therapy have been studied in several clinical situations. Best estimates are that savings of at least

Table 19.2
Reimbursement and Allowable Lengths of Stay
for Selected Infectious Diseases[a]

DRG[b]	Condition	ALOS[b] (days)	Reimbursement
89	Simple pneumonia, age over 69	7.5	$3497.00
96	Bronchitis, asthma, age over 69	6.0	$2834.00
126	Acute and subacute endocarditis	18.1	$8951.00
238	Septic arthritis	9.7	$4369.00
242	Osteomyelitis	11.1	$4941.00
277	Cellulitis, age over 69	7.3	$2658.00
416	Septicemia, age over 17	8.3	$4855.00
418	Postoperative or posttraumatic infections	7.5	$3007.00
419	Fever, unknown origin, age over 69	6.1	$2792.00

[a]Adopted from the *Federal Register* 1986; 51:31561–31574.
[b]DRG, diagnosis-related group; ALOS, allowable length of stay.

$140.00 per day or $3000.00 per treatment course can be realized, even after considering the cost of the outpatient program.[13–15] Average length of each treatment regimen is 20–42 days.[13,16]

Physicians in several geographic areas have become increasingly comfortable in initiating office-based intravenous antibiotic therapy for selected infections and arranging home therapy thereafter. Thus, the patient may never require hospitalization. This has been noted especially in selected HMOs, where the capacity to administer the initial dose of antibiotic in the office setting exists. Selected forms of skin and soft tissue infection are quite amenable to this strategy. Over the past several years many newer antibiotics have been developed that are considered to be "safe" and to possess pharmacokinetic properties that allow infrequent dosing. Several agents now exist that can be administered either once or twice daily and can be easily utilized outside of the hospital.

Other factors have emerged that also influence the use of home intravenous antibiotic therapy. Patients have become increasingly sophisticated with regard to their knowledge of medications, hospitals, and their expectations of treatment. People increasingly recognize the risks of hospitalization, and the rise of prepaid health plans has impacted on cost containment. It is usually in the best interests of health maintenance organizations to treat people out of hospital. It has also been realized that hospitalization is the single largest component of the cost of treatment of many illnesses. Advances in medical technology have allowed the manufacture of new delivery products, including those that can be programmed to deliver medications reproducibly with a diminished likelihood of adverse reactions.[17] Finally, many individuals wish to return to their normal life style as soon as possible.

CONSIDERATIONS FOR A HOME ANTIBIOTIC THERAPY SYSTEM

Individuals of all ages are now considered candidates for home i.v. therapy. Recent data document its safety for children as young as 18 months and show that up to 93% may be able to return safely to school.[18] Alternatively, data available from a home therapy company (Protocare, Waltham, MA) demonstrate that approximately 25% of patients treated with antibiotics at home were at least 61 years old.

However, before patients can be safely discharged to home i.v. therapy, several issues must be considered.[19] Hospitals would be wise to develop strategies to identify suitable patient candidates as early as possible during hospitalization. Individuals hospitalized with diagnoses that include osteomyelitis, infective endocarditis, and septic arthritis should be individually assessed for home antibiotic therapy after appropriate consultation with the attending physician. Other patients could be identified through pharmacy records of patients who have received more than 5–7 days of parenteral antibiotic. At least one hospital has initiated a team approach to further evaluation of those patients initially identified as being candidates based on their underlying disease.[20] The implementation of a team that includes an infectious disease specialist, a pharmacist, and representatives of both social service and a home i.v. therapy company allows for the expeditious assessment of patients. Issues to be evaluated include (1) insurance considerations, (2) trainability/stability of the patient, (3) optimal venous access, (4) availability of support persons in the home environment, (5) the most cost-effective antibiotic for home i.v. use, (6) length of therapy, (7) assessment of risk of abuse of the line, and (8) considerations for medical follow-up and laboratory monitoring for toxicity and adverse reactions.

Training of the patient and (usually) an additional family member is usually initiated in the hospital and can be completed within 24–48 hr. Choice of venous access is dependent on factors that include estimated length of home i.v. therapy, quality of peripheral veins, phlebitogenic qualities of the medication to be employed, and availability of site-changing teams. In general, patients who require treatment in excess of 2 weeks benefit from the placement of central access. Usually Hickman or Broviac catheters are employed, and the patient is instructed in depth on management issues. Recent data demonstrate that the unusual cases of central-catheter-related sepsis can often be successfully managed in the outpatient setting with prompt initiation of appropriate antibiotics and low-dose thrombolytic therapy.[21] In this investigation, 21 septic episodes in 16 patients were successfully managed without removal of the central line.

In all instances the medication to be utilized at home should be first initiated in a controlled health care environment that enables management of immediate untoward reactions. Initial drug administration (if different from that which the patient has been receiving in the hospital) may be begun either by hospital personnel or by representatives of a home i.v. therapy company. The patient must be familiar with all aspects of the infusion setup, including maintenance of asepsis, reconstitution of the antibiotic, and site preparation. Actual ''hands-on'' experience is important prior to hospital discharge.

Suitable facilities for the delivery of therapy must be in place. This should include a mechanism for dispatching medications to the residence, personnel to monitor the intravenous line and to change i.v. sites regularly, people on call at all times to deal with emergencies, and availability of a mechanism to allow for drawing and testing of blood for appropriate tests, as indicated by the physician. It is vital to identify a specific physician who is charged with patient follow-up and assessment of laboratory data used to monitor home infusion therapy. In practice, these issues can be met in a variety of ways, depending on the facilities of a given hospital and the availability of other resources in a geographic region. Some hospitals have developed their own outpatient antibiotic pharmacies. Alternatively, numerous companies now exist (with highly variable levels of expertise, professionalism, and interest) for the dispensing and management of patients on home intravenous therapies. Nursing and phlebotomy services can be provided either by hospitals, by visiting nurse associations, or by the private companies established to render home therapy.

ROLE OF THE PHYSICIAN IN OUTPATIENT INTRAVENOUS THERAPY

The clinician cannot and should not be passive in issues related to home intravenous therapy. The quality of services rendered at home should be as important as that of those in the acute care hospital or nursing home. For this reason, physicians, especially those who are most likely to utilize home intravenous therapy services, must actively participate at all levels of home health care delivery and must be certain that the quality of home health care in no way compromises quality of care. However, any entrepreneurial involvement of physicians must never impact on patient care. There is no reason why doctors cannot become financially involved in home health care so long as it is done in a moral and ethical manner that does not allow remuneration solely on the basis of numbers of patients who utilize the service. Indeed, authorities advise that physicians become more actively involved in home health care in order to help insure the quality of service.[22] Physicians should be able to insure that the care rendered by home health care delivery systems meets their needs for quality, that good modes of communication exist between ''the system'' and the individual physician, and that oversight for quality assurance and utilization review by practicing clinicians and other health care workers exists in the community. Finally, the home health care system must take into account local ideas and practice patterns rather than base its role on centrally promulgated operations that may not be relevant to an individual geographic area.

CHOICE OF ANTIBIOTIC

Although virtually any antibiotic can theoretically be employed at home, practical considerations mitigate against many of them. In general, the trend has been toward the use of monotherapy when possible, and toward the utilization of long-half-life products that allow infrequent dosing. The medication employed should be relatively safe and not likely to result in significant adverse reactions. Thus, considerations for home intravenous antibiotic therapy may differ somewhat from those employed for hospitalized patients. It is the author's opinion that efficacy, safety, and ease of administration are of paramount importance for choice of agents administered out of hospital. Many agents fulfill these criteria, although some authorities have been uncomfortable utilizing agents such as pentamidine isethionate or amphotericin B outside of a health care facility. Recent needs, based on an enlarging population of patients with the acquired immunodeficiency syndrome (AIDS), have shown the ability to render even these products safely at home. And large anecdotal experiences now demonstrate that, by using appropriate written criteria for use and monitoring, amphotericin B and pentamidine can be safely administered in the home-care setting.

From a practical viewpoint, the administration of agents more frequently than every 8 hr is infeasible. This has reduced somewhat the appeal of agents such as penicillin, ampicillin, and the extended-spectrum penicillins, which are usually dosed at 4- or 6-hr intervals. However, the recent availability of prolonged-half-life agents, many of them cephalosporins, has greatly aided the management of many infections and allows treatment regimens that employ either 12- or 24-hr dosing. This greatly enhances patient compliance and allows return to previous life style. Because of this, it is not uncommon to initiate an agent for outpatient therapy that differs from that employed during hospitalization.

Three agents have proven to be particularly useful to the author in the intravenous outpatient management of infections. Ceftriaxone (Rocephin®, Roche Pharmaceuticals) has become immensely popular as an agent for home i.v. therapy because of its prolonged serum half-life, excellent blood levels, broad spectrum of activity, safety, and ease of administration. Several studies have been published that demonstrate the outpatient efficacy, safety, and cost-effectiveness of this compound for a variety of clinical infections that include bacteremia and bone/joint infections.[16,23–25] The half-life of ceftriaxone is approximately 6–8 hr, thus allowing once- or twice-daily dosing for most infections.[26] Usual dosage in adults is 1–2 g each 24 hr. Its spectrum of activity is that of usual third-generation cephalosporins and includes most strains of *S. aureus,* most streptococci (with the exception of enterococci), *H. influenzae,* neisseriae, and most enteric gram-negative bacilli. No significant activity is demonstrated against *P. aeruginosa, B. fragilis,* or several of the most resistant gram-negative organisms.[27] Mixed infections with suceptible organisms (e.g., selected cases of osteomyelitis) could be ideally treated with this agent. Additionally, many individuals have begun to utilize it for other infections. These include bone and joint infections caused by *S. aureus* and other single pathogens where it is felt that the advantages of once-daily dosing outweigh the broader-than-necessary spectrum of this agent.[16,24] Many strains of *S. aureus* and other gram-positive cocci are quite suceptible to this agent *in vitro,* with MIC_{90} of approximately 4 μg/ml.[26]

Vancomycin (currently generically available through at least three vendors) has demonstrated efficacy against infections caused by *S. aureus* and most other gram-positive cocci where bactericidal activity is indicated. An important exception is *S. faecalis,* where bactericidal activity requires the addition of an aminoglycoside, usually gentamicin. The primary examples have been endocarditis, septic arthritis, and osteomyelitis caused by *S. aureus* or *S. epidermidis,* although infections caused by other gram-positive cocci have also been successfully treated at our institution. Treatment of infective endocarditis caused by *S. epidermidis* should usually consist of vancomycin in conjunction with a second agent, often rifampin. Vancomycin is extremely useful in patients with significant allergies to β-lactam antibiotics and can be administered in doses of up to 1 g every 12 hr.[28–31] It is usually well tolerated, although care must be taken to avoid too-rapid administration, which can result in the "red-neck" or "red-man" syndrome.[31] The author recommends that blood counts and renal function be checked at least weekly during administration of this product.

Cefazolin (Kefzol®, Eli Lilly and Co., or Ancef®, Smith Kline & French) is a "first-generation" cephalosporin with pharmacokinetics that usually allow every-8-hr dosing.[32–34] Its spectrum of activity includes many strains of *S. aureus,* most streptococci (except enterococci), and common gram-negative bacilli such as *E. coli,* most *Klebsiella,* and *P. mirabilis.*[33] This agent is stable after freezing and has been used extensively in home infusion therapy with apparently good success for infections caused by suceptible pathogens.[16,18,23,35]

Many other products have also been utilized extensively for home infusion therapy. Most extended-spectrum cephalosporins have been successfully employed for infections caused by susceptible pathogens. These include cefoperazone, cefoxitin, and cefuroxime.[36,37] Aminoglycosides such as gentamicin and tobramicin may also be utilized when necessary, although the need to monitor closely for efficacy and toxicity makes them less attractive choices when alternatives are available.

CLINICAL EXAMPLES

Example 1. A 55-year-old insulin-dependent diabetic was hospitalized for low-grade fever and pain in the foot. Physical examination revealed an oral temperature of 100°F and a small ulcer on the plantar surface of the right foot overlying the first metatarsophalangeal (M-P) joint. Pain was noted on deep pressure. Pulses below the femorals were diminished bilaterally, and sensation was similarly decreased bilaterally below the knee. X rays of the right foot and subsequent bone scan revealed evidence for osteomyelitis in the area of the first right M-P joint. Surgery was undertaken for debridement and bone culture. Osteomyelitis was confirmed at surgery, involved bone was debrided, and cultures demonstrated *S. epidermidis* sensitive to vancomycin and rifampin. Therapy was initiated in hospital with vancomycin, 1 g i.v. every 12 hr administered over approximately 60 min, and rifampin, 600 mg orally daily. After 4 days of hospitalization, assessment revealed that the wound was healing well without evidence of infection, white count, renal function, and glucose were stable, and the patient was tolerating medications without difficulty. The patient was discharged on the fifth postoperative day to complete a 6-week course of home intravenous therapy. Monitoring of complete blood count and renal function was carried out weekly, with the responsible physician apprised of results in a timely fashion. The patient returned to work approximately 2 weeks after surgery, completed therapy without difficulty, and is clinically cured at 6-month follow-up.

Comment: This patient had biopsy-proven *S. epidermidis* osteomyelitis that usually is treated for up to 6 weeks with parenteral therapy. Succeptibility patterns demonstrated the need for vancomycin. Availability of home i.v. therapy allowed early discharge from hospital and saved approximately 5 weeks of hospitalization for an individual who was otherwise healthy and would have been hospitalized solely to receive intravenous medication. Twice-daily infusions allowed this individual to return to work and a reasonable life style at least 4 weeks earlier than if he had remained hospitalized.

Example 2. A 30-year-old male was hospitalized for assessment of drainage from the distal portion of the index finger of the left hand. This was initially noted several days after an industrial accident involving cutting equipment. Initial treatment consisted of oral amoxicillin administered for 10 days with significant improvement. Thereafter, hospitalization was advised when x rays revealed changes consistent with early osteomyelitis. Physical examination was normal except for a temperature of 101°F and a swollen second digit of the left hand associated with non-foul-smelling yellow drainage from a nonhealed laceration on the distal portion of the finger. Gram stain revealed gram-positive cocci in clumps, and culture ultimately demonstrated *S. aureus*. After operative debridement of bone (where subsequent cultures also revealed *S. aureus*), the patient was begun in hospital on oxacillin, 2 g i.v. every 4 hr. After 5 days of therapy, clinical improvement was noted, the operative wound was deemed satisfactory, and plans for home i.v. infusion therapy were initiated. Laboratory studies demonstrated that the *S. aureus* isolated from bone was highly sensitive to ceftriaxone, with an MIC of less than 2 μg/ml. The patient was switched to this antibiotic in a dose of 1 g i.v. every 24 hr, was observed for 2 days in the hospital, and was subsequently discharged to complete a 4-week course. He went back to work after only 1 week at home. Laboratory data that were routinely monitored consisted of complete blood count weekly, with results reported to the attending physician in a timely fashion. No complications were noted, and the patient made an unremarkable recovery with clinical cure continuing at 9-month follow-up.

Comment. This patient was demonstrated to have *S. aureus* osteomyelitis. Classical therapy would have consisted of up to 6 weeks of intravenous antibiotic administered to a relatively healthy individual in a hospital setting. Availability of home infusion therapy allowed for timely discharge and rapid return to work and family. Under "hospital" circumstances, oxacillin or nafcillin administered on an every 4- to 6-hr basis would typically have been employed. However, such a regimen is virtually impossible to administer at home. Ceftriaxone was chosen primarily because of its capacity to be administered once daily and its relative safety, despite the fact that it is of far broader spectrum than needed for the organism identified. One-gram once-daily dosing is extremely cost effective in this clinical situation. Although the question of emergence of resistant organisms can be raised in view of the use of an agent with a spectrum far broader than clinically indicated, this has not been identified as a problem in home i.v. therapy. Additionally, it would be anticipated to be far less of a problem for patients who remain outside of the hospital.

Example 3. A 23-year-old heroin addict was hospitalized with a history of chills, fever, and anorexia of 2 weeks' duration. Physical examination revealed a fever of 102°F, many noninfected needle tracks, a mitral regurgitant murmur, and subconjunctival petechiae. After cultures were drawn, the patient was begun on oxacillin, 2 g i.v. every 6 hr, and gentamicin, 100 mg i.v. every 8 hr. Three blood cultures subsequently grew *S. viridans* species. The patient was switched to penicillin and streptomycin to complete a 2-week course. She required the placement of a central line for venous access and completed her course of treatment without difficulty. Clinical cure has been documented at 6-month follow-up.

Comment. This heroin addict developed *S. viridans* endocarditis and was treated with an approved 2-week course of therapy. Despite the fact that she was clinically stable, it was decided because of her acknowledged active drug addiction to continue treatment in hospital rather than to discharge her with venous access in place.

CONCLUSIONS

Home antibiotic infusion therapy provides a safe, cost-effective mechanism for antibiotic delivery for many patients. Communities are encouraged to develop and utilize this service as an alternative to prolonged hospitalization solely for antibiotic administration. Strategies for patient identification and selection, training, antibiotic supply, and patient management after hospital discharge must be incorporated into any plan. Physicians should actively participate in these issues. Once effected, data show that major cost savings can ensue without evidence of increased clinical failure or adverse drug reactions.

Antibiotics chosen for home management may differ somewhat from those that would otherwise be utilized during hospitalization. Choice is guided primarily by efficacy, safety, and ease of administration and may consist of agents with longer half-lives and broader spectra of activity than classically employed for hospitalized individuals. Such measures, however, will often allow the patient to resume meaningful employment or return to school.

REFERENCES

1. Rucker BB, Holmstedt KA: *Home Infusion Therapy Industry*. San Francisco, Hambrecht and Quist, 1984.
2. Koren MJ: Home care—Who cares? *N Engl J Med* 1986; 314:917–920.
3. Hambrecht and Quist 1987 Report: Home infusion therapy industry to maintain 34% growth while small companies reshape market, stimulate demand. *Home Health Line,* 9 Feb 1987.
4. Nelson JD: A critical review of the role of oral antibiotics in the management of hematogenous osteomyelitis. In: Remington JS, Swartz MN, eds. *Current Clinical Topics in Infectious Disease,* vol 4. New York, McGraw-Hill, 1983:64–74.
5. Siegel D: Management of community-acquired pneumonia in outpatients. *West J Med* 1985; 142:45–48.
6. Scheld WM, Sande MA: Endocarditis and intravascular infections. In: Mandell GL, Douglas RG Jr, Bennett JE, eds. *Principles and Practice of Infectious Disease,* ed 2. New York, John Wiley & Sons, 1985:504–530.
7. Norden CW: Osteomyelitis. In: Mandell GL, Douglas RG Jr, Bennett JE, eds. *Principles and Practice of Infectious Disease,* ed 2. New York, John Wiley & Sons, 1985:704–711.
8. Levison ME, Pontzer RE: Peritonitis and other intra-abdominal infections. In: Mandell GL, Douglas RG Jr, Bennett JE, eds. *Principles and Practice of Infectious Disease,* ed 2. New York, John Wiley & Sons, 1985:476–503.
9. Rucker RW, Harrison GM: Outpatient intravenous medications in the management of cystic fibrosis. *Pediatrics* 1974; 54:358–360.
10. Antonisdis A, Anderson BC, van Volkinburg EJ, *et al:* Feasibility of outpatient self-administration of parenteral antibiotics. *West J Med* 1978; 128:203–206.
11. Stiver HG, Telford GO, Mossey JM, *et al:* Intravenous antibiotic therapy at home. *Ann Intern Med* 1978; 89:690–693.
12. Stiver HG, Trosky SK, Cote DD, *et al:* Self-administration of intravenous antibiotics: An efficient, cost effective home care program. *Can Med Assoc J* 1982; 127:207–211.
13. Poretz DM, Eron LJ, Goldenberg RI, *et al:* Intravenous antibiotic therapy in an outpatient setting. *JAMA* 1982; 248:336–339.
14. Kind AC, Williams DN, Persons G, *et al:* Intravenous antibiotic therapy at home. *Arch Intern Med* 1979; 139:412–415.
15. Eisenberg JM, Kitz DS: Savings from outpatient antibiotic therapy for osteomyelitis. *JAMA* 1986; 255:1584–1588.
16. Poretz DM, Woolard D, Eron LJ, *et al:* Outpatient use of ceftriaxone: A cost–benefit analysis. *Am J Med* 1984; 77(suppl 4C):77–84.
17. Kamen BA, Gunther N: Administering a 24-hour supply of antibiotics with a programmable, automated syringe pump. *Am J Hosp Pharm* 1985; 42:2715-2716.
18. Goldenberg R, Poretz DM, Eron LJ, *et al:* Intravenous antibiotic therapy in ambulatory pediatric patients. *Pediatr Infect Dis* 1984; 3:514–517.
19. Smego RA: Home intravenous antibiotic therapy. *Arch Intern Med* 1985; 145:1001–1002.

20. Rehm SJ, Weinstein AJ: Home intravenous antibiotic therapy: A team approach. *Ann Intern Med* 1983; 99:388–392.
21. Schuman ES: Outpatient management of Hickman catheter sepsis. *Infect Surg* 1987; 6:103–106.
22. Health and Public Policy Committee, American College of Physicians: Home health care. *Ann Intern Med* 1986; 105:454–460.
23. Rehm SJ: Home intravenous antibiotic therapy. *Cleve Clin Q* 1985; 52:333–338.
24. Sorbello AF, Echols RM, Condoluci DV: Clinical efficacy of once-daily ceftriaxone therapy. *Infect Med* 1987; 4:69–78.
25. Jauregui LE, Bischoff MC, Hageage GJ: Combined inpatient–outpatient therapy of serious infections with a single daily dose of ceftriaxone. In: *Progress in Therapy of Bacterial Infection—A New Cephalosporin: Ceftriaxone.* Amsterdam, Excerpta Medica, 1983:104–122.
26. Patel IH, Kaplan SA: Pharmacokinetic profile of ceftriaxone in man. *Am J Med* 1984; 77(suppl 4C):17–25.
27. Cleeland R, Squires E: Antimicrobial spectrum of ceftriaxone: A review. *Am J Med* 1984; 77(suppl 4C):3–11.
28. Geraci JE: Vancomycin. *Mayo Clin Proc* 1977; 52:631–634.
29. Woodley DW, Hall WH: The treatment of severe staphylococcal infections with vancomycin. *Ann Intern Med* 1961; 55:235–249.
30. Geraci JE, Hermans PE: Vancomycin. *Mayo Clin Proc* 1983; 58:88–91.
31. Norris SM, Limon L: Vancomycin—new uses for an old drug. *Infect Control* 1984; 5:302–404.
32. Weinstein AJ: The cephalosporins. *Infect Dis Pract* 1983; 6:1–7.
33. *The Medical Letter:* Choice of cephalosporins. *Med Lett* 1983; 25:57–60.
34. Barza M, Miao PVW: Antimicrobial spectrum, pharmacology, and therapeutic use of antibiotics. Part 3: Cephalosporins. *Am J Hosp Pharm* 1977; 34:621–629.
35. Carone SM, Bornstein M, Coleman DL, *et al:* Stability of frozen solutions of cefazolin sodium. *Am J Hosp Pharm* 1976; 33:639–641.
36. Smego RA, Gainer RB: Home intravenous antimicrobial therapy provided by a community hospital and a university hospital. *Am J Hosp Pharm* 1985; 42:2185–2189.
37. Harris LF, Buckle TF, Coffey FL Jr: Intravenous antibiotics at home. *South Med J* 1986; 79:193–196.

Index